C000212593

Proteins, Pathologies and Politics

Also available from Bloomsbury:

Anxious Appetites, Peter Jackson
Food, Power, and Agency, Jürgen Martschukat and Bryant Simon
Italy and the Potato: A History, 1550–2000, David Gentilcore

Proteins, Pathologies and Politics

Dietary Innovation and Disease from the Nineteenth Century

Edited by
David Gentilcore and Matthew Smith

BLOOMSBURY ACADEMIC
LONDON • NEW YORK • OXFORD • NEW DELHI • SYDNEY

BLOOMSBURY ACADEMIC
Bloomsbury Publishing Plc
50 Bedford Square, London, WC1B 3DP, UK
1385 Broadway, New York, NY 10018, USA

BLOOMSBURY, BLOOMSBURY ACADEMIC and the Diana logo are trademarks of
Bloomsbury Publishing Plc

First published in Great Britain 2019

Copyright © David Gentilcore, Matthew Smith and Contributors, 2019

David Gentilcore and Matthew Smith have asserted their right under the Copyright,
Designs and Patents Act, 1988, to be identified as Editors of this work.

Cover image: Ephemera Collection, showcard advertising Melhuish's New Harvest, 1930s.
(© Wellcome Collection)

All rights reserved. No part of this publication may be reproduced or
transmitted in any form or by any means, electronic or mechanical,
including photocopying, recording, or any information storage or retrieval
system, without prior permission in writing from the publishers.

Bloomsbury Publishing Plc does not have any control over, or responsibility for, any
third-party websites referred to or in this book. All internet addresses given in this
book were correct at the time of going to press. The author and publisher regret any
inconvenience caused if addresses have changed or sites have ceased to exist, but can
accept no responsibility for any such changes.

A catalogue record for this book is available from the British Library.

A catalog record for this book is available from the Library of Congress.

ISBN: HB: 978-1-3500-5686-2
ePDF: 978-1-3500-5689-3
eBook: 978-1-3500-5687-9

Typeset by Newgen KnowledgeWorks Pvt. Ltd., Chennai, India
Printed and bound in Great Britain

To find out more about our authors and books, visit www.bloomsbury.com
and sign up for our newsletters.

Contents

Illustrations

Figures

Tables

Contributors

Agnes Arnold-Forster is a Wellcome Trust-funded postdoctoral research fellow at the University of Roehampton, United Kingdom. Her PhD is from King's College London and her most recent article, 'Mapmaking and Mapthinking: Cancer as a Problem of Place in Nineteenth-Century England', came out in *Social History of Medicine* in 2018.

Francesco Buscemi teaches media history at the Catholic University of Milan and the Insubria University of Como, Italy. He is a member of the International Society for Cultural History and has published on food and media in the twentieth century. His most recent study is *From Body Fuel to Universal Poison: Cultural History of Meat: 1900–the Present* (2018).

Bryce Evans is Associate Professor in History at Liverpool Hope University specializing in food history. His previous books include two political biographies and an economic history of Ireland during the Second World War. He keeps a research blog at www. drbryceevans.wordpress.com. The research underpinning his chapter was funded by the Wellcome Trust.

Kirsten Gardner is Chair and Associate Professor of History at the University of Texas at San Antonio, United States. She has published on histories of women, cancer, and diabetes, including *Early Detection: Women, Cancer and Awareness Campaigns in the Twentieth-Century U.S.* (2006) and recent work in the *Journal of Medical Humanities and Literature and Medicine*.

David Gentilcore is Professor of Early Modern History at the University of Leicester (United Kingdom) and has published widely on the social and cultural history of medicine and on food history in early and late modern Italy, including the impact of food plants from the New World. His most recent book is *Food and Health in Early Modern Europe* (2016).

Clare Gordon Bettencourt is a PhD candidate in History at the University of California, Irvine, United States. Her article, 'Encouraging a Broader Narrative of American Pure Food Legislation: Understanding the Federal Food, Drug and Cosmetic Act of 1938', can be found in *Retrospectives: A Postgraduate History Journal* (2015).

Silvia Inaudi, PhD, is Tutor of Contemporary History at the University of Turin, Italy. She has published several books, including *A tutti indistintamente. L'Ente opere assistenziali nel periodo fascista* (2008), and numerous articles on modern Italy, with a particular focus on welfare, childhood and women's history.

Rachel Meach is a PhD candidate and history tutor at the University of Strathclyde in Glasgow, United Kingdom. Her thesis, titled *A Spoonful of Sugar: Diet and Diabetes in Britain and the United States, 1945–2016*, utilizes oral history testimonies collected in Britain and the United States to uncover the contributory factors leading to rise in type 2 diabetes and the social and cultural factors impacting on changes in treatment in the second half of the twentieth century.

Peter Scholliers is a professorial researcher at the Social & Cultural Food Studies Unit (FOST), Vrije Universiteit Brussel, Belgium. He specializes in the food history of Europe since the late eighteenth century and has recently published 'Norms and Practices of Children's Diets in Brussels Hospitals, 1830–1914', in the *Journal of the History of Childhood and Youth* (2017).

Mircea Scrob is a teaching fellow in the Liberal Arts and Natural Sciences programme at the University of Birmingham, United Kingdom. He has published extensively on developments in food consumption in twentieth-century Romania and his most recent study is 'Does an Early Socialization into a Food Culture Condition Lifelong Food Preferences? Evidence from a Retrospective Study', published in the journal *Appetite* (2016).

Matthew Smith is Professor of Health History at the University of Strathclyde's Centre for the Social History of Health and Healthcare, Glasgow, United Kingdom. His publications in food history include *Another Person's Poison: A History of Food Allergy* (2015).

Maiko Rafael Spiess teaches in the Department of Social Sciences and Philosophy at the Regional University of Blumenau, Brazil, where he is also a coordinating member of the Nucleus of Studies of Technoscience (FURB). He obtained his PhD from the State University of Campinas and has published on the nature of risk in public health.

Introduction

If the 1980s may have been the high point of food additives – with Coca-Cola able to double the sales of 'Tab' in test markets by fortifying the fizzy diet drink with calcium[1] – one of the more recent food trends has been not of additions but subtraction. We have all seen it on our supermarket shelves. A whole range of foods, from soy milk to sausages, are advertised as 'additive-free'. This conveys a positive and healthy image to a public interested in health and well-being but anxious and suspicious about the nature of food additives. The expression has taken the place of abused terms like 'natural' or 'all-natural' on product packaging. It also makes it easier to rationalize the consumption of less healthy foods, which are at least perceived to be free from added artificial ingredients. Why not have another sausage; after all, it has 'no synthetic preservatives' and 'no artificial flavours'? Additives we are understood not to like or approve of are thus removed (even while being simultaneously replaced with others).[2]

But the process of subtraction goes still further. We increasingly shop for products whose key components have been removed, now perceived as unhealthy. Lactose-free dairy products have spread from the lactose-intolerant to those who believe they are and to those who believe that the products are in any case healthier and more digestible, with a global market in excess of $4 billion.[3] Similarly, gluten is seen as such a threat to health by some that foods that have never contained gluten are advertised as being 'gluten-free'. In a range of popular health books and blogs, gluten – associated with newer, high-yielding varieties of wheat, increased fertilizer and pesticide use, as well as modern bread-making processes – has been linked to autism, depression, Alzheimer's, multiple sclerosis, diabetes and some skin diseases. Better to avoid gluten altogether, it is argued. The quite real intolerance of a small minority (coeliac disease, affecting 1 per cent of the population) has not only spawned a whole new clinical entity, 'non-coeliac gluten sensitivity' (NCGS),[4] but it has also become the latest health-related 'lifestyle' trend, fuelling a worldwide gluten-free industry valued at $15 billion per year.[5] This, despite the fact that products labelled gluten-free often turn out to be higher in fats, sugars and salt (in order to mimic the properties of gluten),[6] thus not only negating some of the health benefits in the process, but also countering subtraction with addition. Confused?

The link between dietary innovation and change, on the one hand, and health and disease, on the other, is nothing new. Up until the mid-nineteenth century, dietary innovation had primarily consisted of the introduction of novel foods and cooking techniques from different parts of the world as a result of imperial expansion or the development of new trade routes. From at least the time of the Roman Empire, established tastes and traditions battled with the prestige value of the new and exotic.[7] In a recent article on food and identity, Stephen Shapin has described how Ancient Greek and Roman medical traditions emphasized that such exotic foods could put bodies at risk.[8] Although novel foods imported from afar could impart some 'magical' benefits, it was considered wiser to opt for traditional and 'natural' foods and cooking methods. Such thinking continued to be influential throughout the early modern period in Europe, especially as many new foods and drinks, including many items that became dietary staples – for example, potato, maize and tomato – were introduced via the Columbian exchange with the New World.[9] This way of thinking about traditional or natural foods, rooted in the Galenic humoral tradition, was based upon an understanding that it was the qualities of foods, rather than their constituents, that mattered.[10] In other words, it was the cold, wet nature of a cucumber or the hot, dry nature of a chilli peppers that influenced one's health, not the chemicals that combined to form a cucumber or a chilli pepper.

The rise of chemical and mechanical medicine from the seventeenth century brought substantial changes in the way people thought about foods, physiology and digestion. Medical authors began to look at foods in new ways, measuring quantities and investigating their constituent elements, making use of a new language. This was a transitional phase away from the Galenic focus on the qualities of food. For Shapin, real change came during the nineteenth and twentieth centuries, with the shift towards a materialistic emphasis on the chemical constituents of food – specifically, proteins, carbohydrates, vitamins and other components. Food became 'understood as a bag of chemicals; you are a bag of chemicals, organized into physiological systems; eat the right chemicals and you will enjoy good health; eat the wrong ones, and you will suffer disease and shortened life'.[11] Gyorgy Scrinis has described this reductionist approach to understanding nutrition as 'nutritionism', short for 'nutritional reductionism', whereby food is not only perceived in terms of its component parts, but nutrients – whether they be vitamins, proteins, fats, carbohydrates or whatever – are firmly linked with specific states of health and disease.[12] As a number of the chapters in this volume demonstrate, the dominance of nutritionism in the twentieth century has led to many protracted debates about the health benefits or dangers of particular foodstuffs, sometimes even pitting one nutrient against another.

The transition from perceiving food in terms of their qualities, based largely on sensory perceptions, to thinking about them as admixtures of chemical constituents, was precipitated in part by the emergence of technologies that allowed scientists to analyse and experiment with the components of various foods in new ways. Similar technologies allowed the food industry to transform how food could be processed. For instance, milling techniques allowed maize to separate it into its protein, oil, fibre and carbohydrate components and permitted the creation of pearly-white rice. This facilitated the introduction of a vast array of chemicals into the food supply, such that, in some cases, food really was no more than 'a bag of chemicals'. While some of these developments, such as the introduction of new food preservation techniques and the fortification of foods, could be seen as reducing the risk of disease, the propensity for food processing to increase the profit margins of food manufacturers raised suspicions.[13]

At the same time, there were significant changes in agriculture that transformed the diets of millions of people. For example, the rise in maize cultivation, with its very high yields, seemed full of promise, but when consumed in the form of polenta and corn meal, in parts of Europe and the United States, brought with it the debilitating disease pellagra.[14] Even when the cause of pellagra was finally identified (in the 1930s), concerns began to emerge later in the century about the increasingly widespread use of maize in food processing, with high fructose corn syrup only the most recent by-product to be targeted.[15] Similarly, when new milling techniques to produce white rice were introduced in Japan, the result was 'the fearful national disease' of beriberi.[16] Finally, technological developments in transportation, refrigeration and food preservation, ranging from pasteurization to canning, allowed food to become an ever more global commodity.[17] The combination of these factors during the late nineteenth and twentieth centuries – the shift to emphasizing the constituents (rather than the qualities) of food and the increasing variety of foods available – complicated the relationship between diet and disease. In addition to creating or bringing new foods to Western consumers, many of these dietary innovations in manufacturing and production processes, new food additives and evolving agricultural practices initially came with the promise of improved diet and health, only to become ultimately associated with ill health – either real or imagined. On the demand side of the equation, where populations became increasingly industrialized and urbanized, and there resulted a weakening contact with agricultural production, working-class food choices became limited to what was cheap and readily available in the fast-expanding cities.[18] If mid-nineteenth-century English working-class diets have recently been characterized 'as a superior version of the Mediterranean diet',[19] somewhat optimistically, there was undeniably a marked decline in the second half of the century. A paradox ensued of lowering food standards, variety and nutrition, even while life expectancy (and social conditions more generally) improved.[20]

Central to concerns about dietary innovation and health are fundamental questions about the ideal human diet. Is it possible to perfect our diet through technological innovation, looking forever forwards? Fortifying foods with added nutrients was justified as a necessary and effective process in countering nutritional deficiency diseases, such iodine in salt, vitamin D in milk and niacin in flour.[21] And today we have the promise of 'nutriceuticals' and 'functional foods' (even if their promise seems to be held back by a consumer preference for foods that are 'natural' – that word again! – at least in Europe).[22] Or should we instead look backwards, aiming to consume a local, 'natural', preagricultural diet? The assumption here is that modern Western diets are themselves pathogenetic, figuring among the causes of certain chronic illnesses – 'diseases of civilization'. The question here is a bit like the restoration of period properties: how far back do you go, stripping away the different layers in search of the building's 'real' essence? The 'Paleolithic diet' encourages us to return to the eating habits of our preagricultural, hunter-gatherer ancestors.[23] Supporters of the gluten-free diet argue that the rot set in 10,000 years ago when we (i.e. humankind) started eating wheat, even though for the previous 2.5 million years we had been doing well enough without it. Or is it enough simply to go 'pre-modern', returning (as has been suggested) to an idealized diet sometime before the onset of industrialization and urbanization, when people supposedly enjoyed their food and were all the healthier for it.[24] Perhaps the solution is geographical rather than chronological, ordering the 'Mediterranean option' instead, which at least bears the imprimatur of UNESCO.[25]

What do these recent food trends say about our changing relationship with expertise, as both consumers and patients? In their scepticism of professional expertise, non-coeliacs self-diagnosing a gluten sensitivity upset the doctor–patient relationship, in which food intolerance appears to exemplify a distinct form of contested illness experience.[26] And what are the economics of dietary change? For example, the expansion of the lactose-free market has been exponential, but far from catching the dairy industry off-guard, it has reacted with glee.[27] Who are the historical actors – political, medical, technological – involved in innovation (on the one hand) and what are the social responses to it (on the other)? As an example of the ongoing cycle of action and reaction, let us return to high-fructose corn syrup: while the blogosphere protests about our over-reliance on it and sales of products containing it decline, scientists argue that, from a metabolic point of view, one sweetener is more or less like any other, and the producers propose a name change ('corn sugar') to distract the public, and fast food and fizzy drink manufacturers trumpet their return to 'natural sugar' (paradoxically being able to use sugar as a selling point).[28] What should be the role of government in all of this? Today, the food industry is among the most vociferous lobbyists in the new trade deals being negotiated in an on-again-off-again way by the world's governments, despite popular protests about the secretive nature of the negotiations and the food industry's lack of concern for issues of public health.[29] And indeed to what extent is dietary health itself a cultural construct, a product of history? Far from being neutral, the emerging nutritional science of the early twentieth century came wrapped in a moralizing packaging, where dietary health was linked to self-control, work and the avoidance of excess.[30]

As the chapters in this volume demonstrate, dietary theories of health and disease have proliferated during the past century or so, often fuelled by broader political, social, cultural, philosophical and economic factors that were, at times, far removed from nutrition science and, at others, intrinsic to the development of the science itself. The historiography and other literature related to dietary innovation and disease that has emerged over the past 30 years has similarly revealed how nutrition science and food policy has been highly contingent upon such factors. Building on the earlier work of the late social historian James Harvey Young on the US Pure Food and Drug Act (1906), sociologist James Haydu has emphasized the vital role of progressive women's groups in changing the way 'pure food' was understood by the American public, thus spurring further the need for legislation.[31] The Pure Food Movement emerged during the 1870s as a response to the development of industrialized food production in the United States. Many pure food advocates, including government chemist Harvey Wiley, saw pure food as essentially a consumer issue: when processors adulterated or disguised beef, for example, they took advantage of trusting, innocent consumers (and, to a lesser extent, farmers who wanted a fair market for their product). Representatives of women's groups, such as the General Federation of Women's Clubs, however, were concerned about the health implications of adulterated food. As Haydu describes,

> although unscrupulous urban bakers, dairy operators, and distillers had been putting harmful additives in their cheapest products for a long time, modern food production prompted new anxieties over safety. How could consumers judge the hazards of novel products like margarine, unfamiliar techniques like factory canning, or untested preservatives like benzoate of soda?[32]

The Pure Food Act of 1906, therefore, was made possible by 'political consumerism' and 'maternalist politics' working in tandem, along with the publication of Upton Sinclair's *The Jungle* – which was written to flag up the abysmal working conditions in Chicago's meatpacking industry, not to send Americans into a panic about processed food.[33]

Historians have explored the political aspects of dietary change in other contexts. The organic food movement may be primarily associated with left-wing politics today, but many (though not all) British proponents of organic farming during the 1930s came from the opposite side of the political spectrum, including Jorian Jenks and Henry Williamson, both of whom were members of the British Union of Fascists.[34] For Jenks, organic approaches were seen not only to produce improved food quality and, therefore, better health, but were also part and parcel of a reactionary return to the land and to the 'natural' order.[35] By the 1960s, the organic movement had shifted left and food became a central platform in the counterculture movement.[36] Recent research has further complicated the story. Ian Mosby's analysis of 'Chinese Restaurant Syndrome', for example, has revealed how racist attitudes imbued the debates about the risks about monosodium glutamate (MSG) that began in the late 1960s.[37] Such findings echo the nativist sentiments of some of the founders of organic farming in the United Kingdom. Others, including Michael Mikulak, have highlighted how, despite its counterculture connections, organic food production in the United States is dominated by massive food corporations more concerned with profits than producing healthier or more environmentally friendly food.[38]

The politics of breastfeeding, brought about by the introduction of formula milk in the late nineteenth century, have been similarly intricate. Formula milk has been seen as indicative of how mothers were expected to secede authority over motherhood to male scientists during the first half of the twentieth century, but can also be interpreted as a tool that liberated mothers and allowed them to return to work whenever they desired during the post-war period.[39] Debates about infant feeding have highlighted conflicting scientific advice about which approach is healthiest for babies. While the World Health Organization advocates exclusive breastfeeding for at least the first 6 months of an infant's life and continued breastfeeding until the age of 2, others have argued that the consistency of infant formula (notwithstanding any scandals about adulteration) may make it a healthier option for some children when their mother's breastmilk might be compromised by various factors.[40] Related advice about whether mothers should or should not eat peanuts during pregnancy and lactation has similarly been contentious and has vacillated in recent years.[41]

Establishing clear causal connections between changing dietary practices or novel foods and specific disease states has long flummoxed scientists and policy makers, let alone the consumers who ultimately decide what is to go on the table. Although the increasing amount of sugar in Western diets has been blamed for rising rates of type 2 diabetes, linking other foods with chronic diseases is not straightforward, as a number of historians have shown with respect to cancer and heart disease, and as we shall further in Part One of this book.[42] When the disease state itself is highly contentious and caused by multiple factors, as in the case of attention deficit hyperactivity disorder, it becomes even trickier to establish a connection.[43] During the early 1970s, for instance, San Francisco allergist Ben Feingold developed a food additive-free diet for the treatment of hyperactivity in children. Although many trials were designed to test the Feingold diet, most were undermined by the difficulty in controlling for the many other factors believed to influence child behaviour, as well as the difficulty in diagnosing the disorder itself.[44] Moreover, the food industry, under the vestige of a lobby group called the Nutrition Foundation, took an active role in the trials, funding some and publishing a summative report that downplayed Feingold's hypothesis.[45] Amidst all of this confusion, families tended to resort to their own observations and the experiences of others.

The power of corporations and other vested interests in shaping the debates about dietary innovation and disease is difficult to underestimate. When micronutrients began to be identified in the early twentieth century, it did not take long for food and pharmaceutical companies to market vitamins and vitamin-enriched products, quickly creating a billion-dollar industry.[46] Although diseases such as rickets, scurvy, pellagra and beriberi provide ample evidence of the deadly potential of vitamin deficiency, by the second half of the twentieth century millions of Western consumers – often middle-class individuals with access to vitamin-rich diets – became convinced that they and their children's health rested on taking a daily multivitamin or 'Flintstone's' vitamin (a subconscious plug for a 'Paleo diet' or just a moment of marketing genius?). In the 1980s and 1990s, the food industry similarly took advantage of (now contested) scientific claims about the dangers of high-fat and high-cholesterol foods.[47]

Perhaps looming over everything in the debates about dietary innovation disease are two separate, but related, factors. The first is that food fads, fears and fantasies all make a great story. We are routinely fed a diet of news stories and popular literature dealing with the health implications of diet, resulting in an overload of advice about what we should eat. In spite of this, as David Smith and Jim Phillips have described, 'Everyone thinks that they are an expert on their own diet.'[48] Despite the onslaught of information, we still ignore some of the most established nutrition advice. Michael Pollan's suggestion to 'Eat food. Not too much. Mostly plants.' may be all the advice most of us need, but that does not make it any easier to follow.[49]

Proteins, Pathologies and Politics aims to unpack these current concerns by historicizing and contextualizing the relationship between dietary innovation and health in the past. We have divided the book into three parts, each with a different underlying theme, although the themes themselves are closely interconnected. Part One explores the interplay between chronic disease and diet, focusing on cancer, diabetes and allergies. Diet has been seen as both the cause and, possibly, the cure (or at least treatment) of chronic disease. In a precursor to modern notions of the Paleolithic diet, Agnes Arnold-Forster looks at how the cancer 'epidemic' was viewed in late-nineteenth-century Britain as a direct consequence of dietary change brought about by social and economic progress. Investigators wondered why 'Negro' communities (in nineteenth-century parlance) appeared to be immune to the disease, whereas the 'Anglo-Saxon' races seemed particularly prone. Might the answer lie in their food? Perhaps the broad chronological sweep of civilization, from hunter-gatherer to Western industrialization, had made certain races more susceptible to cancer. At the same time, more short-term shifts in diet also appeared dramatically to affect the cancer incidence of certain countries. In fact, Arnold-Forster suggests, by arguing that differentials in disease propensity were bound up with diet, Victorian medical writers were putting forward a more labile and less inherent concept of racial difference than we might expect.

Dietary shifts were also perceived to have a role in increasing rates of food allergies during the twentieth century. In his chapter, Matthew Smith shows how industrial food production and the emergence of a global food economy provided possible explanations for food allergy sufferers and their doctors. Some allergists suspected that a few of the ingredients used in modern food processing – in particular, maize and synthetic food dyes – were also potent allergens. At the same time, the production of food was becoming further removed geographically from consumers so that it became more difficult for food allergy sufferers to identify harmful allergens, thus making accidental exposure more likely. These explanations were just as controversial as those linked with the rise of cancer a century earlier. Yet they mirrored deeper concerns about escalating rates of autoimmune disease, which merit further analysis, Smith suggests, for what they might be able to tell us about why such diseases are on the rise.

If food and dietary changes have been historically linked to some chronic diseases, food and diet might also provide the answer to others. Around the same time as medical writers in Britain were seeking to explain cancer, doctors in the United States were developing the idea of the 'American diet'. This foundation for dietary recommendations based on food composition and nutritive measurement fed directly into diets recommended for diabetics, as recounted by Kirsten E. Gardner. In the era before insulin, diabetic diets tended towards restrictive models that frequently limited carbohydrates and calories, the most extreme of which being Frederick Allen's so-called 'starvation diet'. It promised to extend life but at great cost. With the advent of insulin in 1921, diabetic diets, and the practice of measuring food, became a foundational recommendation in diabetic treatment, as Gardner shows. Works on the subject devoted much space to nutritive information, and insulin dosing was frequently based on a prescribed diet, often perceived as the closest thing to a cure.

In Part Two, we return to the study of how changing diets have brought about disease from the second half of the nineteenth century, but shift the focus to the scientific controversies that erupted over the nature of the relationship. Once the problem has been identified – whether it be chronic diseases in the 1950s or deficiency diseases like pellagra in the late nineteenth and early twentieth centuries – more often than not, the bone of contention concerned causation. Thus, by the mid-nineteenth century all the medical actors studying pellagra in Italy agreed on the link between maize and the epidemic. As David Gentilcore points out in his chapter, what they disagreed on was the exact causal nature of that link, propounding two divergent, indeed mutually exclusive, explanatory models. Gentilcore's chapter seeks to understand how cultural dominance of one explanatory model (Cesare Lombroso's toxic maize theory), at the expense of another (Filippo Lussana and Clodomiro Bonfigli's deficiency theory), came about; what this dominance can tell us about the nature of Italian medical science in the last few decades of the nineteenth century; and what it meant for the pellagra victims themselves.

When it came to pellagra, a change in approach ushered in by a growing understanding of the role of vitamins in the second and third decades of the twentieth century ought to have led to a complete overturn of the dominant paradigm. And yet, as Mircea Scrob demonstrates in his chapter, it did not quite turn out this way. Scrob's analysis of the writings of Romanian, Italian and US medical researchers on pellagra and the early research on vitamins demonstrates how technological, methodological and/or empirical developments do not automatically lead to a re-evaluation of pre-existing knowledge. Indeed, as in this case, a process of 'sedimentation' can occur, in which knowledge produced under different paradigms can coexist.

Even where the scientists do agree, as Maiko Rafael Spiess demonstrates in his chapter, economic interests and lobbies, scientists' reputations and politics are frequently as important as the scientific method and evidence. His focus is on the Framingham Heart Study, an ongoing cardiovascular epidemiological investigation begun in 1948, and its role in contributing to the risk factor approach to diet taken in official government guidelines. Spiess describes how large population studies on cardiovascular diseases helped to establish the 'diet-heart hypothesis' and US government intervention on dietary habits, especially regarding fat and cholesterol. His conclusion is that, in this case, scientific methods, large-scale studies and new conceptual frameworks helped to blur other societal influences and interests, and at the same time, foster the ideal of neutrality and rationality of dietary recommendations.

Today, sugar seems to have replaced fat as the main culprit, at least when it comes to obesity and diet-related disease, such as type 2 diabetes. However, as Rachel Meach argues in her chapter, the argument is not a new one. And an argument it certainly was, pitting American nutritionist Ancel Keys (fat) against the British nutritionist John Yudkin (sugar) during the 1950s. In an outcome that is strangely redolent of the Italian pellagra debates reconstructed by Gentilcore, Keys and his critique of fat won the debate (evident in the dominance of 'low-fat' dietary recommendations that followed), whereas Yudkin's warnings about sugar lay dormant until revived in recent years. Meach explores the factors that shaped Yudkin's ideas about sugar and how he propagated these to the public. In the process, she traces the rise of nutrition science, the emergence of the state as a nutritional authority, the role of gender and cultural ideals in prescribing dietary advice and the influence of commercial and professional interests in shaping public information concerning diet.

The role of politics on both diet and health, evident in several of the above-mentioned chapters, becomes the focus for Part Three. By 'politics', we mean the state and national governments, political movements and ideologies. War marks the twentieth century and it could not but have significant effects on the changing relationships between food/diet and health/disease. In the case of the First World War, the food shortages that resulted not only impacted on ideas concerning the nature of food itself but on the way that food was served to the public. In his chapter, Peter Scholliers explores how food shortages boosted the popularization of the still new concept of 'calorie', to which recurring media attention actively contributed. Mixing quantitative and qualitative analysis, Scholliers traces the way 'calorie' appeared in Belgian newspaper and magazine articles during the war, as a way of understanding how the general public was exposed to new notions about healthy food. If, prior to 1914, 'calorie' needed to be clarified for a lay audience, during the war definitions became rare. And if some newspapers criticized the concept, it nonetheless easily permeated different levels of society, to judge from the nature and readership of the various publications. In particular, food aid was increasingly expressed in calories, especially when the press called upon the Belgian authorities to improve the supply.

In Britain, the authorities took an active and surprisingly public role in food provision. Bryce Evans discusses the nutritional and cultural effects of a short-lived experiment in public dining. With warfare disrupting food imports, in 1917 the government opened a network of centrally funded public cafeteria known as 'national kitchens' serving cheap yet nutritious food. Part of a wider European drive towards communal dining in wartime, these state canteens 'for all' mushroomed in popularity, eventually surpassing 1,000. Evans demonstrates how anxieties soon emerged, however, centred on the revolutionary potential of large numbers of people gathering all at once in the same place and with an influential trade lobby opposed to national kitchens as antithetical to British patriotic values.

The link between political regimes and food culture is taken in a different direction by Francesco Buscemi, in his study of how three different dictatorships constructed meat-eating as a moral disease, and abstention from it as a means of achieving sacred purity. Whereas the vegetarianisms already widespread in the West were linked to physical and spiritual health, food security or animal care, what Buscemi terms the 'sacred' vegetarianism of the Italian Regency of Fiume (1919–1920), Italian fascism and German Nazism went hand-in-glove with political ideology. From the propagandistic representation of vegetarians as more ascetic during the Fiume Regency, to the use of meat abstention to historically and religiously legitimate Benito Mussolini's regime, and culminating in the Nazi transformation of pre-existing vegetarian philosophies and cults linked to purity and primordial naturism into racist theories, sacred vegetarianism transformed a food practice into a food ideology in support of the three regimes.

With the massive disruption, privation and widespread hunger in Europe following the Second World War, national governments found themselves pressed to intervene in different ways. One of these is examined by Silvia Inaudi in her chapter, in the context of food programmes promoted in Italy in the long aftermath of the Second World War for the alleviation of malnutrition and the improvement of child health. In its public policies, the Amministrazione per gli Aiuti Internazionali (Administration for International Aid), a government body, sought to combine social solidarity with the promotion of the science of nutrition and food education. Inaudi focuses on measures and programmes taken to encourage milk-drinking among Italian schoolchildren. Due to the low and segmented levels of consumption and linked to scientific beliefs as well as material factors, the emphasis on milk remained a central part of food assistance to children for a long time. As Inaudi demonstrates, the case of milk is emblematic of both the potentialities and the limitations of nutrition policies, in the way it mixed the motives of child health and welfare with economic and political interests.

At the same time as the Italian government was seeking to promulgate milk-drinking among schoolchildren, the entire way of eating in the United States was being radically transformed. Clare Gordon-Bettencourt examines the role of the US Food and Drug Administration and its policy response to the proliferation of food additives in the marketplace, from the 1940s and through the post-war period, by means of food identity standards provision. From milk, the focus here shifts to bread, and in particular the use of chemical emulsifiers in bread, as a means of investigating the health implications of these ingredients and the broader cultural significance of processed convenience foods. In the process, Gordon-Bettencourt surveys the forces that shaped the framing of bread standards as a case study for the industrialization of America's food, outlines the proliferation of food additives in food standards following the adoption of emulsifiers in the bread standards and analyses the long-term health effects of additives and consumer relationships to processed foods.

What would an Italian peasant, a Scottish crofter or a New England farmer from the 1850s have made of a modern supermarket? The aisles upon aisles of choice and abundance would undoubtedly mesmerize and entice. So, what would they say then if we informed them that such a cornucopia was also thought to spawn disease and death? From consisting of staples and seasonal fare to encompassing the marvels of chemistry and the delicacies of every corner of the globe, the diet of the average North American and European has undergone unprecedented change during the last century and a half. Concurrently, chronic diseases mediated by lifestyle factors (not least of all diet) have come to replace the infectious diseases that once dominated mortality statistics. But while politicians, health policy experts and the media are quick to point out the links between dietary change and diseases such as type 2 diabetes, cancer and heart disease, the chapters in this volume also highlight how contested and politicized ideas about food and health have been. None of our contributors question that some dietary changes have indeed been pathological, but they all assert how both diet and disease exist in a complex context that is marinated in history, ideology, economic imperatives and cultural traditions. When we forget this, we are bound to overemphasize both the dangers and the benefits of some foods and downplay the effect of other factors. Although this may be the first volume to address the history of the tangled relationship between dietary innovation and disease in Europe and North America, we certainly hope that it is not the last. As twenty-first-century consumers come to contemplate cloned meat, edible water bottles, 3D-printed cheese and, possibly, the Star Trek promise of a meal in a pill,[50] the need to ask such questions will be no less pressing.

Acknowledgements

The chapters in this volume represent the selected output from a conference held on the Island of San Servolo, Venice, in June 2016, organized as part of the Economic and Social Research Council-funded project 'Rough Skin: Maize, Pellagra and Society in Italy, 1750–1930' (PI David Gentilcore). The editors would like to thank all of the conference participants for making it such an exciting event, in particular those who took the additional step to turn their conference papers into book chapters; Egidio Priani for his unflagging enthusiasm and organizational assistance; the ESRC for funding the conference; and the Society for the Social History of Medicine, which provided travel bursaries.

Part One

Responding to Chronic Disease

1

The Pre-History of the Paleo Diet: Cancer in Nineteenth-Century Britain

Agnes Arnold-Forster

Dr Loren Cordain describes himself as the 'world's foremost authority on the evolutionary basis of diet and disease' and as 'one of the world's leading experts on the natural human diet of our Stone Age ancestors'.[1] He is the self-proclaimed founder of the Paleo Diet Movement and champions a way of eating that mimics that of our hunter-gatherer forbears. As its online advocates perform their commitment to this arcane way of eating through the very modern mediums of blogging, Twitter and Instagram, the popular Paleo diet and its cousins seem closely tied to the peculiarities of the twenty-first century. And yet, the Paleo premise is not new. In 2014, Cordain published an article on his website, titled 'Breast Cancer and Other Cancers: Diseases of Western Civilization?'[2] In it, he claims that cancer was 'rare or non-existent in historically studied hunter gatherers and other less westernized peoples'. In support of this, he quotes various early-twentieth-century authorities, including the Nobel prize-winning physician Dr Albert Schweitzer, who wrote on his arrival in Gabon in 1913, 'I was astonished to encounter no case of cancer . . . This absence of cancer seemed to me due to the difference in nutrition of the natives as compared with the Europeans.'[3]

This quotation, which Cordain takes as near-irrefutable evidence, provokes him to insist at the end of the article, 'Any way you look at it, the Paleo Diet is a good remedy to prevent cancer.'[4] It is unusual for someone positioning themselves as a contemporary scientific authority to make use of, and directly quote, historical sources – not as errors to be refuted but as evidence for their claims. What are not unusual, however, are the assumptions that underlie the cancer-preventing claims of the Paleo diet. It is a well-known, if ill-supported, trope that cancer constitutes a 'pathology of progress' – an unintended consequence of modernity. Or, as Charles Rosenberg puts it, 'The notion that the incidence of much late-20th-century chronic disease reflects a poor fit between modern styles of life and humankind's genetic heritage.'[5] His seminal article on 'the idea of civilization as risk' identifies a tendency on behalf of late-twentieth-century critics to point to the 'structured asymmetry between a body evolved in Paleolithic conditions and the late-twentieth-century environment in which that body must maintain itself'. However, he suggests that the conventions of this argument – that the 'change from savage to settled rural and then to urban life brought with it conditions increasingly inimical to the body's requirement for diet, exercise, and stable emotional surroundings' – were already established by the end of the eighteenth century.

However, while Rosenberg devotes considerable attention to the nineteenth-century origins of the ideas about the perceived health dangers of urban, industrial society, he focuses on infectious diseases and emotional disorders. Cancer and other chronic diseases, he argues, are instead assumed to be products of the last 50 years, 'At the end of the twentieth century, many of the same themes and anxieties have recast themselves in rather different form. Our most invisible anxieties have surfaced in regard to chronic disease, not neurosis or hysteria.'[6] Rosenberg is not alone in locating our preoccupation with cancer as a problem of civilization in the late twentieth century and neglecting its nineteenth-century genesis. While Roy Porter called cancer 'the modern disease *par excellence*' and Siddhartha Mukherjee described it as 'the quintessential product of modernity', they locate that modernity firmly in the post-war period.[7] Thus, cancer in the nineteenth century – in general – also remains understudied.[8] What work that has been produced on the disease's history has predominantly focused on the twentieth century. This asymmetry can be partly explained by the ways in which cancer has been constrained by a version of periodization that serves to tie certain maladies – or malady-types – to specific epochs. Medical historians, epidemiologists and demographers have conceptualized the nineteenth century as the 'epidemic century', with infectious diseases and their control occupying the forefront of historical investigation. This periodization is most clearly articulated by Abdel Omran's 'citation classic', published in 1971, on the theory of epidemiological transition.[9] He posited three phases: 'the age of pestilence and famine' – roughly corresponding to medieval and early modern Europe; 'the age of receding pandemics' – the long nineteenth century; and 'the age of degenerative and man-made diseases' – intimately associated with civilization and the development of 'modern' healthcare and medicine.[10] Diet is at the centre of this narrative. Civilized ways of living bring civilized ways of eating – which, in turn, bring civilized diseases.

Yet, and as Cordain has noticed, the idea that 'civilized' ways of eating made certain races more susceptible to cancer has its roots in the nineteenth century. The collection of vital statistics in Britain from the 1840s onwards suggested to troubled observers that cancer's incidence was increasing exponentially. This perceived 'cancer epidemic' captured the medical and lay imagination, and provoked intense debate. Even the fashion magazine *Vogue* despaired, 'It is sad news indeed that cancer is increasing at such a rate.'[11] This chapter thus explores *fin-de-siècle* debates about the relationship between industrialized or civilized life and cancer incidence to address this historiographical lacuna. Specifically, it argues that British discourse about the 'cancer epidemic' orbited around anxieties over social and economic progress and attendant dietary change. This discourse centred on two questions. First, had the broad chronological sweep of civilization – from hunter-gatherer to Western industrialization – made certain races more or less susceptible to cancer? 'Negro' communities (in nineteenth-century parlance) appeared to be immune to the disease, whereas Anglo-Saxon races – situated at the apex of Victorian conceptions of civilization – seemed particularly prone. Could the answer to this hierarchy be found in their food? Second, had more short-term shifts in diet dramatically effected the cancer incidence of certain countries? For example, had changes in diet following the Irish famine (increase in processed food and low-quality American meat) accelerated Ireland's cancer susceptibility?

Various historians have observed that this period witnessed an increased awareness of food as a potential vector for disease.[12] Moreover, some scholars have recognized the close historical relationship between diet and cancer. For example, David Cantor has argued that for many early-twentieth-century Americans, cancer was a disease of nutrition and particularly a product of meat consumption.[13] Similar ideas circulated in *fin-de-siècle* Britain. Like Cantor, I argue that the close connection between cancer and diet was in part a product of how practitioners and the public understood the disease's pathology and character. However, while he suggests that this association proved troublesome for later-twentieth-century public health and awareness-raising campaigns, I contend that the causal relationship between food and malignancy appealed to, and was reassuring for, a professional community otherwise despairing at their impotence in the face of this 'dread disease'.

This chapter is divided into two parts. Part One clarifies what cancer was in late-nineteenth-century Britain and delineates how Victorian practitioners and the public conceptualized its causes, characteristics, and cures. It also provides context to explain the broader connections made between food, diet and malignancy in this period. Part Two shows how *fin-de-siècle* medical men constructed expansive spatial and temporal hierarchies and argued that the broad chronological sweep of civilization – from the Stone Age to late-nineteenth-century modernity – had structured races' susceptibility to cancer. Specifically, it looks at how, as diets moved further from 'nature', they were thought of as increasingly 'cancer causing'. Finally, it zeroes in on a specific case study – Ireland after its famine – taken up by late-nineteenth-century observers as an example of how declining quality of food and the increase in the importing of foreign produce were undermining the cellular integrity of a population.

Nineteenth-century cancer

Cancer in the nineteenth century was identified and diagnosed according to its observed adherence to a set of characteristics. It was, like today, defined by its long duration and its irreversible capacity for growth and spread. Those surgeons who felt surface cancer with their hands were well aware that these masses could be later-stage manifestations of an internal disease; or that breast cancer, for example, could spread to the liver or lungs. Crucially, too, it was a material entity – an 'object' that could be identified by hand or eye.[14] Cancer was evidenced by the presence of a tumour, accompanied by pain, physical degeneration and disability, and marked by its inexorably increasing magnitude.[15] These identifying characteristics were codified following cancer patients' admission to the nineteenth-century hospital, after two cancer-specific institutions were set up in 1792 and 1802.[16] The context of the clinic allowed medical men to trace cancer through its life course, making possible extended observations of its duration and its tendency to grow and metastasize. Then, practitioners watched their subjects die with depressing regularity. Thus, the hospital confirmed cancer as an incurable disease that was distinct from other maladies. Early-nineteenth-century surgeon Thomas Denman insisted, 'Of all diseases deemed *incurable*, that which is denominated *Cancer* has been most generally allowed to be so.'[17]

While many of these identifying features of the disease might be alien to us today, we can nonetheless meaningfully speak of 'cancer' as a broadly coherent and stable disease category in the nineteenth century and before. Historian Alanna Skuse argues that while cancer in the early modern period was predicated on an entirely different way of interpreting the human body and its afflictions, it nonetheless had much in common with our twenty-first-century malady: cancer then is recognizable to us now. She claims that 'cancerous disease "existed" in the early modern period, in the sense of there being a distinctive malady known as "cancer" which was broadly contiguous with the illness sharing that name today'.[18] In the nineteenth century, too, cancer was a distinct pathological entity that shared physical characteristics with the malady in both the sixteenth century and the twenty-first. This stable profile over time, at least in terms of its meaning if not its experience, only makes cancer's relative absence from the historical literature more surprising.

While many other diseases ended in death in the nineteenth century, cancer was articulated as superlative – as the most extreme case on a spectrum. The language used by medical men and the laity alike repeatedly reinscribed this special status. Cancer was synonymous with 'malignancy' – an evocative term that meant both the ability to metastasize and a being with malevolent intention. Cancer was positioned as a disease that was not only deadly, but also cruel. It was a 'pernicious' malady, synonymous with death and decline and feared by doctor and patient.[19] It was, 'of all the ills to which the human frame is liable', the 'most poignant'.[20] It was repeatedly designated the 'crudele opprobrium medicorum' – the cruellest challenge to the medical profession.

The terms here have a moral inflection, and it was common for commentaries on cancer – or commentaries that used cancer metaphorically – to describe the disease as something with agency and independence of thought. These metaphors also inscribed a connection between malignancy, food and eating. For centuries, cancer had been conceptualized as a parasitical being – a creature occupying the body and consuming it from within. In her article on malignancy in early modern England, Skuse describes how in the seventeenth century, the disease was imagined as 'quasi-sentient, zoomorphising the disease as an eating worm or wolf'.[21] This idea that cancer was an animal, distinct from its host, persisted into the nineteenth century. It was endowed with character, temperament and disposition – with needs in direct competition with those of the body it occupied. In 1841, a Member of Parliament claimed, 'The unjust and miserable system of paying wages out of rates – the discouragement of industry, and the premium which was offered to improvidence and sloth – the cancer which has got such a powerful hold of the southern provinces, was gradually *eating* its way to the heart of England [my emphasis]'.[22] Metaphors and analogies are rhetorical or analytical techniques, but they also articulate actual scientific and medical understanding.[23] In other words, for these cancer metaphors to 'work' in the political context of Parliament, they needed to have some widespread purchase on the collective imagination. That MPs could deploy such language to rhetorical effect was dependent on a general understanding of cancer as having intention and being animal-like.

This notion that cancer was a parasite was intimately linked to a prevalent idea that the disease was much affected by the diet of its host. In the 1890s, a doctor called cancer 'an independent organism, like many a protozoon; that lives a life which is wholly independent and proper to itself'.[24] Not only was it conceptualized as a semi-independent life form, one that required its own system of sustenance, but the disease was frequently described using metaphors of food and consumption. In 1910, Charles Walker, from the Glasgow Royal Cancer Hospital, pointed out that 'cancer cells derive their nourishment from the cells forming the body of the organism in which they exist'.[25] Their 'vitality' was well known, so 'any change of diet must affect the [cancer] cells'.[26] It was therefore unsurprising to a *fin-de-siècle* commentator that after the 'female secondary sexual organs', cancer of the stomach was the 'commonest form of the disease in both sexes'.[27]

Thus, the connections drawn between cancer and diet were not just metaphorical. Towards the end of the nineteenth century, food and drink were increasingly offered as explanations for the cancer's origin. For while practitioners had made substantial headway in observing and codifying the disease, its causes remained largely unknown. This acknowledge limitation to medical knowledge, combined with the fear and anxiety associated with the incurable 'dread disease', prompted a wide-ranging search for explanatory models for its aetiology. In 1902, Dr James Braithwaite suggested in the *British Medical Journal* that cancer was caused by an 'excess of salt in the diet'.[28] Similarly, a pair of contemporaneous colonial doctors claimed that tea drinking was to blame for the disease's incidence in New Zealand.[29] The second half of the nineteenth century witnessed diet becoming an increasingly popular explanatory mechanism for cancer and its origin. This was no coincidence and depended not only on a widespread perception that the incidence of cancer was increasing, but also on persuasive contemporary anxieties over racial difference, the unintended costs of civilization and dietary innovation.

The cancer epidemic

The 1840s and 1850s saw the British populace increasingly quantified. This practice derived in part from the development of statistical methods and epidemiology, and grew alongside a numerical study of people and their activities more generally.[30] The main source of vital statistics was the *Annual Report of the Registrar-General on Births, Deaths and Marriages in England*, first presented to Parliament in 1838.[31] The General Registry Office (GRO) calculated the annual mortality by each cause and the proportion of deaths in 100,000 effected by each class of disease in each region. Narrative prefaces to each annual report situated individual investigations within a broad chronology and enabled doctors and public health professionals to comment on yearly shifts in the disease profile of the nation.[32] From the *Fourth Annual Report* causes of death were recorded, alongside the person's sex, age and profession. The causes were divided into 'Epidemic, Endemic, and Contagious Diseases', 'Sporadic Disease of Uncertain or Variable Seat', 'Sporadic Diseases of Special Systems and Organs' and 'External Causes: Poisoning, Asphyxia, Injuries'. Cancer was categorized within 'Sporadic Disease of Uncertain or Variable Seat'.[33] In 1879, the narrative preface to the *Forty-Second Annual Report* reported that there appeared to be a new 'cancer epidemic' in Britain, and that the disease had 'maintained the increase to which it has been gradually mounting for many years'.[34] This new 'cancer epidemic' prompted an array of rival explanatory models and investigative strategies, including spatial configurations of the disease on a global scale.

Thus, and in part because science and medicine were key components of British imperial expansion, by the closing decades of the century, a dynamic and interactive network of scientists and doctors was working in colonial contexts. Men like W. Renner, medical officer of Freetown; Sierra Leone; and Sir William MacGregor, lieutenant-governor of British New Guinea, compiled data and anecdotes about cancer incidence in their respective countries and reported them back to the metropole.[35] London-based journals like the *British Medical Journal* and *The Lancet* acted as nexuses of cancer information, sent in from across the empire. This information fed into conceptual cartographies of cancer that covered the globe. Commentators theoretically plotted populations on a gradient – from immune to cancer-riddled – with sub-Saharan African communities at one end and Anglo-Saxon or Teutonic races at the other. 'Observation has shown that cancer has a certain geographical distribution. It prevails extensively in some parts of the globe, and is scarcely known in others.'[36]

This 'mapping' suggested that England and its Anglo-Saxon inhabitants suffered the greatest burden, 'Englishmen may be regarded as unfortunate; for within the geographical area of these islands cancer asserts largely its malignant and fatal influence.'[37] In contrast, cancer incidence in British colonies was low, even non-existent. In 1906, the *British Medical Journal* reported, 'There can be no doubt that cancer in natives of British Central Africa is of the utmost rarity.[38] Repeated efforts made by Government medical officers throughout the country for some time past have so far resulted in the discovery of but a single case.'[39] The situation in Sierra Leone was similar, 'Cancer as a disease is very rare among the aborigines . . . I would rather not say that the aborigines are immune from the disease, but that the disease is rare among them.'[40] Dr A. J. Craigen, writing from Port Moresby in New Guinea in 1905, reported 'that during his stay of nearly four years in the Possession he has not yet seen a single case of cancer among the native population'.[41] Cancer rates were slightly higher in Hong Kong. 'The returns made to the Registrar-General show that the total number of deaths among the Chinese in the period 1895–1904 was 11, giving an annual death-rate from cancer of 4.45 per 100, 000 of population.'[42] However, as Dr Francis Clark, acting principal civil medical officer, pointed out, this compared 'very favourably with the death-rate from the same cause in England'.[43] These colonial observations of cancer proved troubling to social and medical commentators. Not only was the disease on the increase, but the epidemic seemed to be confined to nations that were conventionally understood as biologically, culturally and economically superior.

The observation that so-called 'primitive' races were relatively immune to cancer required explanation. The idea that certain groups were inherently more or less vulnerable to certain diseases was a common concept in Victorian medicine and it was in part dependent on a version of biological anthropology that structured strict and impermeable boundaries between different races.[44] This period witnessed a concretization of racial distinctions and a heightened commitment of the importance of biology in dictating behaviours and tendencies. This coincided with, and was causally linked to, an increasingly rapacious and fretful imperialism. Late-nineteenth-century anthropology dictated that race was 'no arbitrary idea, no abstraction'– and practitioners toyed with the idea that cancer was also a product of inherent biology. Surgeon Leo Loeb reflected, 'Whether those differences in the cancer morbidity are primarily questions of race or whether they are due to the external conditions under which the races live.'[45]

However, and as demonstrated by discourses of dietary innovation, for most *fin-de-siècle* commenters cancer was less a product of the civilized *body* and more of the civilized *way of living*. Director of the Imperial Cancer Research Fund, E. F. Bashford, insisted that there was nothing intrinsic in the biology of 'Negroes' that made them immune to cancer – nor, as some people suggested, had they been infected by contact with cancer-carrying colonialists – but rather it was due to their conditions of life. He wrote, 'I venture to assert that the prevalence of cancer among the negroes of America was not brought about contact with cancer-infested white men . . . Cancer was inherent in the negroes when they were shipped from their native Africa, where it probably existed as it still does to-day, in natives removed from civilisation.'[46] Eating was central to ideas about the civilized versus the uncivilized lifestyle. The army surgeon William Hill-Climo wrote in 1903, 'There is a strong presumption that it is the food which is at fault.'[47]

Hill-Climo and his co-professionals understood 'uncivilized' people as less vulnerable to malignancy because they lived in harmony with the natural world and pursued simple, abstemious habits. These communities tended to avoid decadent or artificial food, tracked closely to nature and so avoided cancer. Surgical registrar to the Middlesex Hospital, W. Roger Williams wrote in 1902, 'The reputation of Egypt for comparative immunity from cancer is well founded . . . The conditions of existence are unfavourable to the development of cancer. If I am asked to define these conditions, it may be answered that they comprise extreme frugality in living; open-air existence, and last – but not least – an alimentation which includes but little animal food.'[48] The low incidence of cancer in Egypt could be explained by its inhabitants' uncivilized lifestyles – its stable cancer epidemic was a product of the country's static relationship with nature and its stationary position on the gradient of societal progress.

A key aspect of nineteenth-century racial anthropology was that difference was not just spread spatially, but temporally as well. 'Primitive' races did not just exist in far-flung places, but showed 'civilized' observers how their own societies had once been. They were 'survivals' from bygone eras and revealed the stages of human development. Thus, the geographical distribution of cancer incidence helped explain the increasing rates in Britain. Hill-Climo argued that the increasing death rate from cancer in all European countries, and in the United States, could not be 'ascribed to local or accidental causes', but must instead be 'sought for in the growth of new conditions . . . common to all the affected countries, which the people themselves have produced.'[49] The new epidemic was a product of 'new conditions' – and they were conditions of the societies' own making. Hill-Climo's comments relied upon, and in turn confirmed, pervasive contemporary anxieties over the degeneration and decline of 'civilized' societies and the inherent dangers of modernity. Coupled with the observed rise in cancer incidence, global geographies of cancer fed into anxieties about the unintended costs of civilization.

The idea of degeneracy, hereditary or otherwise, suffused *fin-de-siècle* culture and the discourse of Europe's urban elite – and with it the idea that prosperity, industrialization and urbanization brought with them a plethora of physical and emotional complaints. Anxieties over the dangers inherent in industrialized, artificial and urban life were widespread and much has been written about the late-nineteenth-century preoccupation with 'diseases of modern life'. Dr James Crichton-Browne spoke in 1860 of the 'velocity of thought and action' now required, and of the stress imposed on the brain by being forced to process in a month more information 'than was required of our grandfathers in the course of a lifetime'.[50] Charles E. Rosenberg has argued that concern for the 'psychic dangers of an artificial and emotionally fevered life' had become conventional by the mid-century.[51] Commentators observed an increase in diseases from worry, overwork, mental or physical strain, excess, self-abuse, stimulants and narcotics. They diagnosed neurosis, hysteria and melancholy on a mass scale, and articulated modern, urban life as inherently risky. This body of literature dealt with the 'apparent paradox' that civilization itself 'might be the catalyst of, as much as the defence against, physical and social pathology'. In an early-twentieth-century *New York Times* article entitled 'Is Race Extinction Staring Us in the Face?', the author recounted how 'the possibility of the extinction of the human race is predicted by many present-day scientists. They insist that tendencies toward race degeneracy are actively at work.' The author interviewed the founder of the popular cereal brand John Harvey Kellogg, who responded in frantic terms, 'In many large centres of population, Manchester, Eng., for example, it is impossible to find men big enough to serve as policemen.'

These ideas of social and somatic decline in *fin-de-siècle* Europe and North America primed practitioners to express cancer as a consequence of social and somatic degeneration. Historians have described a society preoccupied with inheritance, atavism, evolution and eugenics, and the cancer story can be mapped on to these anxieties. Indeed, much of Kellogg's fretful commentary centred on cancer as a 'by-product of civilisation'.[52] He wrote how, over the past 30 years, 'the mortality from chronic diseases has doubled' and cited 'the rapid spread of cancer in both man and the lower animals as an instance of a degenerative malady characteristic of civilization'.[53] There was, therefore, something carcinogenic in civilized habits and ways of eating.

However, there was some disagreement over what precisely constituted the carcinogenic element of civilized dietary change. There was a popular strand of thought that located the cause of cancer – and its increased incidence – in the consumption of meat, and various doctors, food scientists and social commentators – including Kellogg – advocated for vegetarianism as a preventative measure against malignancy, as well as against a whole range of other maladies.[54] Others found fault not in the type of food, but in the volume. An article published in the *British Medical Journal* in 1900 argued, 'The abundance of food, which is one of the results of our national prosperity, is on the whole a most powerful factor in the improvement of the public health. But the high standard of general nutrition thus maintained appears to be not without its drawbacks.'[55] Thus, the increase in the number of deaths from cancer was due to the 'overeating which is almost universal even among the poorer classes of the population'.[56] Some suggested that the increasing incidence of the disease in civilized nations was because the societies that inhabited them had departed from nature and 'natural' ways of living. This was evidenced by cases of 'primitive' people who appeared to have contracted cancer after deviating from their 'primitive' existence. William Macgregor wrote, 'Dr Johnson . . . tells me that in Lagos during a practice of fourteen years' duration, he has five times seen cancer in native patients, and that in each case the sufferer had lived as Europeans live'.[57] Thus, Kellogg recommended that while 'we need not return to savagery to be healthy', we 'must see that the air we breathe is as clean as that which the savage breathes, that the food we eat is as wholesome and pure as the water we drink'.[58]

Ireland offered an intriguing case study for late-nineteenth-century commentators on the relationship between dietary innovation and malignant disease. The Great Famine, or the Great Hunger, was a period of mass starvation, disease and emigration in Ireland between 1845 and 1852. As Ian Miller has argued, Irish eating habits changed dramatically between the famine and the country's independence in 1922.[59] A perceived increase in the incidence of cancer is an underexplored consequence of this change. Army surgeon William Hill-Climo mulled over the relatively low, but nonetheless rising, cancer incidence in Ireland. For while the disease was less common among Celtic communities than its English counterparts, it nonetheless appeared to be increasing: 'It is clear that two questions require to be investigated; the first is that cancer has steadily increased in Ireland during the past 40 years, and the second is that the mortality is much lower than in England and in Scotland'.[60] His answer to both these questions, 'paradoxical as it may appear', was the '*poverty* of the Irish people'.[61] He harked back to an imagined, prelapsarian phase in Irish history: 'Before the Irish famine the Irish lived on oatmeal porridge, potatoes, eggs and milk, with fish and home-cured bacon occasionally'.[62] Hill-Climo believed that this simpler, less decadent diet was less likely to initiate cancer.

However, he lamented that the Irish had lost touch with their wholesome culinary past; 'Now, cheap American bacon and flour pancakes cooked in bacon fat, Indian meal porridge sweetened with chemically-coloured beet sugars, and boiled tea are the stable food commodities of the people'.[63] This quotation reveals a complex coalescing of anxieties over food, cancer, national borders and imperial coherence. Some were concerned by the potentially pathological results of importing refrigerated meat to the British Isles from overseas dominions and other countries. In 1897, the MP for Dorset North, Mr Wingfield-Digby, proclaimed in the House of Commons that 'the consumers of frozen meat were liable to cancer and other terrible diseases'.[64] Hill-Climo shared in this specific anxiety over meat and argued that 'cancerous diseases . . . are caused by the long-continued consumption of unwholesome animal food'.[65] Although it was unclear what he thought had corrupted this animal food – was it something inherent in the animal-ness of the product, its overseas passage or its foreignness?

The bacon, porridge and tea that Hill-Climo was worried about were all foreign products, imported into Ireland across expanses of land and sea. He was distressed at the 'want of variety' in the food and its unwholesomeness. He argued that the imported flour was 'inferior' and 'wanting in freshness'.[66] This could reveal a generic anxiety over anything alien and introduced from elsewhere. However, it is telling that he noted that the process by which these goods had arrived in Ireland was dependent on 'modern economic conditions'. He blamed technological change, claiming that the shift in diet had 'been facilitated by steam transport'.[67] Hill-Climo was evidently troubled by the possibility that communication and transport technologies – the very fabric of British success and imperial dominion – may well be the source of its undoing. The Irish departure from their 'natural' diets, facilitated by technologies that imported civilization and its attendant consumables from countries like the United States, had made them vulnerable to cancer.

Conclusion

By 1914, the notion that cancer was an unintended consequence of civilization was well-travelled terrain. A range of observers concluded that not only did a society's location on the global hierarchy of social development determine its susceptibility to malignancy, but also recent transformations in the way inhabitants of the British Isles ate had contributed to a new 'cancer epidemic'. These ideas depended on a variety of interweaving threads of nineteenth-century medical and cultural thought. Cancer was conceptualized as a parasitical being, with its own demands on the host body's system of nutrition. The *fin de siècle* witnessed widespread anxiety over 'diseases of modern life' and particularly over the role of food as a potential vessel and vector of ill health. Moreover, cancer's stubborn incurability and the persistent mystery over its aetiology made the disease an attractive subject for debate. Its identity, although fixed in some ways, was malleable in others and could be co-opted to support a range of conceptualizations about bodies, societies, and disease.

Moreover, this explanatory model – that negatively correlated 'nature' and the natural with cancer – was powerful if paradoxical. While cancer – with all its attendant horror and suffering – should be an unequivocal negative, it seemed, in the nineteenth century, to imply positive things about the societies in which it flourished. Mapping the global distribution of cancer had suggested that 'Negroes' – biologically inferior in every other way – were almost immune to the disease. Cancer incidence thus subverted the conventional hierarchy between colonizers and colonized and found in 'savage' lifestyles a fundamental redeeming feature. Nineteenth-century medical practitioners and Dr Loren Cordain alike tie cancer to modernity – and to a modernity of our own making. Our reckless decadence has made chronic disease common. You might think this critique of civilization – this celebration of non-Western diets – would work to upset conventional hierarchies. However, and as Kellogg pointed out, no one wants to return to 'savagery'. Instead, we live in a strange world in which cancer is a marker of social progress and civilization – an inversion of the expected order. It is not uncommon for public health practitioners today to comment on increases in chronic disease in low- and middle-income countries as a 'sign of success'.[68] This strange world is a Victorian inheritance, an inheritance that Cordain, for all his flaws, acknowledges.

2

Nutrition, Starvation and Diabetic Diets: A Century of Change in the United States

Kirsten E. Gardner

Innovations in the way we consume, measure and interact with food influence daily life, but few lives are as affected by food and food innovations as diabetic lives. For diabetics, the intersections of food, its impact on the body and its intersection with personal identities are particularly pronounced. US Supreme Court Justice Sonia Sotomayor, a diabetic of more than 50 years, recently made this point. When asked how diabetes impacted her life, Sotomayor explained that from the moment she awoke each morning until the moment she slept, she considered every morsel she ate and how it impacted her body.[1]

Nineteenth-century nutritional science created a foundation for contemporary discussions of nutrition by designing food tables based on terms familiar today – including protein, carbohydrate and fat content. This offered diabetics a common vocabulary for comparing 'diabetic diets' and opened the gates for consistent measurement of food across the nation and throughout the world. As Frederick Allen thoroughly documented in the first chapter of his 1919 study, *Total Dietary Regulation in the Treatment of Diabetes*, dozens of diets had been heralded as the key to curing diabetes in medical journals, offering diabetics recommendations that seemed helpful at best, but often absurd.[2]

For centuries, medical texts had emphasized the potential of treating diabetes with food innovation. Beginning the in the late nineteenth century, however, the United States joined a transnational conversation about quantifying food composition with household measurement. The science of 'American food products' offered building blocks for diabetic diets and became the foundation of dietary texts that targeted diabetics by promising dietary innovations to improve health. As examples, in diabetologist Elliot Joslin's texts, diabetics learned that 'the diet of a diabetic need not be severe or conspicuous.'[3] In the midst of a mid-century awareness of rising rates of diabetes, especially within the African American population, Nation of Islam leader Elijah Muhammad promised that 'sugar diabetes can be controlled and cured if you only eat correctly.'[4] More recently, Dr Richard Bernstein's *The Diabetic Diet* claimed, 'It is no exaggeration to say that the Diabetes Diet is a lifesaver.'[5] By tracing dietary innovations in the United States for little more than a century, this paper suggests that food innovation has deep roots as a powerful treatment for diabetes and the belief in the power of food persists into the twenty-first century.

Measuring food

The 1893 Chicago World's Fair captured the marvels of modernity in the late-nineteenth-century United States. Audiences flocked from near and far to participate in this moment in history and to consume the knowledge, entertainment and beauty it offered. The fair's celebration of architecture, machinery, art and its stunning esplanade resonated with the audience's imagination and highlighted notions of advancement within the United States and throughout the world. Although much attention has been directed to the splendours of the exhibit, it also launched many scientific innovations. As a case in point, a laboratory housing approximately fifteen scientists, whose space stretched across three campuses, could be found nestled in a corner of the neoclassical, carefully constructed 'White City'.[6] Within that laboratory, scientists worked feverishly to quantify the 'American diet'. After decades of borrowing nutritive information based on European food studies, US scientists promised to analyse 500 American food specimens. This study, and the subsequent nutritional studies that followed, quantified the American diet in a clear and consistent manner by enumerating the grams of food, carbohydrate content, protein content, percentage of fat and more – ultimately creating metrics that allowed medical specialists and others to better understand the intersections of American diet and health.[7]

The beginning of the World Fair's food measurement laboratory began with Dr Wilbur Olin Atwater, who served as a special agent for the US Department of Agriculture. He joined the Chicago World's Fair by promoting how much consumers might learn about the 'American diet' during this measurement project. Food composition analysis promised to unpack the nutritive value of different foods, the costs associated with each food and its essential components.[8] Atwater's professional reputation and his affiliation with Wesleyan University paved the way for his invitation to join Chicago World's Fair exhibit in 1893. Once in Chicago, he invited chemists, assistants and apprentices to join the project; obtained the necessary appliances; secured additional space from the University of Chicago; and ordered multiple apparatus that would facilitate this ambitious project. Atwater and his team tapped into turn-of-the-century faith in the value of measurement to construct encyclopaedic knowledge about American food products and their nutritive value. Perhaps most significant in this story on the history of the diabetic diet, Atwater's work allowed scientists to study the intersections of disease and nutrition with more consistent measurements and greater accuracy. Although Atwater did not focus on diabetes exclusively, his work became foundational in creating the metrics that would assess 'diabetic diets' in the century to follow.[9] Nutritive data allowed for a range of therapeutic recommendations that targeted the American diet in the pre-insulin and insulin era alike.[10] As the *Dietetic and Hygienic Gazette* noted, 'This was the most extensive single inquiry of the sort which had been undertaken up to that time.'[11]

Within a few years of the 1893 Chicago World's Fair, Atwater published food composition data and he became an authority on the 'food of man' for decades to come. The tabular summaries created during the exhibition offered a measurement model that still dominates nutritional science today.[12] Such texts provided tools for patients to better negotiate dietary adjustments and may have modified recipes to create diabetic-friendly recipes, maintain preferred food choices and more. Through this lens, the diabetic diet of the early twentieth century may have seemed more curative than punitive and food may have been attributed as medicinal.

By shifting our lens to dietary innovations in the nineteenth century and beyond and placing diabetic diets at the centre of this analysis, the importance of food measurement comes into sharp focus. Historians of diabetes have noted that early-twentieth-century diabetic diets urged restriction, undernutrition and starvation if necessary.[13] Made most famous by US practitioner Frederick Allen, it was quickly dubbed a 'starvation diet', as there were no bounds to the restrictions it required. Allen's 1919 text *Total Dietary Regulation in the Treatment of Diabetes* reflected Allen's faith in restrictive dietary treatment as well as his appreciation for European research on the topic. He reviewed countless publications on diet modification for diabetes from ancient history to the present, focusing particularly on medical debates about carbohydrate restriction, animal diet and vegetarian diet.[14] He had a keen eye towards practitioners who gained adherents. As he described John Rollo's nineteenth-century animal diet for diabetes, it 'never gained general adoption by the medical profession of any country' yet had 'eminent supporters'.[15] He appreciated the strictness demonstrated by Italian scientist Arnaldo Cantani whose 'treatment set an entirely new standard of strictness; this was the essential contribution made by Cantani. He isolated patients under lock and key, and allowed them absolutely no food but lean meat and various fats.' And he seemed to applaud those who took a stand and supported scientific evaluation of food and diet. German practitioner Naunyn was a 'champion of strict carbohydrate-free diet in a German medical congress where most of the speakers opposed it'. Allen celebrated US diabetologist Elliot Joslin by explaining, 'No other American clinician has followed the scientific study of diabetes so long and so intensely.'[16]

Historians have turned to Allen's text as an indication of the European influence in dietary innovations for diabetes in the pre-insulin era. Michael Bliss's path-breaking work *The Discovery of Insulin* outlines the European origins of restrictive diabetic diets. By the early twentieth century, diet modification was the single most effective means to treating diabetes.[17] French physician, Apollinaire Bouchardet, urged periodic fast days, carbohydrate restriction and exercise.

Food mattered, and the nutritional tables of the turn of the century offered a vocabulary to discuss food, diet and the daily practice of eating (or not eating) as a daily therapeutic act. Nutritive data offered metrics to patients and practitioners seeking ways to compare, quantify and assess the power of food. As early as 1915, we see the optimism infused in this possibility of dietary treatment. As a 1915 advertisement for Battle Creek Sanatorium promised, at its Health resort, 'dieting is not only possible but delightful. Exact knowledge of the nutritive values of each dish enables the patient to choose each meal intelligently without too much restriction of individual taste.'[18] In addition to measuring carbohydrates, fats, proteins and calories, diabetics would adopt measurement practices to quantify sugar in the urine. Later in the century diabetics would measure blood sugar, and still later tests for haemoglobin A1C would become over-the-counter tools for patients to collect data, measure their disease and perhaps modify therapy. As this essay will demonstrate, dietary innovations offer a constant thread to consider competing diabetic remedies, but they also reflect the century-long practice of measuring diabetes – and turning to such measurements as a lens for improved treatment and quality of life.

The pre-insulin era

The connections between food and health have roots in the earliest medical records. As Riddle noted in a recent review of diabetic literature, 'A polyuric state, presumably diabetes, was described more than 3,500 years ago.'[19] Curiously, however, the late-nineteenth-century food studies sponsored by the US government seemed largely inspired by economic considerations. In particular, discussion of the cost of labour, food and the value of nutrition offered new formulas for thinking about labour costs. Realizing that more than 50 per cent of wages went to food costs, food scientists argued that better nutritional consumption could help with one's budget, as well as one's health.[20] As secretary of agriculture for President McKinley, Sterling Morton wrote in 1896, 'In connection with studies of the food of man in this country a standard table of analyses of American food products is very much needed.'[21] Turn-of-the-century science and economics intersected in material ways as economists and others analysed labour's spending patterns and the percentage of wage dedicated to food.

Food studies opened the door for much more extensive analysis in a variety of disciplines. For diabetic practitioners, nutritional studies offered a much-needed comparative lens for examining the intersections of diet and diabetes. As a diabetic text of 1924 captured, 'It is only within the last few years that the constituents of foods have been given their proper place in the estimation of food values.'[22]

Although the association of food and diabetes was well known, the cause and effect of diet's impact on blood sugar varied widely. Some doctors urged calorie restriction, while others advanced a specific 'nutritive-rich' dietary regime. Still others had advanced a diet rich in certain foods such as the 'oat-cure diet' and 'milk diet'. Although not explicitly written for diabetes treatment, nineteenth-century Mexican cookbooks included general *Dietas para Infirma* as a way of prescribing diets for the ill.[23]

In the pre-insulin era (pre-1921), diabetic therapy centred on food and quantified diets became the most effective therapy for diabetes. Published medical texts with recommendations for 'diabetic diets' circulated in the United States, England, Germany, Australia, Scotland and beyond. Many diets had transatlantic audiences, such as the late-nineteenth-century diabetic text written in German, translated into English and republished in Philadelphia, which advised diabetics, 'Articles of food which have an immediate strengthening and nourishing effect . . . are to be allowed.'[24] As historian Michael Bliss has summarized, such diets reflected the 'notion that a diabetic needed extra nourishment to compensate for the nutritive material flowing out of the urine.'[25] Such global advice, often supported with anecdotal evidence, was common. At the same time that some practitioners preached a nutritionally rich diet, others advocated restrictive practices. In the late nineteenth century, many diabetic diets focused on carbohydrate restriction. A popular 1880 newspaper column, *Doctor, What Should I Eat*, advised diabetics to gradually adopt a diet with less starch and carbohydrate.[26] *The First Texas Cookbook* echoed this advice with numerous examples of low-carbohydrate meals. A handwritten 'Bill of Fare for Diabetics' can be found in the back of a first edition of this 1883 text and read, 'Breakfast – Oysters steamed, without flour. Beefsteak, beefsteak fried with onions, broiled chicken, mutton or lamb chops, kidneys boiled, stewed, or devilled.'[27] US practitioner Dr Elliot P. Joslin was experimenting with a range of restrictive dietary therapy and was especially keen to determine the value of fasting, cutting carbohydrates and eliminating fat. As he explained in 1916 in the *Canadian Medical Association Journal*,

> So strongly have a been impressed by the stormy career of the diabetic patients in whose diets carbohydrates have been suddenly restricted and fat increased . . . that whenever I am asked to see a new case of diabetes I beg the physician either not to change the diet at all, or simply to omit the fat until the consultation takes place, and when the patient actually comes for treatment I first omit all the fat in the diet, after two days the protein as well, and then halve the carbohydrate on successive days until 10 grams are reached unless the patient is already sugar-free, and thereafter fast.[28]

As these dietary innovations suggest, diabetics learned about particular diets in popular newspapers, cookbooks and shared recipes, and through medical practitioners.

This close attention to food was part of larger shift taking place generally in American health practices and culture. Returning to 1893 and Atwater's food composition project at the Chicago World's Fair reminds us that food studies garnered increased attention from the public, the government and scientists. Atwater highlighted how these scientific projects would be synthesized into a text that could become an American domestic fixture. As he explained, at the end of the fair, he planned to

> put the gist of the matter in a little book or pamphlet so simple that the ordinary man or woman would understand it, and so practical that the average intelligent housekeeper would apply it, and so useful that the Government would print copies by the hundred thousand and out them into households throughout the country, and so let this be one of the products of the Fair to be permanently useful in the homes of the people – if you could help us to do this we should accomplish exactly what we want to do.[29]

Atwater also argued that for far too long, Americans had turned to Europe for authoritative information about food composition.[30]

Atwater pioneered nutritive studies and urged greater consideration of the composition, value and healthful dimensions of food. For those advising diabetics about diet, nutritive tables offered comprehensive and standardized measurements of food. By the twentieth century, practitioners offered diabetic and dietary advice with greater confidence, consistency and scientific endorsement. As one example, Dr Elliot Joslin's research at the Carnegie Institute yielded food measurements that categorized foods by carbohydrate composition – distinguishing those with less than 5 per cent carbohydrates (lettuce, celery and Swiss chard); those with 10–15 per cent carbohydrate content (squash, oranges, apples, lima beans) and those with 20 per cent or higher carbohydrate content (bananas and potatoes) (see Figure 2.1). By measuring how diets impacted diabetics' sugar levels, Joslin could recommend particular dietetic therapy. Advising patients to eat as little bread as possible, to balance carbohydrate, protein and fat intake, and recommending exercise as therapy, Joslin and other twentieth-century practitioners embraced nutrition as a means to a cure. As the second edition of Joslin's popular *A Diabetic Manual for the Mutual Use of Doctor and Patient* made clear, 'Certain articles of food should be selected whose composition is simple and well known; that the quantity of these food taken in each twenty-four hours should be weighed or measured; that the facts so obtained should be reported to a physician, and finally, in order to show the result of the diet, a specimen of the urine saved.'[31]

Nutritive studies offered a new lens for diabetologists struggling to better understand how diabetes and diabetic symptoms intersected with diet. Atwater's 1896 and 1906 food composition books allowed for simple measurement, fostered dialogue of dietary practices between physicians and patients and allowed for increased analysis of comparative and restrictive diets. As one diabetic manual explained, 'The more a patient knows about the composition and heat values of foods the wider range of food he will have and the better health he will enjoy at the same time . . . if the patient thoroughly masters the diet problems for diabetes, and follows his particular diet faithfully, he can consider his diabetes practically cured.'[32] Throughout the twentieth century, diabetic manuals have included foundational information about American food products, their composition and nutritional function. Diabetic manuals have encouraged diabetics to record an array of data including consumed calories, carbohydrates, proteins and fats. Although many diabetic diets circulated in the pre-insulin era, none epitomized the trend towards measurement, quantification and scientific rigour more so than Dr Frederick Madison Allen's studies.

Allen first introduced his ideas about diabetes, animal studies and the impact of nutrition in his 1913 publication, *Studies Concerning Glycosuria and Diabetes*.[33] Curiously, this publication, which would frequently be cited as the basis for his subsequent 'starvation diet' to treat diabetes, merely summarized three years of animal study, conducted at the Harvard Medical School, and largely self-funded. In this 1,179-paged text, Allen summarized his animal-based diabetes experiments and concluded that 'diabetes is now a feasible experimental problem'.[34] *Studies* reflected Allen's meticulous research practices, detailed experimental approach and impressive review of previously published diabetes, but it offered little evidence on dietetic therapy. As geneticist and scholar, Allan Mazur makes clear in his important 2011 review of Allen's research practices, 'In this book, Allen gives no prescription for calorie deprivation as a therapy for human diabetes, nor does he describe any felicitous effect of starvation on his animal subjects.'[35] However, the book made an impression that Allen's faith in dietary innovation, in the form of dietary restriction, indeed offered most effective

37

Composition of American food products—Continued.

Food materials.		Number of analyses.	Refuse.	Water.	Protein.	Fat.	Carbohy drates.	Ash.	Fuel value per pound.
				Per ct.	Per ct.	Per ct.	Per ct.	Per ct.	Per ct.	Calories.
VEGETABLE FOOD—continued.									
Bread, crackers, and pastry—Continued.									
Crackers, pilot bread		1		7.9	12.4	4.4	74.2	1.1	1,795
Crackers, soda		1		8.0	10.3	9.4	70.5	1.8	1,900
Doughnuts	Min	5		11.6	5.1	16.4	45.8	.6	1,880
	Max	5		25.8	7.6	25.7	63.2	1.4	2,155
	Avg	5		17.9	6.6	21.9	52.6	1.0	2,025
Jumbles		1		24.8	6.3	15.7	51.9	1.3	1,745
Pie, apple	Min	3		41.8	2.6	7.7	40.3	.9	1,180
	Max	3		45.5	3.8	11.3	43.3	2.8	1,295
	Avg	3		43.2	3.3	9.8	41.7	2.0	1,250
Pie, cream	Min	2		27.8	5.6	6.9	54.1	1.1	1,430
	Max	2		30.9	7.0	9.3	55.8	1.5	1,535
	Avg	2		29.4	6.3	8.1	54.9	1.3	1,480
Pie, custard		1		62.4	4.2	6.8	26.1	1.0	830
Pie, lemon		1		47.4	3.6	10.1	37.4	1.5	1,190
Pie, mince	Min	2		34.1	5.5	9.7	30.4	1.3	1,115
	Max	2		51.1	7.5	14.5	44.0	1.9	1,530
	Avg	2		42.6	6.5	12.1	37.2	1.6	1,325
Pie, squash		1		64.2	4.4	8.4	21.7	1.3	840
Average of all pie	Min	10		27.8	2.6	6.3	21.7	.9	840
	Max	10		64.2	7.5	14.5	55.8	2.8	1,535
	Avg	10		44.8	4.6	9.5	39.6	1.5	1,220
Pudding, tapioca	Min	2		52.0	3.0	2.6	21.9	.9	570
	Max	2		71.6	4.2	4.8	38.1	.9	990
	Avg	2		61.8	3.6	3.7	30.0	.9	780
Wafers, vanilla		1		5.8	6.8	15.7	71.2	.5	2,115
Sugars.									
Honey, strained	Min	30					68.1		1,265
	Max	30					80.7		1,500
	Avg	30					75.1		1,395
Molasses	Min	12		19.6			58.8	1.4	1,180
	Max	12		33.6	5.1	.1	73.2	7.2	1,400
	Avg	12		25.7	2.7		68.0	3.6	1,315
Sugar, extra C and similar sugars							95.0		1,765
Sugar, granulated							100.0		1,860
Sugar, maple	Min	17					74.0		1,375
	Max	17					95.2		1,770
	Avg	17					82.8		1,540
Sirup, maple	Min	50					45.9		930
	Max	50					81.9		1,525
	Avg	50					70.1		1,305
Starches.									
Tapioca	Min	2		10.8	.3	.2	86.6	.2	1,635
	Max	2		12.3	.6	.3	88.4	.5	1,660
	Avg	2		11.6	.4	.3	87.5	.2	1,650
Starch							98.0		1,825
Vegetables.[1]									
Artichokes, as purchased	Min	2		77.5	2.2	.1	15.3	.9	330
	Max	2		81.5	2.9	.2	18.3	1.1	395
	Avg	2		79.5	2.6	.2	16.7	1.0	365
Asparagus, as purchased	Min	3		93.6	1.6	.2	3.1	.5	100
	Max	3		94.0	2.1	.3	3.6	1.0	110
	Avg	3		94.0	1.8	.2	3.3	.7	105
Beans, dried, as purchased	Min	9		10.4	19.9	1.4	57.2	2.7	1,540
	Max	9		15.5	26.6	3.1	63.5	4.4	1,690
	Avg	9		13.2	22.3	1.8	59.1	3.6	1,590
Beans, Lima, dried, as purchased	Min	3		9.9	12.8	1.6	61.6	3.6	1,600
	Max	3		12.2	20.9	1.9	70.1	4.7	1,645
	Avg	3		11.1	15.9	1.8	67.1	4.1	1,620
Beans, Lima, green, as purchased		1		68.5	7.1	.7	22.0	1.7	570
Beans, string, as purchased	Min	2		83.5	1.7	.3	6.2	.7	165
	Max	2		91.0	2.8	.4	12.6	.8	300
	Avg	2		87.3	2.2	.4	9.4	.7	235
Beets	Edible portion. Min	17		83.0	.9	.1	4.0	.7	115
	Edible portion. Max	17		92.9	1.9	.2	13.7	1.3	300
	Edible portion. Avg	17		87.6	1.6	.1	9.6	1.1	210
	As purchased Avg	17	20.0	70.0	1.3	.1	7.7	.9	170
Brussels sprouts	Edible portion	1		88.2	4.7	1.1	4.3	1.7	215
	As purchased	1	15.0	75.0	4.0	.9	3.7	1.4	180
Cabbage	Edible portion. Min	7		86.0	1.4	.1	3.4	.6	100
	Edible portion. Max	7		94.3	2.9	.7	8.0	2.7	225
	Edible portion. Avg	7		90.3	2.1	.4	5.8	1.4	165
	As purchased Avg	7	15.0	76.8	1.8	.3	4.9	1.2	140

[1] Such vegetables as potatoes, squash, beets, etc., have a certain amount of inedible matter, skin, seeds, etc. The amount varies with the way they are prepared, and can not be accurately estimated. The figures given for refuse under vegetables approximately represent the average amount of refuse in these foods as ordinarily prepared.

Figure 2.1 'Composition of American Food Products', table in W. O. Atwater, *The Chemical Composition of American Food Materials* (Washington, 1896).

diabetic therapy of the era. Within a few years, the *British Medical Journal* claimed that the popular US diabetic diet had international appeal: 'It is clear that Dr. Allen's treatment has proved most successful in America, and it is much to be desired that it should be given a full trial in this country.'[36]

In 1913, after the publication of his study, Allen joined the Rockefeller Institute for Medical Research (now Roosevelt University) and gradually started testing his restrictive diet therapy on human subjects. Between 1915 (when his human studies moved beyond a pilot phase of eight patients) and through 1922 (when insulin became available), Allen collected data on approximately 100 diabetics proscribed the Allen diet.[37] In short, Allen reduced patient diets until they were sugar-free, even if this meant several days or even weeks without food. Allen also urged patients to adopt a weekly semi-starvation day, to boil veggies three times to reduce carbohydrates and to exercise. While it is impossible to know the impact and application of Allen's remedy, it is clear that the diet gained recognition on a global level. As explained in the *British Medical Journal*, 'The patient should be up and about during the period of starvation and not confined to bed.'[38] As one indication of its impact, the first edition of his text can be found in libraries throughout the Unites States, as well as libraries in Australia, Canada, France, Lebanon, the United Kingdom, the Netherlands, Germany, Switzerland, Denmark, New Zealand and South Africa.[39] As Dr Jeffrey Friedman, geneticist and investigator for Rockefeller University, concluded that in the pre-insulin era, 'Allen was the first to realize that diabetes was a general disorder of metabolism and that acidosis and death could be forestalled in caloric intake was restricted.'

Perhaps the premier US diabetologist of the early twentieth century, Dr Elliot P. Joslin, also endorsed the Allen plan or 'starvation diet' as therapeutic. Joslin is recognized as the first diabetes specialist in the United States, opening a clinic in Boston in 1898 after training at Harvard Medical School. In the pre-insulin era, Joslin had established a diabetic practice that attracted patients from near and far and published three significant diabetic studies and a manual dedicated to diabetic treatment that was so popular that it is currently in its fourteenth edition. Joslin had a great reputation in the field then (and now) and likely his support secured Allen's fame. As Joslin pronounced in one ringing endorsement of the Allen plan, 'Thanks to Dr. Frederick M. Allen we no longer nurse diabetics – we treat them!'[40] The pre-insulin era of diabetic therapy focused almost exclusively on dietary innovation as a therapy or 'cure' to the chronic disease, diabetes (see Figure 2.2). The turn-of-the-century shifts in thinking about diet, especially the creation of American food composition tables, offered a way to make the measurement of food more accessible, meaningful and foundational in healthcare. For diabetics, diets could be measured in terms of carbohydrates, proteins and fat and the intersections of food and blood sugars may have become more apparent. The early-twentieth-century diabetic diets, epitomized by the Allen plan, also accentuated the power of food as a therapy. Practitioners and patients alike practiced dietary innovation as the most powerful way to treat diabetes. In the early twentieth century, the discovery of insulin would have a profound impact on ways of thinking about and treating diabetes.

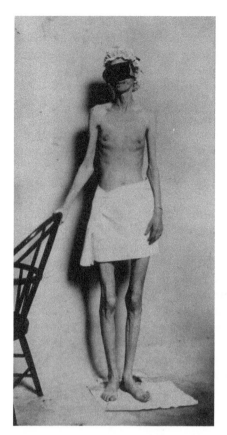
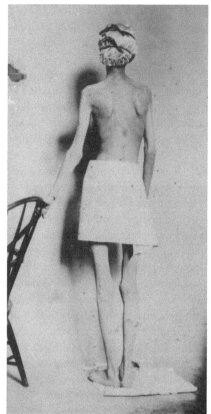

Figure 2.2 'Treated' diabetic before insulin to illustrate extreme nature of therapy. Photo credit: The Thomas Fisher Rare Book Library of Toronto.

The insulin era

The discovery of insulin at the University of Toronto in 1921 instantly transformed therapy for severe diabetics.[41] Insulin offered effective treatment for the harshest cases of diabetes which tended to afflict children, lead to early death and devastate the body regardless of dietary therapies. As Bliss's foundational history of its discovery described it, 'A medical fairy tale come true of the lone doctor and his partner overcoming all obstacles to realize an idea and save the lives of millions and millions of people.'[42] In the early 1920s, science did not distinguish diabetes by type, yet all practitioners recognized a severe form of the disease (now labelled type 1 or insulin-dependent diabetes mellitus) and recommended insulin without hesitation for patients at the brink of death. Because Allen's diet had required the greatest calorie restriction among those with the most severe form of the disease, his treatment quickly fell from favour. However, the diabetic diet persisted, as illustrated in the following example.

In 1928, Henry John published *Diabetic Manual for Patients*, an accessible text written for diabetic patients in simple, practical and clear instruction. The book illustrated some painful memories of severely restrictive diets, likely referring to the Allen plan explicitly when it described diabetes in the late 1920s and post-insulin era: 'No longer do we see the dragging, emancipated men, women, and children with a hopeless outlook, constantly suffering from the torturing pangs of hunger.'[43] John then shared a 'striking story' with readers. A year after the discovery of insulin, a formerly emaciated patient entered his office, appearing as a 'strapping fellow, looking like a star football player' and unrecognizable to John. When the patient revealed his identity, John exclaimed, 'It seemed like a miracle! Today that young man is leading an active, useful life; he is married, and is carrying on a regular medical practice.' However, John concluded the story with a serious reminder, echoed in other diabetic manuals of the era. 'Can one take an unlimited amount of food and, so to speak, balance it with sufficient insulin? No! Eve with insulin the diet still is and will always be the principal factor in diabetic treatment. Dietary control constitutes about 80 per cent and insulin 20 percent of the treatment.'[44]

Insulin offered medication for diabetes, but as John's story makes clear, diet remained a powerful intervention point for diabetic care. Scientific literature reinforced this point. A 1931 *Scientific Monthly* article emphasized that 'education in measured diets has become the cornerstone in the treatment of an increasing number of disorders.'[45] Authors Gray and Stewart explicitly discussed diabetes, recognizing the increased opportunities for dietitians and the centrality of food tables that could be obtained by mailing 10 cents to the government.[46] Gray and Stewart analysed competing diabetic models of the post-insulin era defining each as the low-carbohydrate diet, the diabetic diet and the high-carbohydrate diet.[47]

Dieticians and education material emphasized the importance of measurement, linking it to household 'terms' that fostered a sense of familiarity. 'This quantification may be begun in simple household terms of ounces or tablespoons.'[48]

Also evident in the 1930s, some diabetologists, such as Karl Stolte (Germany) and William Samsum (United States), began collecting evidence that calories mattered and increased caloric intake might be a path to improved diabetic outcomes. This theory stood in opposition to the restrictive patterns of the pre-insulin era, many of which persisted in the insulin era. By the late 1920s, Stolte questioned the strict limits of diabetic diets in the post-insulin era and adapted a therapy that called for three insulin shots daily. Along with multiple injections, Stolte advocated free choice of foods for diabetics.[49] This approach, often labelled a 'free diet', may have been a backlash to the restrictive ethos of the early twentieth century that lingered long after the discovery of insulin. In fact, although these diets were not quite as liberating as their name implies, they offered an early departure in therapy that mapped out a path for considering collaboration between insulin and nutrition practices and, moreover, embracing a broader vision of insulin's transformative potential. Stolte advocated particularly for children with diabetes whose lives seemed overly restricted on diabetic diets.[50]

Simultaneously, Dr Edward Tolstoi, a leading diabetologist in the United States, started advocating a free diet for his patients with diabetes. After 15 years of this practice and collecting data from more than 4,000 patients, he 'abandoned the strictly regulated and weighed diets' and shared his finding in his manual named *Living with Diabetes*. As Tolstoi explained, he encouraged 'the diabetic to eat a self-selected, unweighed, unmeasured diet in a quantity to satisfy his hunger, and of a quality to satisfy his tastes'.[51] Although a variety of diabetic diets had always coexisted, Tolstoi's claim to a 'new' approach was valid, as it strayed far from the conventional approach of moderation, restriction and measurement. Instead, as he described in his practice, 'My patients eat normally while being treated with a new (protamine) insulin'.[52]

Hans Christian Hagedorn discovered the aforementioned protamine insulin in 1936. One of the original founders of Nordisk Insulinlaboratorium of Copenhagen along with August Krogh and Hans Hagedorn (who had been given the rights to insulin in 1923), he discovered that the addition of protamine zinc prolonged the life of insulin. Its significance here, however, is that as insulin assumed greater flexibility, conversations emerged about more flexibility in diabetic diets. Long-acting insulin ushered in an era of possibility – and coupled with free diet – offered a departure from restrictive and standard approaches that lacked flexibility.

In the United States, this played out in dramatic ways. Most clearly, the expanding presence of the Joslin clinic for diabetes care and its consistent emphasis on diabetic diets stood in opposition to trends to move towards a free diet. In the end, clinical studies would affirm Joslin's approach which was dependent on both dietary modification and medical treatment. As Chris Feudtner has clarified about the mid-century debate in competing diabetic standards of care, 'In many ways, what has compelled physicians to align themselves on one side or another of the control issue has never been a simple assessment of physiological efficacy, but rather a complex set of ideas and ideals. The Joslin group structured their diabetic management around the ideal of seizing control of the disease, preventing all complications, and extending life at virtually any cost'.[53]

To be sure, mid-century diabetic manuals also persisted in devoting substantial sections of text to diabetic-friendly recipes, nutritional recommendations and guidelines. 'Diet is still the backbone in the treatment of diabetes, while insulin is used as an adjunct in a large percentage of the patients', explained Dr Abraham Rudy in the 1947 introduction to his *Simplified Diabetic Manual* that included 180 recipes. His text, like many manuals of the era, offered instructions of household measurement, nuanced discussions about how and why portion size mattered and emphasized the value of food and nutritional measurement. He explained to readers, 'In the prescription of the diabetic diet the physician usually allows a definite, calculated amount of carbohydrate, protein and fat. It is therefore essential to have charts from which these diets can be computed'.[54] In fact, by mid-century, diabetic manuals offered some of the most sophisticated information about contemporary ideas of food content often defined by carbohydrate measurement, fat content analysis and measurements of protein. Joslin's 1941 manual read, 'The task of the modern diabetic is not so much to learn how to live comfortably upon less carbohydrate and more fat, but rather to balance the carbohydrate in his diet with insulin so that he can utilize it and thus keep his urine sugar-free'.[55] On the same page, Joslin inserted a table with recommendations for carbohydrate, protein and fat consumption. Likewise, his subsequent chapter, 'Foods and their Composition', filled nearly two dozen pages with data about popular food and drink.

In the decades that followed the discovery of insulin, diabetologists abandoned a fixed discussion of restriction and adopted a new and innovative framework for thinking about the intersection of food, medication and patient practices. As Joslin's trajectory from the pre-insulin to post-insulin era demonstrated, food still mattered deeply, but diabetics could abandon undernourishment routines. The adoption of insulin therapy also allowed the quality of patients' lives to assume a more prominent place in the conversation of diabetic treatment. In short, the restrictions of the early twentieth century seemed barbaric by mid-century.

The final topic of this chapter speaks to the more recent resurgence of restrictive diets – both to treat diabetes and to lose weight. In the late twentieth century, Dr Robert C. Atkins gained a cult following for his weight loss strategy. Commonly labelled a 'fad diet', Atkins' low-carb approach, in fact, echoed many early diabetic therapies. The historical memory of diabetic restrictive diets had faded by the end of the century, however, and instead his diet gained a huge number of devoted adherents. By 2002, *Time* magazine labelled Dr Atkins one of the ten most influential Americans of the year.[56]

This late-twentieth-century resurgence of calorie and restrictive approaches to diet circled the globe, once again capturing the transnational phenomenon of food studies. Many described restrictive diets as innovative or even revolutionary. Consider the titles of popular diabetes diet books of the twenty-first century: *Atkins Diabetes Revolution*, *The New Diabetes Prescription*, and *The PhD Miracle for Diabetes*. In fact, the diets dominating contemporary discourse build from the foundation of early twentieth century trends – there is little new, revolutionary and miraculous about them.

In an alternate model, Luz Calvo and Catriona Rueda Esquibel proudly claim the dietary knowledge of ancestors and urge readers to learn this history as a path to health. In their cookbook *Decolonize Your Diet*, they argue, 'U.S. born Latino/a communities are facing a health crisis, most notably with diabetes . . . We believe that it is time to reclaim our cultural inheritance and wean our bodies from sugary drinks, fast food, and donuts. Cooking a pot of beans from scratch is a micro-revolutionary act that honours our ancestors and the generations to come.'[57] Reclaiming ancestral practices, the authors urge audiences 'to build an awareness of the relationship between food and community offers one way to claim indigenous knowledge.'[58]

Conclusion

Dietary innovations are an intimate part of the history of diabetes. Food intersects with a person's life and identity in a much more personal way than the daily medication of a pill or even of insulin injections. A century of medical and popular descriptions of the 'diabetic diet' reveals its elasticity and fluidity. There has never been one 'diabetic diet', nor has there ever been a medical consensus on the best 'diabetic diet'. With that recognition, an examination of recent history of diabetic therapy offers a rich lens for thinking about competing ideas of chronic illness, the power of food and the prescriptive nature of diets.

Diabetes is a metabolic disorder closely linked to food; however, unlike deficiency diseases, diabetes cannot be cured by diet modification alone. Dietary innovation remains a very powerful tool for treating diabetes, even since the introduction of insulin and oral hypoglycaemic agents. As transnational ideas about the impact of diabetic diets circulate the globe rapidly, a historic analysis reminds us that nutritive studies, restrictive diets and measurement have defined diabetic care for many generations and persist – in spite of many difference of opinion on best practices – in large part because of the shared belief in the power enfolded within dietary innovation.

The nutritional insight gleaned from food composition studies of the late nineteenth century offered a key – for patients and practitioners alike – to unlock the daily intersections of food and medicine in American diabetic management. By the twentieth century, 'diabetic diets' moved into the realm of clinical science, with diets increasingly supported with evidence.[59] The practice of food measurement proved particularly useful in the post-insulin era, when patients were now expected to measure diet, sugar levels in urine and insulin doses. Although food measurement practices became standardized, competing theories on the most effective diabetic diet continued.

The popular press celebrated the tools of patient knowledge about food and its intersection with disease. As one journalist explained, 'The educating of the patient himself is most important, for he is impressed with the idea from the first that he is merely correcting errors of diet, changing the intake of fuel for his furnace, and that he may, therefore, not be suffering from an inherently progressive disease.'[60] In a pattern that was typical of the pre-insulin era, the shifts in nutritive studies allowed for calculated decisions about diabetic therapy, urging patients to 'keep careful watch over his meat and drink day by day – not in a brooding, introspective way, but with the mood of one who, seeing a defect due to a quite preventable mistake in practice, devotes himself to removing its cause'.[61]

Mid-century diabetic advice continued to advocate for patient knowledge about nutrition. Dieticians rearranged data of the early twentieth century to construct food tables and exchange lists designed to simplify measurement for patients.[62] The American Dietetic Association and others imagined food tables and exchange lists as an innovative way for patients to have greater control of their diet. Additionally, the American Diabetes Association helped direct much attention to diabetic diets and to broaden its audience by identifying the large population of 'undiagnosed diabetics'.[63] To be sure, food remained a pathway for good diabetic care, but debate continued about the best diabetic diets. Many critics of diabetic diets questioned the need for constant measurement and surveillance of food.

Medical uncertainty about the merit of diabetic diets disappeared in the 1990s, however, with the release of a 10-year randomized clinical study, the Diabetes Control and Complications Trial (DCCT), that evaluated intense diabetic control defined in part by strict dietary measures.[64] The results definitively demonstrated a positive long-term impact of intense diabetic control, and once again, diabetic diets increased in popularity. The DCCT also made clear that diabetic care is about more than the day-to-day indicators. In other words, intense management and effective diabetic diets (indicated by diets that improved stable blood sugars) prevented many long-term complications. Perhaps most compelling, the DCCT demonstrated that diabetes was not progressively worse, but instead with intervention, outcomes could be improved.

The diabetic diet assumed new potential as it offered the potential to diabetes and also to improve cardiovascular health, general wellness and more.

Innovative dietary practices offer a tool for disease intervention. Throughout history, diabetic communities have adopted food and herbal remedies for diabetes. Often labelled, folk remedies, such practices capture a shared practice of turning to food for its curative powers. In a recent collection of essays dedicated to *Embedding Education into Diabetes Practice*, Massimo Porta has written that 'patient education has long been considered the Cinderella of diabetes care, often considered non-scientific, non-evidence-based, non-standardized: in two words almost non-serious'.[65] However, if we focus more closely on dietary innovations in twentieth-century American history, patient education and measurement practices have offered tools to patients that make clear the power of food and its potential in treating diabetes.[66] By focusing more on the power of food and the innovations it fosters, the nuances and tensions of diabetes diets can be reimagined as important tools for patients seeking a myriad of ways to gain more control of this vexing chronic illness.

3

Allergic to Innovation? Dietary Change and Debate about Food Allergy in the United States

Matthew Smith

Introduction

The expert on nutrition is not the nutrition expert, but the man who has studied nutrition by the ultimate method of research, the struggle for survival. The Eskimo, living on the ice floes of the North Pole, the Red Indian travelling hard and far over wild lands in hunting or war, the trapper in the Canadian forests, the game hunters in Africa – these men must find food that gives the greatest nutritive value in the smallest bulk [. . .] All these men have found that a diet of meat and animal fat alone, with no carbohydrates, with no fruit or vegetables, with no vitamins other than those they get in meat, not merely provides them with all the energy they need, but keeps them in perfect health for months at a time. Seal meat and blubber for the Eskimo, pemmican for the Indian and the trapper, biltong for the hunter, have proved to be the perfect diet.[1]

In the search for the ideal diet, is it best to innovate? Or is it better to look to the past, perhaps even the distant past?[2] In his foreword to the bestselling *Eat Fat and Grow Slim* (1958), a diet book written by British psychiatrist Richard Mackarness (1916–1996), Sir Heneage Ogilvie (1887–1971) opted for the latter. Both argued that the protein- and fat-rich diets of early humans, which still endured in existing hunter/gatherer communities, were clearly superior to anything that had been developed since. Or, once humans began to develop agriculture 12,000 years ago, cultivating carbohydrate-rich grains and rearing animals for dairy products, dietary problems started to emerge. Reflecting this connection with early human diets, what Mackarness described rather clumsily in 1958 as the Eat-Fat-Grow-Slim diet in *Eat Fat and Grow Slim* became the Stone Age diet in an article that appeared the following year.[3]

The purpose of *Eat Fat and Grow Slim*, as indicated by the title, was self-evident. But by the 1970s, Mackarness, psychiatric registrar at Park Prewett Mental Hospital in Basingstoke, had begun to associate a much broader range of chronic health problems with diet, eventually describing his findings in *Not All in the Mind: How Unsuspected Food Allergy Can Affect Your Body AND Your Mind* in 1976.[4] Mackarness, in other words, had stepped into the controversial world of food allergy. Coined in 1906 by Austrian paediatrician Clemens von Pirquet (1874–1929), the term 'allergy' was originally defined broadly as 'any form of altered biological reactivity' and incorporated both functional immune reactions and dysfunctional allergic reactions, but was chiefly associated with asthma, hay fever and idiosyncratic reactions to animals, insect stings and food.[5] The subject of food allergy quickly divided allergists.[6] While self-described food allergists believed that it was a common and underdiagnosed explanation for a range of chronic health problems affecting virtually every system of the body, ranging from asthma and eczema to flatulence and migraine, orthodox allergists claimed that it was much less ubiquitous and that many patients were better served seeing a psychiatrist. In other words, the symptoms of many so-called allergy sufferers were presumably psychosomatic, as the historian Mark Jackson has discussed.[7] In turn, many food allergists believed that psychiatric symptoms were caused by food allergy. The complex relationship between allergy and mental health helps to explain why a psychiatrist such as Mackarness would have become interested in allergy, though he clearly already had a clinical (and possibly financial) interest in dieting and diet books. Making matters more complicated is the fact that allergists (then and now) struggle to explain what ultimately causes food allergy. While theories about genetics, infant feeding and excessively clean domestic spaces abound, no definitive explanation has emerged. Into this vacuum, dietary theories have abounded.

Mackarness's influences included von Pirquet and his 'wide, biological view of allergy', but chiefly the more recent work of American food allergists, including Herbert Rinkel (1896–1963), Arthur Coca (1875–1959), Albert H. Rowe (1889–1970) and especially Theron G. Randolph (1906–1995). All of these Americans emphasized that food allergy was the cause of countless undiagnosed chronic symptoms in Americans (including themselves). Combining the ideas of his American mentors with his own clinical observations at Park Prewett Hospital, Mackarness eventually concluded that eating a modern diet rich in carbohydrates, dairy products and chemicals could cause a wide array of health problems in the hypersensitive.[8]

As its title and his vocation suggested, Mackarness was particularly interested in how reactions to foods could trigger psychiatric symptoms. The motivation of Mackarness and many like-minded physicians was largely due to the struggle to diagnose and treat patients suffering from depression, mania and other mental health problems who were ill-served by prevailing psychiatric treatments, such as psychoanalysis, psychopharmacology, electroconvulsive therapy and lobotomy.[9] Underlying such clinical issues, however, were more fundamental concerns about modern diets and their propensity to cause chronic, otherwise unexplained, health problems.

Historians, such as Jackson, Gregg Mitman and Michelle Murphy, have begun to examine the history of allergy and immunology, but few have explored in detail the relationship between changes in food production and the proliferation of allergy.[10] More emphasis has been placed instead on the role of pollutants and chemical products. Similarly, food historians have researched the emergence of food processing but have not fully examined ideas about the health implications of such changes.[11] The connections that have been made between the rise in food production and the emergence of allergic disease have typically not been made by historians, resulting in analyses that are disconnected from the broader and deeper contexts of developments in allergy, food production and consumer practices.[12] In this chapter, I attempt to bring together these areas of historical inquiry together to explore how the relationship between food processing and allergic disease has been conceptualized in the United States during the twentieth century. While Mackarness's advocacy of a Stone Age diet may have gone further than most in critiquing dietary innovation, he was not alone in asking questions about the association between modern diets and disease.[13] Many food allergists linked the emergence of processed food during the twentieth century with increased numbers of allergies. I begin by explaining why the emergence of food processing posed particular challenges to people with food allergies, and then provide two examples of foodstuffs that were indicted as particularly problematic, namely, corn (maize) and synthetic food colours. Although such ideas were highly controversial – and remain so – they nonetheless mirrored deeper concerns dating back to the early modern period about the emergence of diseases of civilization and, more recently, escalating rates of autoimmune disease.[14] Rather than dismissing these ideas as quackery, outdated or fanciful, we should engage with them more deeply in the hope of explaining why such diseases are on the rise.

Processing allergy

In the historian Harvey Levenstein's recent apologia for the state of American food, he cites the emergence of large-scale food processing as one of the catalysts for concerns about the food supply.[15] Food production moved out of American homes during the late nineteenth and early twentieth centuries as society urbanized, industrialized and took advantage of the rapid advancement of transportation networks.[16] While most Americans in 1850 would have primarily consumed food produced nearby by people they likely knew (including themselves), by 1950 Americans ate food produced by large, impersonal food companies and were far removed from any aspect of its production. Distance from food production led to distrust and, according to Levenstein, an irrational fear of modern food and a counterproductive craze for the organic.

Levenstin's reassurances about the state of the American food supply have not been echoed by most other food historians and food writers, who have expressed grave suspicions about the dominance of large corporations in dictating the food we eat, the emergence of global food economies (at the expense of local food systems) and the reductive nature of nutrition science, which privileges industrial food production.[17] Allergic Americans had more reason than most, however, to want to know exactly what was in their food and, therefore, distrust the food industry when ingredients were not clearly identified or left off the label altogether. Concern about accidental exposure to peanuts and the seven other 'major' food allergens has led to at least a little more transparency with respect to labelling the ingredients of processed foodstuffs.[18] Since 2006 and the enactment of the Food Allergen Labelling and Consumer Protection Act (FALCPA), warning labels have to be present on foods containing peanuts, milk, wheat, eggs, fish, tree nuts, soybeans and shellfish. But for Americans diagnosed with allergies prior to the passage of FALCPA and, indeed, Americans allergic to the 150 *other* foods known to be possibly allergenic, some suspicion was well-founded.

Food processing had a bearing on allergy in two ways: first, because the industrial processing of food made it difficult to identify the specific ingredients of food; and second, because food allergists began suspecting some of the core ingredients of food production as particularly allergenic. The emergence of mass food processing after the Second World War made it more difficult for people to know exactly what they were eating. A case from the 1930s featuring pioneering food allergist Herbert Rinkel illustrates how changes in how Americans sourced their food made diagnosis of food allergy more difficult. Rinkel had suffered from allergic symptoms, including a severely and persistently runny nose, throughout his medical training. Nevertheless, he had failed to identify a precipitating cause. After reading the food allergy research of Oakland allergist Albert Rowe, however, he self-experimented to determine if food was the cause of his agony. Eventually, he discovered that the culprit was eggs, which he had eaten in abundance for years. His father was a Kansas farmer and had regularly sent him cases of eggs throughout university. Rinkel immediately stopped eating eggs and the symptoms ceased after a few days. The fifth day, however, was his birthday and, accordingly, Rinkel ate a piece of birthday cake baked by his wife. Within minutes, he had collapsed onto the floor. When he regained consciousness, his wife confirmed that the cake contained three eggs.[19]

In many ways, Rinkel was lucky. Given his ready supply of eggs and their dominance in his diet, eggs were a likely suspect for Rinkel. It is probable that most people suffering allergic symptoms would have similarly pinpointed eggs given similar circumstances, and not have gone to the same lengths as the curious clinician to confirm unequivocally that they were at fault. Compare Rinkel's situation, then, to Americans whose diet included considerable amounts of processed foods. There were far more ingredients in the television dinners, cake mixes and breakfast cereals that came to dominate the American diet, making it much more difficult to identify potential allergens. Even after the Fair Packaging and Labeling Act of 1966, which tightened the laws on listing food ingredients, the sheer quantity of contents and the use of synonyms for describing certain ingredients (for instance, albumin for egg or groundnuts for peanuts) made it difficult for allergic consumers to determine exactly what they were eating.

Despite the difficulties inherent in identifying problematic ingredients, there was some help for allergic consumers. By the 1930s and 1940s, food companies had recognized a market in allergen-free food and had developed products guaranteed to be free of particularly ubiquitous ingredients, such as wheat, eggs and milk. The allergic could now turn to Ditex Oat Crisps, free of egg, wheat, corn and barley, washed down with maple-flavoured milk substitute, Allerteen.[20] But overall, according to Pennsylvania home economist and poet Helen Morgan (1904–1989), the author of one of the first recipe books for allergy sufferers, 'the attention given allergic's dietary needs has been woefully meager'.[21] The subtitle of *You Can't Eat That! A Manual and Recipe Book for Those Who Suffer Either Acutely or Mildly (and Perhaps Unconsciously) from Food Allergy* (1939), which included a foreword by Mayo Clinic gastroenterologist and medical columnist Walter C. Alvarez (1884–1978), neatly revealed how food allergy was conceptualized by many food allergists during the 1930s, the era in which they enjoyed the most legitimacy and respect from their medical colleagues. It suggested that mild sufferers deserved the same support as those who suffered acutely (who likely found it easier to identify the foods to which they were allergic) and also reflected the belief of most food allergists that the condition was much more common than usually acknowledged. Although Morgan admitted that 'some people have taken up allergy as a fad, the way they did mah-jongg and knitting', the overall message of the book was that allergy was widespread and that sufferers needed more help in identifying safe foods and recipes.[22]

Morgan worked with nutritionists, cooks, bakers and the California Health Food Service in order to develop recipes that avoided common allergens. She also received assistance from most, but not all, of the major American food producers with identifying the ingredients of various processed foods. Explaining the need for greater disclosure, Morgan declared, 'This is the age of packaged goods, which are a boon to the average housewife but a bane to the individual on a diet.'[23] While most of the food companies Morgan contacted were forthcoming, some 'did not wish to disclose the ingredients of their products', and others, including the National Biscuit Company, preferred to indicate which of their products did not contain certain ingredients, including egg, yeast, milk and sugar.[24] A subsequent chapter entitled 'Jokers in Cooked Foods', revealed processed and unprocessed foods that tended to contain hidden ingredients; 'chefs and good cooks too, have a distressing habit of putting certain ingredients where you least expect to find them.'[25] Bread could contain fillers such as 'fruit pulps, potato, nuts, all cereal grains, peas, beans, lentils, peanuts, cassava roots, cooked squash, pumpkin, and sweet potato', which were 'used when wheat prices are very high'.[26] Candies could contain eggs, milk, nuts or potato starch.

It is worth remembering that *You Can't Eat That!* was published in 1939, prior to the explosion in food processing that was fomented by technological developments during and after the Second World War.[27] Most of the foods it discussed were staples, such as wheat, milk and eggs. After the war, however, the number of food additives entering the food supply increased rapidly, as did the use of other staples that were ubiquitous in food processing.[28] Concern soon emerged about the allergenicity of these substances. In other words, many food allergists and their patients believed that the very foods and food chemicals that made food processing possible were those that were making an increasing number of people allergic. One of the chief instigators of this idea was the controversial Illinois food allergist turned clinical ecologist Theron Randolph.

A corn-ucopia of allergy

Randolph began training in allergy and immunology in the late 1930s, when Helen Morgan was writing *You Can't Eat That!* and when food allergy had reached its zenith in terms of legitimacy and respectability. Although food allergists and orthodox allergists debated whether to define allergy broadly or narrowly, food allergy was still discussed in a relatively open and friendly atmosphere, and most acknowledged that it was a prominent source of chronic symptoms. The psychosomatic theories that would divide opinion during the 1940s and 1950s, for instance, had not yet emerged.[29] Equally, the ecological ideology that would influence many food allergists during the 1960s and 1970s had not yet been articulated. After the Second World War, however, and paralleling the rapid changes in food processing, food allergists led by Randolph became suspicious of the foods and food chemicals used in food production, associating them with rising rates of food allergy.[30] For Randolph, one of the most problematic of these was corn.[31] As he would discover, however, questioning corn raised the hackles of the food industry and created divisions within the allergy community about the possible perils of food processing.

As Paul Roberts describes in *The End of Food* (which conveniently features a cob of corn on its cover), during the '1920s and 1930s, scientists came out with hybrid strains of corn that not only had bigger, more plentiful ears, but also grew more closely together in the field – all of which meant more corn per acre'.[32] Yields rapidly increased, going from less than 20 bushels per acre in 1935 to just under 100 bushels per acre in 1970, and over 160 bushels per acre in 2010.[33] New fertilizers and irrigation also meant that corn could be grown in new regions, such as the Great Plains. Finally, with the passage of the Agricultural and Consumer Protection Act (1973), corn farmers were ensured of a guaranteed price for their crop which encouraged even more production; today, corn is the most subsidized crop in the United States.[34] Although most of the corn produced was used in livestock feed, it was also increasingly used in food production, where the processes of dry and wet milling broke the kernels up into the constituent parts, which could then be used in a plethora of foods, ranging from candies and sauce mixes to soft drinks and snacks.[35] By the mid-1940s, when he was in private practice and teaching at Northwestern University Medical School, Randolph was beginning to suspect it as a hidden source of allergy, responsible for everything from chronic fatigue and depression to muscle ache and sore throats.[36]

Randolph's opinions about corn as an allergen were highly personal as he, much like many leading food allergists, was a sufferer himself. In 1944, Herbert Rinkel visited Randolph at his practice which had just opened and:

> After an hour or so he commented: 'Ted, I don't think that you are diagnosing your allergy to corn.' Upon answering that I had not seen a case, he pulled from his pocket a small typewritten sheet of not more than a dozen lines of the sources of corn in the American diet. However, all that I had needed was a mirror, for I immediately diagnosed my own allergies to corn, wheat and all other cereal grains by applying what I had recently learned from Herb – details of the individual food test and the corn sources. The avoidance of cereal grains not only relieved my frequent headaches and uncontrollable intermittent somnolence, but also provided a needed boost of energy and returned productive evenings for the first time in several years. Prior to this time, I had only known that I was sensitive to maple and peanut.[37]

Rinkel's list of hidden sources of corn indicates how difficult it could be for patients and allergists to identify it. Moreover, most food allergists thought that reactions to most staple foods such as corn did not typically occur immediately after ingestion, but occurred after a few days and, in other cases, only after the food was ingested repeatedly over many days. Among all the foods likely to cause such 'masked' allergies, the most common and most insidious, given its ubiquity in the food supply, was corn.[38]

Randolph's emphasis on corn did not win him many friends within the food industry or within the orthodox allergy community. Following initial articles on how the use of corn starch in food packaging could cause reactions and on the allergenicity of corn sugar, Randolph was called to appear at the Food and Drug Administration's (FDA's) Bread Hearings in 1949, which were held to discuss the use of additives in bread.[39] During the hearings, Randolph described how the surreptitious addition of corn and corn derivatives to bread caused allergy symptoms in 20 per cent of his patients. This claim triggered heated opposition from orthodox allergists and food manufacturers.[40] According to Randolph, orthodox allergists, sponsored by the Corn Products Research Foundation (referred to Randolph as the 'corn people'), were called to the hearings to negate his testimony and undermine his call for better labels.[41] Undaunted, Randolph would proceed to stress the prevalence of corn as a food allergen again in the textbook *Food Allergy*, which he co-wrote with Rinkel and Michael Zeller (1900–1977) in 1951.[42] The largely sympathetic review of *Food Allergy* by New York allergist Will Spain noted that the book's emphasis on corn would 'be challenged in many quarters', but this proved to be an understatement.[43] Unwilling to back down from his views as demanded by his superiors, Randolph was fired from his position at Northwestern University Medical School in 1951 for being 'a pernicious influence on medical students' and was faced with the prospect of rebuilding his career.[44]

While many of Randolph's close friends and colleagues were sympathetic, the influential, yet controversial, Arthur Coca argued in a 1953 letter that he had gone too far:

> No doubt you realize that you aroused the instinct of self-preservation among the corn-products people by your rather unmitigated and, I believe, statistically exaggerated emphasis upon corn-sensitivity. Their persecution of you was dastardly, yet it might have been prevented if your reports had carefully avoided the implication that corn-products are a specially unwholesome category of food stuffs.[45]

To this criticism, Randolph replied, 'I am obviously disturbed when my efforts to be thorough, as I attempted to be in dealing with the corn question, have been construed as a specific attack. That certainly has not been my intention.'[46] Although a dispute between the two about the allergenicity of Coca's 'Dust-Seal' spray (meant to keep dust out of homes) might partly explain Coca's lack of support, the exchange did highlight how food allergists' observations about reactions to foods used in processing had to run the gauntlet of food industry opposition.[47] Whether it be by producing Ry-Krisp crackers in the 1930s and gluten-free beer in the 2010s or by sponsoring allergy conferences in the hope of influencing allergists in the 1980s and 1990s, the food industry has always had a stake in how food allergy was defined and understood. Indeed, after Randolph's run-in with the 'corn people', he claimed that the Sugar Research Foundation (which represented the cane and beet sugar industries) approached him in hope that he would help them 'regain some of the markets they had lost to corn sugar [. . .] Of course there was nothing I could do.'[48]

In spite of all his detractors, Randolph continued to attract patients and advocates who banded around him and his concept of clinical ecology. A series of letters exchanged by Elizabeth Magner, a patient of Randolph's, Coca-Cola and the American Academy of Allergy (AAA) in 1974 illustrates both the challenges he faced as well as the support he enjoyed. Magner had written to Coca-Cola to complain that corn syrup was not labelled on its bottles. The corporation responded by stating that Magner's letter was the first it had received and that when it consulted with the AAA, it was informed that the refining process used in production made the corn derivatives 'free from offending components and, therefore, such refined corn products would not require special labeling'. Magner followed with the AAA and declared,

> I first cried when I read your letter – then I was tempted to scream [. . .] I am stunned and disappointed to hear that there are board approved allergists who are not aware of the wide spread problems of corn [. . .] Dr. T. Randolph has testified several times over the years to government committees on the wide spread problems of corn, but those reports somehow got buried. None of us want to harm the corn industry! We fully realize the economics of the situation and appreciate the problems of cost and availability of sugar, production problems. What we are begging for is the proper labeling so that products containing any form of corn can be avoided by those who need to avoid such.[49]

Lost somewhere in the vitriol spilled forth about corn allergy were patients such as Elizabeth Magner who did not necessarily want to transform the food industry, but rather wanted recognition for their condition and some basic support in dealing with it.

Allergic to additives

Food allergists believed that nearly every system of the body could be affected by reactions to corn and other foods. Of particular concern to many, however, were neurological symptoms, ranging from headache and fatigue to hyperactivity and psychosis. Since orthodox allergists believed that allergic symptoms were often psychosomatic, claims that foods could cause mental health problems triggered heated debates between food allergists and their orthodox opponents. These debates became more vitriolic during the 1960s, when questions were raised about synthetic food additives and their possible effects on mental health and, especially, hyperactive behaviour in children.

Although Rachel Carson's *Silent Spring* (1962) is often hailed as precipitating fears about environmental chemicals, concerns about the health effects of food chemicals escalated throughout the 1950s.[50] One example of this is the Chemical in Food Products hearings, which began in 1950 and resulted in the Delaney Clause, which banned food additives proven to cause cancer in test animals.[51] For allergists, the most notorious food chemicals were synthetic coal tar dyes, which transformed the food manufacturer's palette (if not doing much for the palate of consumers). Food colours had been used for centuries for decorative purposes and to disguise low-quality foods or foods cosmetically damaged by processing, but up until the late nineteenth century, most of these dyes were natural (such as carmine, saffron or beetroot). Coal tar dyes would replace these natural alternatives primarily because they were cheaper.[52] While there was some justification for some food additives (e.g., preservatives and pesticides) on the grounds that they made food less expensive by reducing waste, food colours were chiefly marketing tools used to target the children and their parents with garish candies, technicolour breakfast cereals and lurid drinks.

The first reports that indicated how food dyes could trigger strange reactions were presented by Pennsylvania allergist Stephen D. Lockey (1904–1985) in a presentation to the Pennsylvania Allergy Association in 1948.[53] Focusing especially on the yellow dye tartrazine, Lockey claimed that such substances could cause allergic symptoms including hives and asthma in children, and published further findings sporadically in subsequent decades. Concurrently, an increasing number of food allergists were also claiming that behavioural problems in children could be caused by food allergies, a phenomenon that had been reported as early as 1916.[54] By the 1970s, these two separate observations – that food colours could cause allergic reactions and that childhood behavioural problems could be caused by food – merged into one in the form of the Feingold diet.

During the late 1960s and early 1970s, San Francisco allergist, Ben Feingold (1899–1982) developed the idea that the behavioural problems of many hyperactive children (hyperactivity had been coined as a distinct psychiatric disorder in the late 1950s) were caused by the ingestion of food additives, including synthetic colours, flavours and preservatives.[55] Writing up his findings in the popular book, *Why Your Child Is Hyperactive*, Feingold would spend the rest of his life promoting his food additive-free Feingold diet and warning Americans about food chemicals.[56] The story of the Feingold diet is described elsewhere, but what is worth emphasizing for this chapter is the broader claims Feingold made about exposure to food chemicals and human health.[57]

Quoting figures provided in 1971 to the US Congress for a set of hearings entitled, 'Chemicals and the Future of Man', Feingold stated that Americans consumed 5 pounds of additives every year.[58] What effects did such consumption have on human health? Mirroring Mackarness's view that humans had simply not evolved to eat such substances, Feingold speculated that food chemicals could be responsible not only for behavioural problems in children, but also for increased levels of violence and aggression in American society, disrupting both neural pathways and mutating genes. The effects, Feingold warned, could be far-reaching:

> In this rude dawn and uneasy period of questioning, it is not too surprising to find that the rapidly developed food synthetics have been introduced into the fuel that operates the human body with little public awareness. Realization often comes only at the precise moment of reading the fine print on a food-package label. The time is now long overdue to look at these chemicals, not in regard to the H-LDs

[children with hyperactivity and learning difficulties] but in regard to the human species as a whole.[59]

Read today, Feingold's words might have the ring of Cassandra to them. But two factors should be taken into consideration before dismissing them. First, while debates were raging about the Feingold diet in the American media during the 1970s, other scientists were making connections between lead exposure in children and a wide range of health problems, including hyperactivity.[60] Forty years on, scientists are investigating broader claims about lead exposure and levels of societal violence during the twentieth century.[61] While the removal of lead from petrol has been far less contentious than the debates about food chemicals (partly because there were broader environmental rationales for reducing atmospheric lead), this has perhaps paradoxically stymied more research into the link between environmental pollutants and mental health. Second, Feingold might have failed in his attempt to convince physicians, food manufacturers and the FDA that food additives were harmful to human health, but his diet won over the parents of thousands of hyperactive children. Thirty-five years after his death, the accumulation of anecdotal reports – along with a handful of positive clinical trials – finally swayed some food manufacturers to remove synthetic dyes from their products and some regulators to issue warnings on labels. Again, these successes, along with the lingering notion that the Feingold diet was nothing more than a food fad, have not prompted much more serious research into the link between food chemicals and behavioural problems. We are left wondering, as did Feingold, if the link between food additives and hyperactivity is merely the tip of the iceberg.

Conclusion

In the last 30 years, debates about food allergy have changed dramatically due to the rapid increase in the rate of peanut allergy. Largely unknown prior to the late-1980s, peanut allergy quickly became the most feared type of food allergy, leading to new labelling legislation, changes in the ways foods are processed and marketed and the creation of peanut-free zones (for instance, in schools, airplanes and sports arenas). Although increases in the consumption in packaged, processed food containing peanut products (possibly as a by-product of processing) in the past few decades may have contributed in small part to the peanut allergy epidemic, many of the dietary innovations with respect to peanuts and peanut butter emerged during the early twentieth century, long before fatal peanut allergy reactions became commonplace.[62] The emergence of peanut allergy transformed food allergy (or, at least, anaphylactic food allergy) from being a pariah subject that divided the allergy community into a topic that commanded attention. The reason for this was simple: unlike allergies to corn and dyes, which caused chronic symptoms that were difficult to substantiate, peanut allergy could and did kill. In order to deal with the dangers posed by peanut allergy, the food industry had to innovate. Companies, such as Mars Canada and Kinnerton Confectionary in the United Kingdom, developed either nut-free facilities or nut-free production lines complete with different coloured uniforms for staff on either side of the dividing line. There has even been research into whether it might be possible to use processing methods to reduce or eliminate the allergenicity of certain foods.[63]

Similarly, the apparent rise in gluten intolerance has also thrust food allergy into the spotlight. While gluten intolerance can be a serious and life-altering health condition (for instance, in the form of coeliac disease), there has also been concern that the prevalence of the condition has been vastly exaggerated in order to sell gluten-free products and cookbooks.[64] Overarching the debates about 'gluten-free lifestyles' has been the same idea that has underwritten many dietary explanations for ill health: specifically, that humans have not evolved to eat many of the foods found in the shelves of supermarkets.

The juxtaposition of a peanut allergy epidemic that has been treated with alacrity and a fashion for gluten intolerance that has been viewed with widespread scepticism glosses over the experiences of the vast majority of allergy sufferers and obscures a great deal of what really matters with respect to dietary innovation and allergy. So, what is the part of the historian in resolving these debates? Ultimately, the history of food allergy is a story of division and discord, where the experts became more strident and stubborn in their views over time. The role of dietary innovation in the broader history of food allergy has been similarly contested. While some have blamed the first agricultural revolution for much undiagnosed chronic ill health, there have been numerous counter claims that modern food production has only been a force for good, lowering food prices and increasing choice.[65] In both cases, personal interest – whether it be ideological or financial – has played a role in entrenching these positions. Recognizing this, historians can help to sort the wheat from the chaff, so to speak, and identify topics that would benefit from more fundamental, objective scientific research. The two cases discussed in this chapter – corn and food dyes – would be good places to start.

Part Two

Scientific Discourses

4

Dietary Change and Epidemic Disease: Fame, Fashion and Expediency in the Italian Pellagra Disputes, 1852–1902

David Gentilcore

Pellagra: From symptoms to causes

On 21 July 1902, the Italian Parliament passed the country's first law dedicated to countering the harmful effects of pellagra.[1] There were an estimated 72,000 victims of pellagra, located chiefly in Lombardy and the Veneto, suffering, as the disease progressed, the telltale effects of severe peeling of the skin, chronic diarrhoea, dizziness, weakness and lethargy, insanity and death.[2] To combat the pellagra epidemic, the law prohibited the sale of unripened or spoilt maize, whether in the form of grain or flour, and trade in all products made from unripened or spoilt maize. It also mandated the installation of public maize-drying ovens in affected areas, authorized the free distribution of salt to pellagrins and obliged municipalities to report new cases of pellagra in a timely fashion and keep up-to-date statistics. A fund of 100,000 *lire* a year was to be set up to allow local authorities to implement these measures.[3]

The law was certainly worthwhile in its intentions. By 1902, maize had transformed much of northern Italy. The arrival and spread of this high-yielding plant from the New World had been dramatic: a 'revolutionary irruption', in the words of one historian.[4] By the time of the law, it was the most cultivated crop (in acreage terms) in Piedmont, Lombardy, the Veneto, and Emilia and Romagna. And, in the form of maize polenta, it was also the cheapest food by far. Maize subsistence came at a price, however. Increased maize cultivation had brought with it a structural shift in the Italian countryside over the course of the nineteenth century. Peasants were transformed from the tenant farmers of the traditional *mezzadria* system to renters (in cash); or else they became field hands, working for a wage rather than for a part of the production – at a time when increasing numbers of people were chasing too few agricultural jobs and too little land.[5] Peasant living conditions had declined as a result, and they had become 'trapped' in an economic system from which the only means of escape was mass emigration.[6] And peasant diets had declined. Maize polenta had become more than a staple; it was the only food consumed during winter and spring by large sectors of the agricultural population. Pellagra was the cruel result.

Paradoxically, and rather perversely, the anti-pellagra law was not only long overdue, combatting a disease that had ravaged maize-growing areas of the country since the middle of the eighteenth century, it also came too late, in the sense that by 1902 pellagra rates had been declining for the previous decade or so, as diets had slowly improved (partly due to emigrants' remittances). Strangest of all, perhaps, the law put the weight of the Italian state and gave legal status to only one of multiple theories explaining the causation of pellagra – which turned out to be the 'wrong' one.

The experience of pellagra in Italy provides an example of how dietary change, in this case the shift to mass maize cultivation and consumption in the nineteenth century, led directly to disease, in this case the very man-made pellagra epidemic. This was at a time when health was perceived in terms of an adequate diet and when much research in chemistry and physiology was attempting to define just what constituted this.[7] There was evidently something potentially very unhealthy about maize, as it was consumed in Europe; by the middle of the nineteenth century, all the medical actors involved agreed on the close link between maize and pellagra. What they disagreed on was the exact causal nature of that link, propounding two divergent, indeed mutually exclusive, explanatory models. The fact that one of these, the more culturally influential one, turned out to be the 'wrong' one, and the other, less culturally successful one, turned out to be the 'right' one – although this would only become evident long after the events narrated in this chapter – allows us to study a history of 'stasis, of delay, of digression', to quote David Wootton, when 'bad ideas [...] triumph over good'.[8] Did this result in what Wootton has controversially called 'bad medicine' – medicine that did far more harm than good?[9] How the cultural dominance of one explanatory model, at the expense of another, came about; what it tells us about the nature of Italian medical science in the last few decades of the nineteenth century; and what its dominance meant for sufferers, is the subject of this chapter.

The historical study of pellagra in English has tended to focus on the US experience of the disease, which has explored pellagra as an exclusively American problem, in search of an American solution.[10] In addition to determining the geographical focus, this has meant a limited chronological one – that is, the first three decades of the twentieth century, when pellagra was epidemic in the parts of the southern United States, culminating in the experimental work of Joseph Goldberger to identify its causation and treatment during the 1920s (which lay the basis for eventual success in defeating the disease).[11] Similarly, Italian historiography has focused on the Italian experience of pellagra, mainly during the nineteenth century. It has tended to do so from a social history perspective, within the context of explorations of agricultural change and the marginalization and impoverishment of the Italian peasantry.[12] If the medical history of pellagra in the United States has been well served, this has been much less the case for Italy.[13]

In order to introduce the medical dispute which is the subject of this chapter, we need to backtrack a bit. Since the 1760s, Italian medical investigators had been debating the nature, causes and treatment of pellagra, which they recognized as a new disease. At the turn of the century, two of them, Francesco Fanzago and Giambattista Marzari, became embroiled in a classic priority dispute over the idea that the disease was at least in part a result of increasing maize consumption by the poor peasants of northern

Italy.[14] They were certainly on to something. This was not their main concern, however, which was in fact nosological – to understand what sort of illness pellagra was and how it could be classified. This could only be achieved by understanding its most prominent signs and symptoms or certain morbid alterations in the body. Thus, when confronted by a disease like pellagra, a medical investigator's question was more likely to be, 'Why does this person now have pellagra?', rather than 'How does pellagra come about?'[15]

At this point, understanding disease causation took a secondary place to understanding the nature of a disease. And this was just as well, given that every disease had a lengthy list of causes associated with it. Pellagra was no exception – climate (the burning sun), hard labour, dire poverty, habit (alcoholism), heredity and, now, diet. To impose a sense of order on the existence of multiple causes for every disease, doctors broke them down into different sorts, such as proximate and remote (with the latter being distinguished into predisposing and occasioning). This range of causes, as well as individual temperament, sex and age, would be brought to bear as variables in understanding, and so treating, individual cases. They also explained to contemporaries how the effects of pellagra could vary so widely from patient to patient.

The result was that, if Italian medical investigators largely agreed on the clinical picture of pellagra, they continued to debate the relative importance of different causes. For example, if Fanzago and Marzari were agreed in excluding heredity and contagion as possible causes of pellagra, two decades later Andrea Bisaglia saw these two factors as the only means of accounting for the way the disease seemed to run in certain families and was concentrated in particular parts of town.[16] Paradoxically, it was around this time, the 1830s, that a few European researchers began to think of several different organic disorders as having single causes that were both universal and necessary. For this to be possible required a radical shift in the way doctors defined diseases – from symptoms to causes. The so-called aetiological approach to disease, championed by Ignaz Semmelweis in his explorations of puerperal fever,[17] meant that every case of the disease had the same cause. And, as a result, any prophylactic or therapeutic measures directed at that cause, which were effective in one case, would be effective in every case. The aetiological approach offered a coherent means of explaining a bewildering range of facts and observations about a disease, while making the search for prevention and cure more focused.[18] This did not mean that there were not disputes over the basic nature of diseases like pellagra, however, as we shall see in the next section.

The dispute: Filippo Lussana, Cesare Lombroso and Clodomiro Bonfigli

When it came to the study of pellagra, the first to shift the focus to aetiology was the community physician, hospital director and later university lecturer, Filippo Lussana.[19] His first (brief) foray into the aetiology of pellagra owed a debt to the quantitative 'animal chemistry' approach pioneered by Justus von Liebig as a means of determining the body's physical needs in terms of food.[20] Four years later, in 1856, Lussana developed this into a book-length study (co-authored with the pathologist Carlo Frua). It begins with a chapter on the aetiology of pellagra, which occupies a full third of the book.[21] If the content here is partly traditional, surveying each of the by-now standard range of causes in turn, it offers a radical departure in singling out a cause which Lussana considers 'essential' – 'a dietary regime of insufficient plastic nutritive regeneration'.[22] For Lussana, the deficiency of a maize-based diet was thus the primary cause of pellagra, with all other factors being secondary. It was key to an understanding of the disease's pathology and therapeutics, as discussed in the rest of the book. We thus have a *necessary* cause, if not yet a single one.

The dispute did not begin until 13 years later, with the work of Cesare Lombroso – the originator of what I referred to above as the 'wrong' theory, which lay at the heart of the 1902 law. If Lombroso is best known today as the originator of criminal anthropology, which brought him international fame (the infamy came later), some of his first published works were on pellagra and he continued to investigate and write on the subject for the rest of his life – some 200 publications in all.[23] Lombroso first noted a link between the consumption of maize and the spread of pellagra in the Italian region of Lombardy in 1863, while he was a lecturer in mental illness at Pavia University and director of the insane ward at the town's hospital. This first period of research culminated 6 years later in Lombroso's monograph on the 'clinical and experimental study of the nature, cause and therapy of pellagra'.[24]

Here Lombroso explicitly espouses the aetiological agenda, in a book intended to identify the factor which, as he puts it, 'is the exclusive cause of pellagra'.[25] And he found it in 'spoilt maize covered with penicillium glaucum'.[26] This idea, which is the focus of the book, is not presented as hypothesis but as fact; there is no room for doubt. 'And so is destroyed, *a priori*, that doctrine which had pellagra deriving from an insufficient plastic diet', referring to Lussana's work.[27] Lombroso spent most of the 1860s and 1870s fleshing out what became known as the toxicozeist or spoilt maize theory of pellagra causation, with laboratory investigations, to counter Lussana's use of Liebig's chemical studies in support of what became known as the deficiency theory. At a time when Liebig's own nutritional theories were being increasingly called into question, Lombroso was a follower of Liebig's main critic in the nascent field of nutrition, Jacob Moleschott.[28]

Lombroso turned a factor or principle discussed by Lussana as a possible, secondary cause of pellagra – spoilt maize[29] – into the necessary, single cause of the disease. Moreover, it was one for which he (Lombroso) now, triumphantly, took sole credit. If Lombroso tended to see pellagra-like effects of spoilt maize everywhere, and if his experiments with penicillium worked better in the lab than in real life, this did not stop him from being surprised and dismayed when people did not replicate his findings and agree with his conclusions. 'You cannot imagine the pains that research on maize have caused me', Lombroso wrote in 1875 in a letter to the political economist Luigi Bodio.[30] By this time, open and direct confrontation was an accepted part of scientific dispute, especially on the Continent, including (on occasion) *ad hominem* attacks.[31] Within the realms of civility (just about), views had to be defended and opponents swiftly and decisively dealt with.

Opposition to Lombroso came in part from Lussana, who in 1872 responded with another study of pellagra. That Lussana too had embraced the issue of causation was evident from the book's title ('on the causes of pellagra'), but he could not share

Lombroso's conviction that the 'common mold' penicillium glaucum underwent a harmful toxic alteration in contact with maize.[32] Lussana used this book to refine his ideas, stressing that maize was not a cereal-based disease, along the lines of ergotism, but the result of a diet deficient in 'azotates' (proteins). He did offer a compromise with Lombroso, in singling out 'poor quality and spoilt maize' as particularly low in azotates.[33] But, in essence, Lussana's work was a refutation of Lombroso's. As Lussana made clear, he could not be convinced of the role of spoilt maize in causing pellagra until this was shown to be a real toxin, which could pass from one generation to the next, remain in the body all life long, whose effects could be felt in all seasons of the year and which could only affect certain people and not others – all features which Lussana considered evident in pellagra.[34]

In response, Lombroso quickly dashed off a thirty-page 'polemical letter' to Lussana.[35] The polemic is not without its humour. In response to Lussana's claim to have ingested as much spoilt maize in a single meal as a peasant family would eat in a single month, without any ill effects, Lombroso retorts, 'I was aware of the ready and powerful digestive powers of professor Lussana, but really that a so gargantuan voracity able to swallow, at a simple breakfast, 150 kilograms of maize, was difficult to conjure up even with the most Rabelaisian imagination.'[36] Then, Lombroso proceeds to the serious point – that the toxin is most harmful when ingested over protracted periods, as Lussana should have known. This was, in fact, Lussana's problem, trying 'to compensate for a lack of method, the essence of sound erudition, with impatient brilliant insights, which are sometimes fertile but are more often erroneous'.[37] Not only was Lussana wrong about pellagra's aetiology, Lombroso seems to be claiming the study of its aetiology for himself, since only he had the right idea and the right methodology. If he has been overly 'resolute' and 'combative' in his rebuttal of Lussana's more 'delicate' approach, he apologises; but how could he respond otherwise, 'When a doctrine [Lombroso's own] has been refined over such a long period of time and when we know that on it depends the wellbeing of thousands of people.'[38]

The dispute continued through the 1870s, even as pellagra rates climbed to 100,000 identified cases.[39] Lombroso and Lussana differed over the key question of whether maize was a sufficiently nutritional food when consumed by hard-labouring peasants as a staple. Lombroso took as a given that it was and concentrated his chemico-toxicological analyses and experimental tests on the effects of humidity, while Lussana focused on analyses of maize samples. In 1878, the director of the insane asylum in Ferrara, Clodomiro Bonfigli, drew on Lussana's theory and his own experience to argue for the 'dietary insufficiency' of maize.[40] When the article was republished in *La Rivista*, Lombroso immediately answered back in the same periodical (no. 44, 1878),[41] which he later amplified into book form.[42] Bonfigli replied in turn with a lengthy article in *Il Raccoglitore Medico*, an important medical periodical which often hosted controversies of this kind. Bonfigli substantiated his findings and directed his fire at Lombroso (which included reproducing verbatim Lombroso's 1878 rebuttal).

In particular, Bonfigli was critical of the strichnoid toxin which Lombroso claimed to have isolated 2 years earlier and promptly baptized 'pellagrozeine'. Bonfigli accused

Lombroso of wanting to establish pellagrozeine as the single cause of pellagra at all costs, even though (as Bonfigli affirmed) peasants refused to eat moldy maize.[43] The gap between the socially orientated Bonfigli and the laboratory-focused Lombroso could not have been clearer. Bonfigli and Lombroso locked horns over everything from the quantities of maize eaten by field hands and the digestibility of maize and its relationship to malnutrition, to the existence of cases of pellagra without maize. They also differed on preventive and therapeutic measures. For Bonfigli, these came down to resolving 'the most serious and urgent social question of the pauperism of the rural classes'.[44] Lombroso countered that this would mean 'a social revolution'; the money Bonfigli proposed spending to improve the diet of the rural poor would be better spent on providing maize drying ovens.[45] Their respective rhetorical styles were also different. Bonfigli adopted the moral high ground and a tone of quiet persuasion; Lombroso characterized Bonfigli's study as 'superficial' (p. 31), making 'comical assertions' (p. 37), 'falsifying' data (p. 72) and perhaps lowest of all, not even up to 'the principal of my adversaries, Lussana' (p. 27).[46]

Lussana did not let that get away and returned to the fray with a short article entitled 'Professor Lombroso's hallucination', which cites a range of studies against Lombroso's toxicozeist theory.[47] Lussana refers to Lombroso's virulent comments against both him and Bonfigli as evidence of Lombroso's unbalanced mental state, diagnosing him (only partially tongue-in-cheek) as a *mattoide*. The irony is that *mattoide* was a term Lombroso himself had coined to label the mad genius – that is, mad on the surface but normal underneath and so distinguished from the criminally insane.[48] Lussana refers to Lombroso as a 'poor delusional' who in his 'frenzied delirium' sees the spoilt maize toxin everywhere. Lussana concluded his article with the rather childish remark, 'If he does not consider my experiments then naturally I will not consider his.'[49]

Scientific controversy and the success of Lombroso

With the benefit of hindsight, it is all too tempting to side with Lussana and Bonfigli in the debate – not only because the deficiency theory would eventually prove to be the 'right' one, but also because Lombroso appears as the bully of the piece.[50] However, on closer reading of the treatises, articles and short notices, it is not immediately apparent why one theory – Lombroso's toxicozeist hypothesis – should have been the influential one at the political level, while the other – the dietary insufficiency hypothesis – was marginalized. The participants disputed both facts and the interpretation of those facts, according to their differing theoretical positions. A history of science approach can help us here, encouraging us to understand the past on its own terms, by reconstructing the 'reasonableness' of the arguments, while also allowing us to appreciate the range of factors involved, such as social interests and political struggles.[51] Even in the most internalist of scientific controversies, broader 'social' aspects come to the fore, including issues like academic status and power relations.[52] In the case of Lombroso and pellagra, we might reduce these aspects to three: the fame, fashion and expediency of this chapter's title.

Let us begin with fame. At an international level, Lombroso was Italy's most read author, hailed as the founder of a new science – criminal anthropology.[53] An adulatory article in *Appletons' Popular Science Monthly* referred to 'a strong intelligence, a robust will, and a keen intellectual curiosity', as well as his 'indifference to the incredulous smile, the sarcasms, that greeted his first efforts at solving problems hitherto held insoluble' (Figure 4.1).[54] In Italy, Lombroso's was an increasingly loud and powerful voice. He was becoming a very public figure: at once doctor, philosopher, anthropologist, sociologist and political commentator.[55] Lombroso worked tirelessly to shape public opinion, mobilize intellectuals and organize a 'school' of followers able to penetrate the apparatus of the state. (The direct political involvement would come later.[56]) As a positivist scientist, he saw himself as the bearer of a mission to educate, inform and influence, especially in the field of public health.

When it came to pellagra, from the early 1870s Lombroso unceasingly and bullishly drove his message home, publishing a seemingly endless flow of long and short articles in both scholarly journals and the popular press, book and article reviews and book prefaces. He combined a populist approach, (over)simplifying complex scientific ideas, with a narrative and provocative writing style. He missed no occasion to expound and defend his theory. As Gaetano Strambio wrote at the time, no one was able to set the

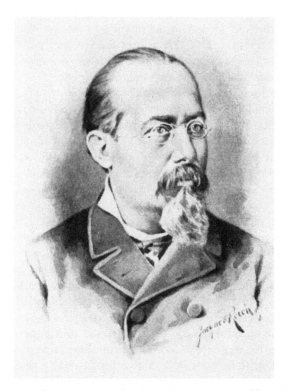

Figure 4.1 Cesare Lombroso. From *Appleton's Popular Science Monthly*, vol. 52, April 1898.

pellagra agenda and fill it with a lot of media 'noise' (*rumore*) like Lombroso, with 'all the conviction of a religious believer and the dialectical savvy of a lawyer'; no one had been able to shift the debate on to his own particular aetiological hypothesis, 'involving public health doctors and chemists alike', like Lombroso; and no one was able, 'reducing a frightful and arduous social problem to the level of the simple regulation of public health', to persuade the authorities of the usefulness of his own proposed solutions and treatments, like Lombroso.[57]

In developing his toxicozeist theory of transmission, Lombroso rode the fashion for bacteriology, the success of which was allowing medicine as a profession to regain the prestige it had lost earlier in the century.[58] The bacterial hypothesis forcefully suggested that each disease was caused by some bacterium; determining causation was thus reduced to a matter of identifying the single bacterium concerned.[59] In the 5 years between 1879 and 1884, the causative organisms for leprosy, typhoid, malaria, diphtheria, cholera and tetanus were identified.[60] There may have been many germ theories of disease (focusing, variously, on chemical poisons, ferments, degraded cells, fungi, bacteria or parasites), but proponents tended to subsume these into a single theory in order to strengthen their position.[61] Lombroso was able to document how the consumption of poorly dried and stored maize – itself a widespread reality at the time – was linked to the development of a pellagra-causing toxin. And he did this by making the most of the educational facilities, licensing standards, medical societies and research periodicals so dear to the positivist, scientific medicine of the day. From Lombroso's new base at the University of Turin, he was able to develop a well-articulated scientific research programme based on laboratory analysis, with followers endeavouring to duplicate his results elsewhere in Italy.

And the science was important, since it allowed Lombroso to be more convincing than Lussana or Bonfigli. Knowledge of metabolism and foods did not allow the latter two to articulate clearly the precise relationship between maize subsistence and pellagra. Their use of generic expressions like the 'meagre nutritive physiological value' of maize did not quite cut it when compared to Lombroso's well-articulated (if ultimately flawed) laboratory methodology.[62] At a time when chemical methods and experimental physiology dominated medical research, influenced by figures like (first) Justus von Liebig and (later) Robert Koch, 'setting up a laboratory for his clinic soon became a point of honour to the clinician'.[63] Not all medical investigators were equal when it came to technical and experimental sophistication; nor were all clinical laboratories, when it came to resources and qualified staff. Nowhere is this more evident than in Lombroso's magnum opus on the clinical and pathological science of pellagra, published in 1892. Its 400 pages detail the numerous experiments on live animals, drug trials on living humans and autopsies on dead ones (113 in all), all made possible by the extensive resources Lombroso had at his disposal, in terms of personnel and funding.[64] Whereas Lussana and Frua provided most of their data – and their book's only illustration (Figure 4.2) – for the section dedicated to the pathology of pellagra, outside of the main aetiological thrust of the book, Lombroso bombarded his readers with detailed tables and illustrations of all sorts, the latter alone covering a range of topics, from the microorganisms of spoilt maize to the gaits of pellagra victims (Figure 4.3).

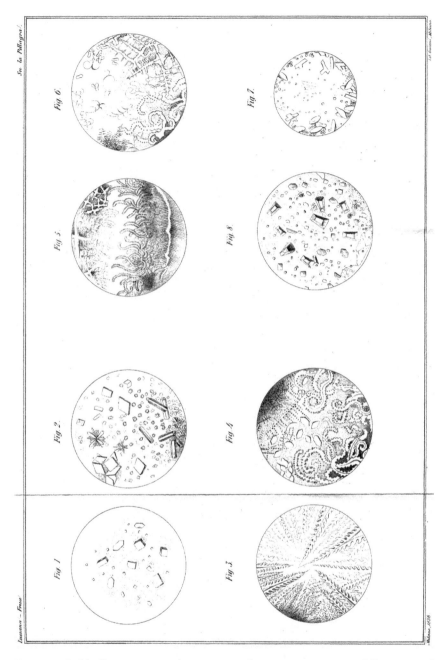

Figure 4.2 'Table illustrating several microscopic observations concerning different animal humours of pellagrous and non-pellagrous subjects'. From: Filippo Lussana and Carlo Frua, *Su la pellagra: memoria* (Milan: Giuseppe Bernardoni, 1856).

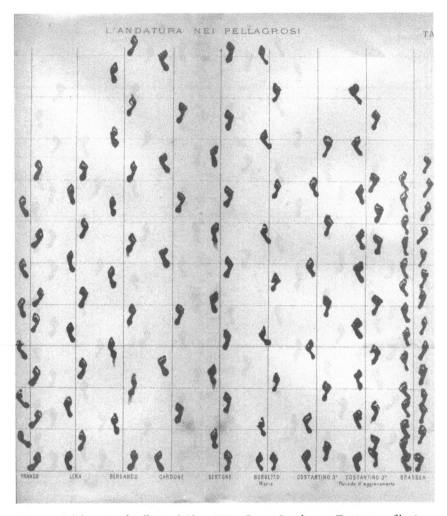

Figure 4.3 'The gait of pellagrins'. Plate 10 in Cesare Lombroso, *Trattato profilattico e clinico della pellagra* (Turin: Bocca, 1892).

In addition to his personal fame and his use of influential bacteriology, expediency had a part to play in the success of Lombroso's aetiological model. It suited government, which sought a clearly identifiable enemy and practicable solutions; and it suited the ruling bourgeois and agrarian classes, in identifying pellagra's origins as 'hygienic' (public health) rather than the ordering of society (peasant poverty). From the 1880s, a series of proposed laws fighting pellagra had failed to receive parliamentary assent, because they interfered with the maize-related interests of landowners, millers and traders.[65] Watering down the legislation, combined with a new liberal-left government in office, more receptive to social issues, allowed the 1902 law to pass. Lombroso's measures brought no social disruption, and the cost to the public purse was minimal.

Conclusion: The dispute's impact on pellagra and pellagrology

In 1892, Lombroso complained that ongoing opposition to his theory – the result of 'caste and personal interests', habit and short-sightedness – had harmed his career, affecting 'my reputation as a doctor, as a scientist and even as a teacher'. It had also meant that 'large sums of money' had been spent on preventing and treating the disease to no effect, by following 'false causes'.[66] We might say that Lombroso was accusing his opponents of practising 'bad medicine'. Paradoxically, it was Lombroso's own 'wrong' theory which can be accused of having had the most deleterious effects on the lives of pellagra sufferers, if not on medical investigation into the disease.

This is because Lombroso dismissed the idea that diet alone could cure pellagra. He relied instead on 'a few medicinal substances, such as arsenious acid and above all like lead acetate, [which] can bring the most resistant pellagrous manias to a complete cure', and salt.[67] In 1883, Lombroso contacted the founder of the town of Mogliano Veneto's Hospice for Pellagrins, Costante Gris, to propose a trial. Gris was to treat forty pellagra sufferers with drugs alone, without modifying their diet. However, after 5 months, with the patients as ill as ever, Gris decided on his own initiative to reverse the experiment. 'By means of the restorative diet alone', Gris later informed Lombroso, 'and without the use of the aforementioned medicines, I obtained much better results than with the first method'.[68] This was 'bad medicine' indeed – Lombroso's treatment was worse than none at all. Not only was Lombroso treating pellagra with what amounted to a dangerous poison, in eschewing a diet-based treatment he effectively eliminated the one effective remedy available (and which was perceived as such, by some, at the time). Moreover, Lombroso stubbornly continued in this conviction until his death, as we have seen.

What impact did the dispute have on Italian medical practitioners more broadly? If Lombroso was able to dominate the pellagra debates at the higher echelons of medical science and government, the situation down on the ground could play out quite differently. A look at the aetiological models adopted by asylum and town doctors, who treated pellagrins on a day-to-day basis, suggests that practitioner responses were not clear-cut. If I have polarized the pellagra dispute hitherto, construing it as a two-sided debate (much as Lombroso himself saw it), in fact it was multisided, almost fluid, as are most controversies in science.[69]

For the Venetian asylum director Cesare Vigna, the aetiology of pellagra saw medical investigators divided into three camps: 'unicists', who favoured either one of the two dominant explanatory models based around maize; 'dualists', who opted for a mixture of the two main theories; and 'pluralists', who continued to acknowledge a wide range of causal factors in the generation of pellagra.[70] These divisions are borne out by work that I and Egidio Priani have carried out on the thousands of diagnoses of the pellagrous insane referred to the Venetian asylums of San Clemente (for women) and San Servolo (for men).[71] Throughout the latter two decades of the nineteenth century, the patient records continue to refer to multiple causal factors – heredity, sunstroke, poverty and hard labour being the key ones. It is not unusual to read, under 'known causes' of a patient's pellagrous insanity, phrases like 'sunstroke, field labours, combined with diet'.[72] This may be throwback to the pre-aetiological age, but it may just as likely refer to the difficulties faced by nascent clinical psychology in coming to grips with causation in a disease like pellagra that mixed physical and mental aspects.[73] There was a tendency still to distinguish between levels of causation, with heredity being a predisposing rather than direct cause of pellagrous insanity. Against this backdrop, there were increasing references to either dietary deficiency or spoilt maize intoxication, but with a preference for the more generic and mixed causation evident in expressions like 'poor nutrition' or 'bad diet'.

Gauging the opinions of community-funded town doctors (*medici condotti*) is more difficult. One possible source consists of the case notes they submitted to the two Venetian asylums when referring a patient for admission. But these are inconclusive. Thus, the patient files of sufferers referred from the province of Rovigo, in 1882, provide examples for both sides of the debate. A Dr Marco Baia used the language of the deficiency theory in noting, for Taddeo A., that his 'usual diet [consists] of foods deficient in azotate substances and in limited quantities'. By contrast, a Dr Renier went to great pains to tow the Lombrosian line, writing in his case notes that the patient may have eaten plenty of maize but it was of 'excellent quality' and was the patient's preferred food.[74] More helpful in gauging the stance of town doctors is a 1912 survey of 242 *condotti* with experience in treating pellagrins. The survey found that they were divided (much like asylum doctors) – eighty-seven town doctors (or 35 per cent) were found to favour dietary insufficiency, seventy-nine (32 per cent) opted for spoilt maize intoxication, sixty-six (27 per cent) preferred a mixture of both of these theories and the remaining fifteen (6 per cent) favoured a range of other causes, including alcoholism and infection.[75]

What were the effects of this conviction on the field known as pellagrology? There is no evidence that Lombroso's predominance here harmed the careers of either Lussana or Bonfigli. Lussana continued his research in the neurophysiology of the brain and was professor of physiology, first at Parma (1860–67) and then at Padua (1867–89), the years of his long-running dispute with Lombroso.[76] Bonfigli likewise continued to publish widely and translated several works of German psychiatry. After a successful tenure in Ferrara, in 1893, he took up directorship of the Santa Maria della Pietà asylum in Rome and the chair of psychiatry at Rome's 'La Sapienza'. He was elected to the twentieth legislature of the Italian Parliament, 1897–1900, where he spoke on issues regarding public health and asylum legislation, and was the founding president of the Lega Nazionale dei Fanciulli Deficienti in 1902. He retired from his asylum directorship in 1905 and died 4 years later, the same year as Lombroso.[77]

Finally, its effects on the research agenda were less than might be expected. If the 1902 pellagra law suggests some kind of 'closure', a defining element of scientific controversies, in fact the Italian dispute over pellagra's aetiology remained open and unresolved, even while the disease continued to decline in Italy. Lombroso's may have been an intimidating presence in the field of pellagrology throughout the last three decades of the nineteenth century and into the twentieth, but this did not actually stifle investigation and debate. The 'success' of his explanatory model – measured in terms of its influence in the public health realm, if not among practising doctors – did not prevent exploration into alternative theories of causation and treatment. The field's main journal, the *Rivista pellagrologica italiana*, may have been a Lombrosian stronghold, founded (in 1900) and directed by one of his former pupils, Giuseppe Antonini; but its pages provide ample evidence of the continuing vivacity, urgency and variety of the investigations into the disease. Indeed, as I have noted elsewhere, the first decade of the twentieth century saw more Italian publications on pellagra than any other.[78]

The second decade of the century witnessed a return to the dietary insufficiency model. In 1911, Aristide Stefani, who had studied under Lussana, wrote of certain 'imponderables' necessary to health but which the body could not manufacture by itself. Stefani argued that while maize was probably adequate in proteic terms, this did not mean that it could be considered a complete foodstuff, containing all the dietary 'principles' necessary to man, in the way of breast milk or wheat.[79] The following year the Polish biochemist Casimir Funk, working in the United States, published his findings on a group of what he termed 'deficiency diseases', of which pellagra was one, all caused by 'monotonous diets'.[80] By comparing pellagra to diseases like beriberi, both caused by foods lacking in 'vital amines' (or 'vitamines') essential to nutrition, Funk put the deficiency hypothesis back on the research agenda (see Scrob chapter in this volume). Funk himself suggested the direction: more research into which specific diets helped the condition of pellagrins improve and discovering a means of inducing experimental pellagra in animals to permit further laboratory work would both help 'ascertain definitively whether or not pellagra is a deficiency disease'.[81]

If this call was quickly taken up in the United States, where pellagra rates were then rising steeply, Italian investigators, with the exception of Stefani, were less enthusiastic. Due in part to the continued influence of Lombroso's toxicozeist research agenda, and in part to the ongoing decline of pellagra rates in Italy, with no new cases, the whole issue became less pressing. Medical investigators turned their sights to other research topics. The First World War, far from increasing pellagra, assisted its decline, as the Italian government imported massive amounts of wheat and sold it at subsidized prices. By 1922, pellagra had all but disappeared, without the Italian public being much aware of it – a 'silent victory', in the words of one journalist.[82]

5

Conceptualizing the Vitamin and Pellagra as an Avitaminosis: A Case-Study Analysis of the Sedimentation Process of Medical Knowledge

Mircea Scrob

Introduction

In 1912, Casimir Funk, a young Polish chemist proposed the term 'vitamine' to refer to a chemical substance which he isolated from extracts of rice bran and yeast and which seemed to be indispensable to maintain the organism in good health.[1] The research summarized by Funk's announcement ushered a paradigm change in the field of nutrition in the typical Kuhnian sense. Subsequent scholars have acknowledged the game-changing implications of this research, not just because it conclusively showed that the established consensus from the past 50 years – that protein, energy (from a suitable mix of protein, fat and carbohydrates) and minerals were sufficient to maintain well-being – was inadequate, but also because it demonstrated the great potential of combining standardized diets and the use of laboratory animals for furthering nutritional knowledge.[2] While acknowledging these claims, my argument is that the early research on vitamins had another, more pervasive influence in that it changed the epistemological standards for evaluating nutritional knowledge. In particular, before the conceptualization of vitamins, it was possible to positively maintain that some recognized nutrients are sufficient to keep an organism in good health although they had never been administered alone or even separated to the extent possible from the many other chemical components found in test foods. Reviewed in retrospect, therefore, this claim had only the characteristics of a working hypothesis, one that ultimately solidified into an unquestioned norm so much so that its underlying assumptions were not revisited even though techniques of separating chemical components in foods had been developed that made possible to (in)validate it. By contrast, after the conceptualization of vitamins, it has been possible only to maintain that a certain nutrient is necessary for good health under specific conditions but not that the chemical components identified at one time are all that are required to keep the organism in good health under all conditions. This epistemological shift is evident in the studies performed from the 1910s onwards, on vitamins and nutrition more generally, and in vitamin research it has been responsible for the rapid differentiation of vitamin types after the concept became established. Most importantly, the two epistemological approaches supported different perspectives on the relation between diet and disease: a closed perspective in which dietary diseases were caused by an insufficient intake of a few known nutrients and an open perspective in which the cause of a disease can be looked for in an insufficient intake of a previously unrecognized nutrient and, if a relationship is discovered, lead to the conceptualization of a new nutritive component.

My chapter discusses how these different perspectives shaped the conceptualization of pellagra as a deficiency disease. The primary purpose is to show how the pre-vitamin established consensus, far from being a mere convention for guiding research, became an accepted dogma which precluded a systematic conceptualization of pellagra as a form of deficiency disease even though compelling evidence seemed to support such an interpretation. The first step in this analysis is to show the hardness of the pre-vitamin scientific consensus, with a special emphasis on how the conceptualization of vitamins actually testifies to this hardness. In this section, I also discuss how nutritional research became epistemologically more open after the conceptualization of vitamins and how this perspective facilitated considerable progress in nutritional knowledge. The hardness of the established consensus is visible also in the research on pellagra, the focus of the second section, most clearly in the attempts of a minority of pre-vitamin researchers to interpret it as a dietary deficiency disease. Their struggle to explain the persistent association between pellagra and maize consumption within the confines of the established consensus, never fully questioning its unverified assumptions even when confronted by their opponents with the claim that 'maize was one of the most nutritious cereals', is suggestive in this sense. Furthermore, the almost immediate application of the vitamin deficiency model to pellagra together with its general acceptance suggest that what had been missing until then was the conceptual framework for interpreting otherwise well-established observations. This discussion will take up the third section of this paper. Finally, a discussion of how the vitamin deficiency model had been applied by members of the Romanian, Italian and US medical communities is included since, I argue, it offers important insights into the wider conditions that facilitated a more sustained engagement with the interpretation that pellagra was due to improper nutrition. This case study analysis illustrates well a process of sedimentation in which knowledge produced under different, sometimes even incompatible, technological, methodological and/or empirical paradigms can coexist side by side in the corpus of knowledge.

From a closed to an open approach to nutritional knowledge

By 1911, two research strands were coming together to show that nutritional knowledge was incomplete: laboratory research on animal feeding using ever more purified foods and the research on the curative properties of rice polishings in beriberi. In the research on feeding experiments, for instance, Hopkins was involved in making sense of experiments performed in 1906 which showed, to his surprise, that rats fed casein/Protene, starch, cane sugar, lard and salts failed to grow despite generous rations.[3] Equally puzzling, a small addition of milk, which contributed insignificant quantities of the then known nutrients, was highly effective at restoring growth.[4] A few years later, McCollum started his own feeding experiments, whose results showed that a diet of casein, lard, lactose, starch, agar-agar and salts, which amply supplied all the known nutrients, was insufficient to support growth in rats.[5] However, if lard was replaced by butter as the source of fat, growth resumed, while if it was replaced by an equally rich source of fat, such as olive oil, no effect was observed suggesting that the growth-promoting factor in butter was not fat. Similarly disruptive for the established consensus, Holst and Frolich and Stepp have shown that vegetables and fruits on the one hand, and alcohol extracts of milk bread, egg yolk and calf brain on the other,[6] corrected diets which otherwise were incapable of keeping guinea pigs and rats in normal health. Besides these studies, earlier experiments in which laboratory animals failed to thrive when fed liberal amounts of protein, calories and minerals, as various combinations of food, and to a lesser extent, the findings of Emil Fischer and Osborne and Mendel on the amino acid composition of proteins and their biological value, were capable of casting doubt over more or less central tenants of the established consensus.[7]

However, it is important to emphasize regarding these experiments that they were not designed to examine the established consensus but were formulated within its conceptual framework, often to determine the biological value of recognized nutrients. What was exceptional about them was that they happened to administer the known nutrients in a less 'contaminated' form, either by having unintentionally selected a nutrient source that was naturally poor in the yet unrecognized nutrients (lard instead of butter for fat) or artificially rendered so (Hopkin's Protene), or by intentionally separating the known nutrients from other chemical components found in food through various chemical processes (extraction by alcohol). It is illustrative for the serendipitous quality of these studies that the most disruptive observations came not from the experimental animals, but from the control animals, their unexpected failure to thrive even though fed a supposedly suitable diet having prompted some of these authors to reconsider and explicitly question the established consensus. For all these reasons, these experiments cannot be taken as examples of challenges to the established consensus and, in fact, the lack of such directed studies together with the limited impact within the research community of the anomalous findings that were reported testifies to the hardness of the established consensus.

It was the discovery that beriberi can be cured through the administration of rice polishings, that the curative substance was effective in minute amounts and that the recognized nutrients cannot account for the curative properties that energized the re-evaluation of the established consensus. Beriberi is nowadays conceptualized as a deficiency disease caused by an insufficient intake of vitamin B1 (thiamine) and was historically associated with the consumption of white rice. At the beginning of the twentieth century, beriberi was becoming endemic in South-East Asia partly following the introduction of mechanical mills which separated more thoroughly the husk from the rest of the grain. Regarding the conceptualization of vitamins, the research on beriberi which had an immediate bearing had been performed by Stanton and Fraser beginning with 1907. In an experiment which is remarkable through its scope and design, the researchers assigned groups of labourers working on a railway in the Malaysian jungle on diets in which the only component which was expected to differ was whether white or brown rice was served.[8] After sufficient cases of beriberi appeared in the white rice group, the diets were switched with the results that beriberi appeared in the previously immune group. The experiments were informed by previous observations which showed that beriberi was associated with the consumption of rice, and in particular white rice, and that the administration of rice polishings can cure the disease. Nevertheless, at the time of Stanton and Fraser's research, one common interpretation was that beriberi was an infection linked with certain features of a locality and the inclusion of a counterbalanced design was intended to address this possibility and show that the type of rice was the only aspect associated with the disease. The two researchers ended their report rather overly cautious by just reaffirming the connection between white rice consumption and beriberi but they were persuaded by the results to conduct a follow-up study to explore the crucial question of what is the curative substance in rice polishings. For this task, it was fortunate that the polishings delivered marginally higher amounts for just two of the recognized nutrients, fat and phosphorus (phytin), compared to white rice.[9] It was thus necessary to design experiments that would show for just two nutrients whether they were responsible for the curative properties before considering the presence of unrecognized nutrients. It was also fortunate that the unrecognized nutrient did not have similar chemical properties to fat or phytin so that when the researchers extracted these substances from polishings to check which one was responsible for the curative effect, they were not 'contaminated' by the missing nutrient. Furthermore, only a small fraction of the content of polishings was found to be active which suggested that ordinary nutritional processes were unlikely to be responsible for the curative properties. At the same time, this finding argued against the interpretation, under the intoxication theory of beriberi, that the polishings contained an antitoxin since within the existing models such substances were needed to be consumed in significantly larger quantities to be effective. Finally, Funk managed to isolate the substance further and show that 1 kilogram of rice contained no more than 1 gram of it.[10]

The vitamin as a new category of nutrients has been, therefore, conceptualized to account for the anti-beriberi properties of rice polishings and, soon afterwards, for the growth-promoting properties of such foods as butter and milk, a chain of events acknowledged by such pioneers as Hopkins, Funk and McCollum.[11] With the conceptualization of vitamins, a new model of deficiency diseases emerged – avitaminoses – that were caused by an insufficient intake of the newly recognized nutrient and the interplay between the two categories powered significant progress in nutritional knowledge over the next decades. In particular, once the conceptual breakthrough had been achieved, researchers became immediately interested, and successful, in identifying types of vitamins and/or in applying the avitaminosis model to puzzling diseases. The procedures used by researchers grew increasingly more complex with each new identified vitamin but the underlying criteria and logic remained consistent throughout – the existence of a new vitamin would be demonstrated either by showing that a health condition can be improved by administering a food component and none of the recognized nutrients could be responsible for it or that a health condition develops on a diet containing all the known nutrients.[12] These standards were conservative as the burden of proof was placed on the proponents of a new vitamin even though the known nutrients were not completely purified, not unlike the standards that were in place when the first vitamin had been conceptualized. What was qualitatively different this time was that researchers considered possible, some even likely, that more vitamin types existed or, at least, that no conclusive answer could be given until all known nutrients were purified.[13]

Indicative in this regard, several researchers have immediately looked for other vitamins, guided by the criteria described above and using established chemical processes to separate potential unidentified nutrients from the recognized ones. For instance, after it was demonstrated that a newly recognized nutrient can cure beriberi and can promote growth and cure xerophthalmia, the question arose whether these effects might be due to one and the same substance. By showing that certain foods (butter) can cure xerophthalmia but not beriberi, while other foods (rice polishings) can cure beriberi but not xerophthalmia, it was shown that the anti-beriberi and anti-xerophthalmia/growth-promoting factors were chemically distinct.[14] Another question was whether fat-rich foods contained one or more active substances since some such foods had been proven effective against xerophthalmia, rickets and in promoting growth. Addressing this question was complicated by the fact that such hypothetical substances would share some chemical properties, for instance solubility in fat and alcohol. Nonetheless, McCollum, Simmonds and Ernestine Becker were able to show that heating cod liver oil and running a stream of oxygen through it destroyed the anti-xerophthalmic factor but left the anti-rickets factor intact, whereas some foods – coconut oil for instance – were highly effective against rickets but much less effective against xerophthalmia, a strong proof that there were at least two different vitamins soluble in fat.[15] Turning to pellagra, Elvehjem proved that it was an avitaminosis by showing that dogs fed a test diet that, Goldberger argued, was pellagra-inducing developed a condition called black tongue which could be cured by administering niacin or tryptophan, an amino acid known by then to be a precursor of niacin.[16]

The central argument of this section is that a closed approach to nutritional knowledge, at least in respect to fundamental principles, has dominated research before the conceptualization of vitamins, whereas an open approach, in which knowledge was continuously questioned and refined, prevailed afterwards. The different approaches are only to a limited extent explained by the availability of techniques and foods required for examining these fundamental principles – simple use of different foods that were equally good sources of a recognized nutrient but would have likely varied in their composition of other hypothetical factors (lard vs butter, cod liver vs coconut oil) or from which more and more of the 'contaminant' factors were excluded through chemical processes (extraction with different substances) have been central to the identification of vitamin types but also available to researchers working under the established consensus. Rather, the relation was the other way around with the change in the epistemological perspective having promoted the proliferation of new and ingenious techniques of purifying foods. Finally, it should be mentioned that the open approach is still dominant today and is most visible in the fact that the list of vitamins remains open in anticipation of the identification of new 'vitamins'. At the same time, the closed approach is most visible in the way diseases such as beriberi, scurvy, rickets or pellagra, which seemed to have a definite relation to food consumption, have been conceptualized within the framework of the pre-vitamin established consensus. The purpose of the next sections will be to explore how the closed and open perspectives on nutritional knowledge have shaped the conceptualization of pellagra as a dietary deficiency disease.

The pellagra conundrum within the established consensus on nutrition

Pellagra is nowadays conceptualized as a deficiency disease caused by an insufficient intake of niacin. Relatively rare today, pellagra became widespread by the beginning of the twentieth century in North America (southern states of the United States), Southern Europe (particularly northern Italy, northern Spain, Moldova and Wallachia) and parts of Africa (Egypt, South Africa). The official statistics on the number of pellagrins for the most affected countries are staggering – roughly 80,000 for the Old Kingdom of Romania in 1902,[17] 72,600 in Italy in 1899[18] and showing a rapid progression in the United States after 1905, and although these statistics have been disputed by some contemporary researchers, what is more important is that pellagra had been perceived as a major public health problem in all these countries. Nevertheless, despite sustained interest from the medical community over almost 50 years, no consensus had been reached over the conceptualization of pellagra as a type of disease. Most researchers, from Lussana to Lombroso, Babeş, Funk and Elvehjem, accepted two crucial epidemiological facts about pellagra – that the disease was endemic only among populations who subsisted on maize and was almost entirely absent from ones who subsisted on other grains and that not everyone who consumed maize suffered from pellagra. Indeed, it was recognized, then as now, that pellagra emerged in Europe following the introduction of maize from the Americas, possibly because the crop was imported without the practice of cooking it by soaking the grains in lime water before grounding and thereby making the contained niacin biologically available or the wider indigenous crop/ dietary patterns which complemented maize by supplying any missing nutrients.[19] Furthermore, it was acknowledged that pellagra generally occurred among persons who lived on diets in which maize predominated while animal foodstuffs were consumed in only limited amounts. Nevertheless, the general consensus vanished when it came to interpreting these epidemiological facts.

The principal theories up to the 1920s that aimed to explain these epidemiological features can be grouped under three broad categories: pellagra as a 'deficiency' disease, as an intoxication or as an infection. Pellagra as a deficiency disease involved either an insufficient consumption of albumins (proteins), of proteins of high biological value or of a 'vitamin', all because maize was nutritionally deficient in one or another respect. The suspicion that pellagra emerged because maize was nutritionally inadequate was first cast into a modern, scientific framework by Frua and Lussana in the 1850s.

They argued that maize-based diets were inadequate because the ratio of proteins to respiratory parts in maize was severely unbalanced towards the latter group, an unbalance rendered worst if maize did not reach maturity for whatever reason.[20] Their theory was formulated, therefore, within the boundaries of the emerging consensus with the overemphasis on proteins and the focus on the ratio of nutritive principles reflecting the 'physiological fundamentals of Human Nutrition' at that time.[21] In fact, the authors firmly believed that the new science of nutrition, together with biochemical analyses of maize performed within its conceptual framework, would finally reveal the specific fault in what was for them undoubtedly a disease of unbalanced nutrition. Nevertheless, just a few years later, Ismael Salas argued, based on the same biochemical analyses used by Frua and Lussana, that the proposed nutritional shortcomings cannot be responsible for pellagra as maize contained as much albuminous substances as the other major cereals and a ratio of albuminous materials to other organic compounds that was not (significantly) worse off.[22] Besides this well-grounded refutation, however, the idea was starting to take shape that the nutritional value of maize was, theoretically, as good as that of any other cereal. Variants of this claim, including that maize is a 'perfect' food or one of the most nutritious articles of diet, would became a mantra[23] for opponents of the dietary deficiency theory from Lombroso[24] to Babeş[25] and Lavinder[26] who were always keen to reference one or another set of biochemical data to argue that maize was no less adequate than other grains. Thus, the availability of biochemical data, together with the closed perspective on nutritional knowledge, has pushed the deficiency theory of pellagra to the margins of what was deemed scientific by some and to a secondary position in relation to the intoxication and infection theories.

The remaining followers of one or another variant of Frua and Lussana's theory were aware of this conundrum and some of the strategies adopted to overcome it had been to rework the hypothesis within the confines of the established consensus or even to question its validity, although most often just half-heartedly. For instance, Ioan Neagoe, a Romanian doctor commissioned by the Romanian government to undertake two research trips in the countries most affected by pellagra (the Balkans, Italy, France and Spain) to identify the best measures for tackling the disease at home, had remained throughout his career a firm believer that regular, unspoiled maize was nutritionally inadequate. Neagoe explained this nutritional deficiency as either due to a lack of potash salts (following Urbeanu)[27] or to the low biological value of albumins in maize (a recasting of the Frua-Lussana theory in light of the biochemical data). From this latter perspective, Neagoe argued that the nutritional inadequacy of maize might be due to the fact that it lacks gluten, 'the plastic nitrogen, the tissue-building nitrogen',[28] a missing ingredient shown by the inability to make leavened bread out of maize flour.[29] However, Neagoe seems to have gone even further by arguing that, because the 'theory of life processes [. . .] is still incomplete, as also is the issue of the chemical and physiological features of the various nitrogenous substances, animal and vegetal',[30] the often referenced sets of biochemical data cannot conclusively settle the question of whether maize was as nutritionally adequate as other cereals. Even more explicitly, when discussing the question of whether maize has all the nutrients found in wheat or rye, which were known not to cause diseases if unspoiled, Neagoe answered, 'It has more of some, less of others while some are completely missing, for instance gluten.'[31] Yet, despite his unorthodox outlook on nutrition, Neagoe stopped short of conceptualizing pellagra outside the framework of the established consensus but instead cautiously concluded that sound maize, as opposed to 'wheat, rye or even millet', was causing pellagra because 'it lacked nitrogenous substances of the quality and, relatively, of the quantity as well needed by the human organism'.[32]

Responses to Neagoe's ideas came swiftly from Victor Babeş, a renowned Romanian bacteriologist, and from Adolf Urbeanu, a Romanian chemist and military pharmacist. Babeş brushed off Neagoe's claims by arguing that they were no longer tenable when detailed analyses 'showed that maize was a complete food, much more nutritious than rice, on which subsists the greater part of humanity'.[33] The reference to rice was significant since this grain lacked gluten as well and, moreover, delivered lower quantities of protein per weight but nevertheless did not cause pellagra, contrary to what would be expected if Neagoe's specific claims were true.[34] Urbeanu, however, took a more nuanced stance by arguing that although the available data recommended the idea that maize was as nutritionally adequate as the other cereals,[35] the question of the relative quality of the proteins in maize remained open and was scientifically justified.[36] He considered necessary for addressing this question to determine the relative biological value of zein, in which form were found the greater part of maize proteins, which was specific to maize and displayed distinct chemical and physical properties. Accordingly, Urbeanu conducted several experiments in which six dogs were successively fed maize flour, zein, wheat flour (one dog) and gelatin (one dog) and four men maize flour for various number of days up to a maximum of 10 days. The chosen outcome was whether maize or zein could keep the organism in nitrogenous equilibrium and the positive finding convinced Urbeanu that 'the nitrogenous substances in maize, especially zein, had absolutely analogous physiological properties to those of wheat' and that, therefore, 'physiologically speaking, maize cannot be inferior to wheat'.[37] With this debate, the question of the nutritional value of maize seems to have been settled in the Romanian context, although Neagoe kept further to his version of the disease.

In the Italian medical community, Professors Albertoni and Tullio were themselves exploring the possibility that the poor quality of proteins in maize caused pellagra and their research received a powerful boost from the finding that the biological value of proteins was determined by their amino-acid composition. In 1906, Willcock and Hopkins published their research findings showing that when tryptophan is added to a zein-based diet the lifespan of rats is increased from 16 to 30 days.[38] This finding conclusively showed that the biological value of proteins varied depending on their amino-acid composition and, in the particular case of maize, that zein was an incomplete protein because it lacked tryptophan. Subsequent and previous experiments showed that the remaining proteins in maize complemented well the amino-acid composition of zein (in the short term)[39] but the supporters of the older deficiency theory appropriated the initial research findings and used them to breathe new life into it. Informed by this early research on zein, Albertoni and Tullio recast pellagra as a protein deficiency due to the inadequate amino-acid composition of maize and set to design experiments to evaluate this claim, including keeping three pellagrins on a strictly maize-based diet and monitoring their nitrogenous balance compared to a meat-based diet – that is, compared to a diet long known to prevent and cure pellagra.[40] Nevertheless, despite the availability of a new conceptual framework, most researchers in Europe remained overall unconvinced by a deficiency model of pellagra which seemed to them unable to explain why a protein deficiency disease would show such a definite relation to maize while being absent in reputedly well-known cases of low protein intake or even during famines. Indicative in this respect, the US researchers who took upon themselves to inform their medical community about the disease which was rapidly advancing in their home country mentioned only in passing the deficiency theory and only to point out that it had been thoroughly discredited while reproducing verbatim the claim that maize was a 'perfect', 'most nutritious' food.[41]

Besides these researchers, who most often discussed the hypothetical deficiency in maize within the conceptual framework of the established consensus, there is some evidence that at least one researcher had been compelled to actively question it in view of the pellagra puzzle. Professor Aristide Stefani, Lussana's successor in the Physiology Department at the University of Padua, presented in 1911 a report on the work of the local Pellagra Commission, extensively excerpted in an issue of *Rivista Pellagrologica Italiana* from 1916,[42] which deserves special consideration because of its disruptive ideas. Stefani admitted that Lussana's original theory that maize did not contain sufficient quantities of proteins could no longer be defended but he went on to argue that this 'in no way proved that maize is a complete foodstuff that contains all the required nutritive principles or in the required quantity'.[43] This was so because while 'chemical analysis could prove that a food contains nutritive principles, it cannot say which are the required nutritive principles that are missing and that is because it is not yet known which are the nutritive principles that are required by an individual'.[44] According to Stefani, therefore, empirical observations and experiments, rather than chemical analyses, were relevant in establishing the nutritional value of a food and the empirical data available on pellagra, from its epidemiological features to the curative effects of a 'good' diet, suggested that maize was nutritionally less than adequate. It is not possible from the available information to retrieve further how Stefani came to question the established nutritional knowledge but what is more important for my argument is that his ideas have not been picked up in any comprehensive survey of pellagra produced by Italian, Romanian or US medical researchers. Rather, they seem to have been recuperated by the authors of the review to argue, retrospectively, that the by then established vitamin theory of pellagra had originated, in spirit if not in details as well, from within the Italian medical community.

The focus on the supporters of the dietary deficiency model is only intended to illustrate the difficulties of conceptualizing pellagra as a deficiency disease within the theoretical confines of the established consensus and should not obscure the fact that this model remained marginal in terms of number of supporters. A further demonstration of the importance of the theoretical framework in conceptualizing pellagra comes from the change in the medical researchers' outlook after the 'discovery' of vitamins but in the absence of any new epidemiological findings.

Towards pellagra as an avitaminosis

The application of the new findings concerning beriberi to the study of pellagra followed almost naturally given that the two diseases had been frequently grouped together either as an intoxication or as an infection based on analogies between their clinical manifestations and epidemiological features. Accordingly, it is perhaps not surprising that beginning with 1911, Durk, Lavinder,[45] Funk,[46] Rupert Blue (surgeon general of the United States),[47] Sandwith,[48] Wilson,[49] Saunders,[50] Voegtlin and Vedder,[51] among others, have explored the possibility of pellagra being a deficiency disease on the model of beriberi with more or less conviction. Funk's ideas on this matter require further presentation not just because they have been the most elaborate among those of the early proponents of the 'deficiency' model but also because they have influenced greatly the US and especially the Italian and Romanian researchers. In a seminal publication from 1912, Funk provisionally included pellagra in the category of deficiency diseases alongside beriberi, scurvy and infantile scurvy, although he admitted that the evidence supporting a dietary deficiency in pellagra rested mainly on 'its similarity in some respects' with other deficiency diseases and on sparse information about the dietary habits of the pellagrins.[52] In subsequent articles, Funk put forward several claims including that pellagra was due to an 'unvarying', 'one-sided', 'monotonous' diet since these diets were more likely, although not necessarily, to be missing vitamins,[53] to an insufficient intake of vitamin C[54] or of an unknown nutrient that was originally present in maize but was lost through excessive milling.[55] All these arguments have been put together in a rather disjointed manner in the book *Die Vitamine*[56] which added only one other argument in support of the deficiency theory: a reference to a possible pellagra outbreak in Rhodesia that was cured through the administration of undermilled maize.[57] Thus, *Die Vitamine* presented readers, mostly from the Romanian and Italian medical communities, with two versions of pellagra as an avitaminosis: a narrow version in which pellagra was caused by the consumption of overmilled maize and a general version in which it was due to an unspecified fault in a 'one-sided' diet that could be corrected through a more varied diet.

1914 is a landmark year in this progression as, on the one hand, Joseph Goldberger published his first of an impressive series of studies which ultimately provided fundamental insights into the etiology of pellagra and, on the other hand, the Romanian and Italian medical communities produced their first systematic assessments of the avitaminosis model of the disease. Their different responses to the avitaminosis model warrant a separate presentation and discussion of the factors which might account for this difference. Joseph Goldberger, under the conceptual influence of the 'comparative recent studies that have definitely established beriberi as a "deficiency" disease [. . .] in a sense hardly dreamed of before',[58] considered pellagra to be due to a 'one-sided', 'unvaried', 'restricted' diet and that, accordingly, a 'mixed', 'well-balanced', 'varied' diet was capable to prevent and cure it.[59] Goldberger submitted, therefore, to Funk's general understanding of pellagra as a deficiency disease and his initial studies had all been designed to prove that pellagra was due to a 'fault' in diet by demonstrating the preventive and therapeutic value of a 'proper' diet,[60] the pellagra-producing property of an 'unvaried, one-sided diet'[61] and the relationship between such diets and pellagra in naturalistic settings.[62] In terms of the specific dietary fault that was responsible for pellagra, Goldberger considered that it might be due to a deficient intake of either proteins (amino acids), inorganic substances, the anti-beriberi vitamin, a yet unknown dietary factor or to a combination of all of them, although at this initial stage he was less concerned with isolating the specific dietary fault than with identifying the most suitable foods to correct it. By contrast, the majority of the Romanian and Italian medical researchers have appropriated and reacted to Funk's narrow understanding that pellagra was caused by the consumption of overmilled maize. Babeş,[63] Rossi,[64] Bravetta,[65] Ramoino,[66] Clementi[67] and Rondoni[68] have all focused on the claim that maize lost part of its vitamin content through fine milling and, because of this, became pellagrogenic and all of them have been swift in dismissing this explanation. Exceptionally among these researchers, Rondoni went beyond Funk's narrow claim that overmilled maize flour was the cause of pellagra and studied the effects of supplementing the guinea pig's rations of finely milled maize flour with either purified protein, cabbage, carbohydrates, alcoholic extracts of liver and cabbage or adrenaline.[69] By 1916 then, Funk's narrow version of pellagra as a deficiency disease and, to a significantly lesser extent, his more general version had been thoroughly debated in the Italian and Romanian medical communities and although the former version failed to gain support, the majority of researchers were in agreement that the discovery of vitamins made imperative the need for a new approach in the study of pellagra.[70]

A question emerging from this overview is why the Romanian and Italian medical communities focused preferentially on Funk's narrow hypothesis at the same time that the US researchers were working with Funk's general hypothesis, especially since these former communities had ready access to relevant information on the 'one-sided' character of the pellagrins diets and on the curative effects of a diet consisting of milk, meat or dairy products. In this sense, Funk himself provided in *Die vitamine* examples of dietary tests such as feeding small quantities of meat, milk or, crucially, yeast that were specific in showing that pellagra was an avitaminosis even within a fragmented theoretical landscape in which several conceptualizations incorporated diets as an important predisposing factor and which were relatively easy to implement. A plausible explanation has to do with the fact that the Romanian and Italian medical researchers had been foremost interested in identifying practical, feasible solutions to pellagra as a public health problem. In this respect, it has to be considered that solutions to pellagra as a public health problem already existed: for instance, replacing maize with wheat was considered capable of preventing pellagra under most understandings of the disease, from the deficiency to the intoxication to the autointoxication theories. Yet, the implementation of this solution, as of others like increasing the consumption of dairy products and meat, was deemed to exceed the limited possibilities of their home states. In switching from maize to wheat for instance, the Romanian authorities had to reckon with the challenges that wheat fetched, on average, 44 per cent more than the equivalent quantity of maize, a significant price difference for a dietary item eaten at every meal and in considerable quantities, that its preparation into bread required more complex assets than the preparation of mămăligă (boiled, cornmeal mush) and that two-thirds of the gross wheat harvest was needed to leave the countryside to feed the urban population and to balance commercial transactions.[71] By comparison, Funk's narrow hypothesis promised a quick fix to pellagra as a public health problem as it required simple recommendations, or at worst administrative regulations, for maize not to be milled too finely in order to effectively manage the disease. It is true, in this regard, that theoretically, any conceptualization of pellagra as an avitaminosis carried with it the prospect of an economical solution to pellagra through the isolation of the missing chemical compound followed by the identification of the cheapest food/ method that would furnish it to pellagrins. This promise would be eventually realized through the production and administration of yeast in the 1920s and of PP vitamin pills in the 1950s Romania. However, as Rondoni admitted in 1915, the prospect of administering the pellagra-preventive vitamin other than through the consumption of foods already known to contain it seemed too distant to have any practical relevance – that is, wheat, meat and dairy products were still the remedies that had to be provided under Funk's general understanding of pellagra.[72] Such considerations of the economic viability of the practical measures inspired by any theory of pellagra appear to have had a strong influence on researchers either by facilitating the reception of theories that offered the most convenient practical solutions or by requiring a relentless search for the most cost-effective variant within the framework of any theory.

Conclusions

In nutritional science during the past 20 years at least, a change in methodological paradigm from observational research designs using complex regression analysis to randomized controlled trials using comparatively simpler methods of analysis has been in progress. This change impacted the standards of evidence with which researchers operate with randomized controlled trials being considered to provide the best-quality evidence followed, at a significant distance, by cohort, case-control and ecological research designs.[73] Theoretically, therefore, knowledge produced under these different methodologies is considered to differ in terms of the degree of confidence they command but, in practice, a process of sedimentation can occur in which they coexist in training manuals, compendiums/encyclopaedias and formal training courses. Not only that, but they may even be assigned equal standing since they are usually presented separated from the relevant methodological context in which they were produced.

The case study discussed in this article illustrates such a process of sedimentation – a working hypothesis concerning the nutritive elements required for maintaining well-being had solidified into an unquestioned dogma which outlived the development of methodological and technological means capable of disproving it. The methodological sophistication evident in Stanton and Fraser's experiments on beriberi and in Goldberger's on pellagra, the elaborate techniques for isolating nutrients that facilitated the early research on vitamin types and the critical appraisal of scientific output displayed by scholarly debates among researchers, together with the findings produced through them, coexisted with a corpus of knowledge which had been produced under a different methodological and technological paradigm and which had not been revisited in light of subsequent relevant developments.

This failure to revisit basic tenets is striking given that epidemiological observations for several diseases, pellagra included, and occasional experiments which returned unexpected results should have additionally prompted researchers to do so. The main problem, in my opinion, is that no efficient mechanism was, or is, in place to efficiently reassess knowledge from the scientific corpus in light of subsequent changes in methodological paradigms in particular. To be sure, randomized controlled trials, when coupled with multifactor analysis of variance (ANOVA), are particularly adept at identifying and shedding erroneous information from the corpus of knowledge because of their experimental and iterative nature. However, powerful use of multifactor analysis of variance requires the implementation of a second intervention which might not seem appealing from a theoretical perspective compared to other alternatives and which carries with it considerable costs. A possible solution to this problem might, then, come from historians who can take on the role of mediators between two different knowledge traditions and thus trace the genealogy of various scientific information back to a context of knowledge which may no longer be compatible with the currently dominant one and, through this, refer it for re-examination.

6

Food and Diet as Risk: The Role of the Framingham Heart Study

Maiko Rafael Spiess

From the 1950s to the 1970s, fat consumption and cholesterol were extensively studied as risk factors for cardiovascular disease. The evidence collected by the Framingham Heart Study (FHS) and similar research became widely known and accepted, and helped to shape official dietary recommendations and guidelines (such as the famous Food Guide Pyramid) giving them a scientific background and credibility. Therefore, our current dietary habits and perception of food as potential health risks are frequently considered to be scientific and based on hard evidence. However, the science of official dietary guidelines is often questioned. The frequent controversies regarding food and diet show that there is more to official dietary guidelines than science – economic interests and lobbies, scientists' reputations and politics are frequently as important as the scientific method and evidence.

This chapter addresses the relation between science, politics and economics for the emergence, evolution, dissemination and public debate on dietary recommendations. It focuses on the case of the FHS – an ongoing cardiovascular epidemiological study started in 1948 – and its role for the risk factor approach of diet on official guidelines. More precisely, it describes how the Framingham scientists built and presented their evidence and conclusions, and how risk factor statements produced in this specific environment came to be widely accepted by the public through official dietary guidelines, at first in the United States and then worldwide.

It describes not only the mundane aspects of daily scientific activity but also the political negotiations for funding the research, building its credibility and making the risk factor approach a substantial part of our current understanding of diet. It suggests that dietary practices and innovations during the last century are deeply influenced and constrained by several cultural, economic, political and technical factors. However, scientific methods, large-scale studies and new conceptual frameworks helped to blur these influences and, at the same time, to foster the ideal of neutrality and rationality of dietary recommendations. The history of the FHS and its importance for twentieth-century dietary guidelines are presented here as a way to deepen the understanding of our current foodways.

Food and diet as risk

Risk factors are a relatively new idea. In fact, there was a time when the knowledge and concepts about coronary heart diseases were radically different. For a good part of the history of medical sciences and health practices, constitutional hypotheses prevailed. In other words, heart diseases used to be attributed to individual, personal traits. Conditions like *angina pectoris* – an acute pain in the chest now understood to be caused by heart muscle ischemia related to atherosclerosis – were rarely linked to heart problems but frequently associated with the personality and mental state of the patient.[1] During the Victorian era, heart disease was often attributed to the passions, disillusions, mental stress and excitement of poets' and intellectuals' minds afflicting their hearts.[2] For most of the experts in the first half of the twentieth century, cardiovascular diseases were seen as a result of ageing and, therefore, a natural phenomenon.[3]

After the Second World War, advancements in epidemiology and statistical techniques helped to change these notions.[4] Between the 1940s and 1950s, several different population-based studies were designed and conducted in order to understand chronic diseases and their causes. Large-scale studies like the Minnesota Business and Professional Men Study (1947), the FHS (1948), the Los Angeles Civil Servants Study (1949), the Albany Civil Servants Study (1953), the DuPont Company Study (1956), the Chicago Western Electric Study (1957), the Chicago People's Gas Study (1958) and the famous Seven Countries Study (1958) proposed new hypothesis and methods for studying chronic diseases. Clinical case studies started to give way to a more collective, quantitative approach in medical science and epidemiology. Accordingly, lay, professional and institutional views started to change and adapt to these new discoveries. Disease, in general, and particularly the cardiovascular diseases, became a matter of personal habits and exposure to risk.

Cardiovascular disease risk factors are now widely known. Some of them are inherent, 'non-modifiable', such as gender, age or family disease history. Others can be changed by individual action. This is the case for raised or altered blood cholesterol and triglycerides levels, high blood pressure, diabetes, overweight or obesity. The more risk factors an individual presents, the greater the chance of developing cardiovascular diseases. These relations are largely based on statistical evidence and, therefore, introduce a rational, mathematical approach to diseases: if risk can be assessed and predicted, then individuals can take steps to reduce their exposure. Cardiovascular diseases are no longer an inexorable, fatalistic condition. On the contrary, risk factors helped turn diseases into a matter of personal behaviour and attitude. This change introduced the current trend of 'secular morality'[5,6] and 'technologies of the self'.[7]

Some risk factors for cardiovascular disease came to be directly related to dietary habits. For example, atherosclerosis is related in a physiological level to low-density lipoproteins. Some of these proteins, like cholesterol and triglycerides, can build up within the arteries forming atheromatous plaques. Cholesterol is naturally produced by the human body but it can also be ingested through habitual nourishment. High cholesterol levels can also be caused by a diet rich in saturated fats (usually found in animal products) and trans fats (mostly from products with high quantities of hydrogenated fats used in processed, industrialized food). Therefore, from a biochemical point of view, there is relation between a diet high in fats and cardiovascular disease (the diet-heart hypothesis). Yet, this causal link is not unequivocal: some people can spend most of their lives with 'risky' dietary practices and still never develop any heart condition. This uncertainty is exemplified by the French paradox, that is, the epidemiological observation that the French people have a relatively low incidence of coronary heart disease, despite having a diet rich in saturated fats.

The risk factor approach bypasses these uncertainties by the use of 'large numbers'[8] and the 'domestication of chance'.[9] That is to say, risk is not determined individually. Instead, risk statements are built from population studies and statistical multivariate analysis. Consequently, they describe correlations between observed variables at a collective level but cannot ascertain causal relationships at the individual level. Nevertheless, risk scores and risk assessment have been providing estimates that are presented and perceived as facts. For individuals, they give a scientifically based guideline for health promotion; for practitioners, risk statements are technical resources for rationalization and standardization of medical advice; and for governments and private organizations, they provide easily identifiable objects for policies and practical actions. Thus, the supposed neutrality of numbers and statistical estimates make risk factor 'black boxes' that can be easily adopted in different social contexts and for different individuals.

Coupled with a nutritional reductionism or 'nutritionism', that is, the 'decontextualization, simplification, and exaggeration of nutrients' role in determining bodily health',[10] risk has changed food and diet significantly. Nowadays, food engineering, regulation, marketing and consumption are rarely approached without considering ingredients or nutrients according to a risk rationale. While, on the one hand, it may promote healthy practices and overall risk reduction, on the other, it mostly ignores the complexities of food processing techniques and food–body interactions. In particular, the focus on risk oversimplifies food and diet, and downplays the broader importance of social contexts and dietary patterns. Yet, throughout the twentieth century, public health experts and policymakers focused mostly on this reductive approach to fight chronic disease, obesity and other related conditions.

Official dietary guidelines are a good example of this tendency. These recommendations have been issued by national governments since the late nineteenth century. At first, they focused on the issues of food scarcity and health conditions related to nutrient deficiencies. The famous *Food for Fitness: A Daily Food Guide* or simply 'Basic Four'[11] is one example of this approach. It recommended a minimum number of daily servings, divided in four food groups: (1) two servings of milk or milk products; (2) two portions of meat, poultry, eggs, legumes and nuts; (3) four servings of fruits and vegetables; and (4) four servings of grains. Little or no recommendation was given at this point regarding fat and sugars, or in relation to caloric intake. At this stage, food had a positive function and was presented as a way to achieve and maintain a healthy state. That is, recommendations were focused on what should be consumed.

During the 1970s and 1980s, this view changed radically. Official dietary guidelines started to adopt a language of food restrictions: certain food groups or nutrients were described as potential risks, and the guidelines began to present negative orientations, that is, indications of food to be actively avoided. The first *Dietary Guidelines for Americans* (1980) and the famous *Food Guide Pyramid* (1992) are examples of this shift to a risk-based approach. Fat-rich foods, and particularly the ones containing saturated fats, were to be avoided or consumed sparingly. Thus, milk, meat and eggs came to be associated with cholesterol and heart disease.[12] At the same time, carbohydrates were considered by medical researchers as the base for a healthy diet. These notions are now largely questioned but for some time they were the basis for a series of important changes in Western foodways. For example, the adoption of hydrogenated vegetal oils as a substitutive for saturated fats (e.g. using margarine instead of butter), despite the available evidence that trans fats actually raise cholesterol,[13] was directly influenced by these risk statements regarding saturated fats as they were then presented by governments and public health experts.[14]

Risk factor approach profoundly changed food and dietary practices. The kind of simplification it provides for the public, experts and policymakers turned risk factors into a central part of our current understanding of food, diet, health and disease. The creation and success of this relatively new way of understanding disease is the result of two simultaneous processes: first, the advancement of nutritional and medical sciences, the development of population epidemiological studies and the emergence of the technical infrastructure needed to process large amounts of statistical data; and second, the growing public and governmental concern with chronic, non-transmittable diseases after the Second World War, particularly regarding heart diseases and obesity.[15] At the centre of this change are several scientific studies designed to further understand disease causality, prevalence and distribution. Therefore, in order to fully grasp the meaning of these recent changes in food and dietary practices, we need to look at the history of the risk factor approach.

The Framingham Heart Study

The FHS, started in 1948, is a central part of our current understanding of risk. For more than seven decades, scientists have been studying the inhabitants of Framingham, Massachusetts, in order to unveil the causes of coronary heart disease.[16] Originally, 5,209 men and women between the ages of 30 and 62 were accompanied for an initial period of 20 years, regularly reporting for medical examinations and interviews. The data from these participants (such as their weight, blood pressure, cholesterol levels, personal habits, etc.) were carefully registered and then analysed by powerful yet primitive computers at the National Institutes of Health in Bethesda, Maryland.[17] Additional cohorts of local residents joined the study in 1971 (5,124 of the original participants' children and spouses), 1994 and 2002. From the observation of this large number of volunteers and thanks to the powerful tools of statistics and computing, the researchers from the Framingham Study were able to propose the probabilistic notion of risk factors as a way to understand and predict coronary heart disease. Up to this day, more than 2,500 scientific papers were published based on the data from the FHS.

The history of the Framingham Study has been told before. In this sense, there are mainly three types of work. First, the accounts produced by the researchers from the study themselves. Understandably, in these cases, the historical narrative is not only rich and detailed but also uncritical, triumphalist or even 'whiggish'. Second, there are studies that describe the evolution of the FHS from a history of science point of view[18] or to highlight its importance for medical sciences and cardiovascular disease.[19] Third, historical accounts produced by historians or sociologists of science and medicine in which the history of the Framingham Study is discussed as a way to understand and explain the emergence of the risk factor approach[20] or the history of specific risk factor, such as cholesterol.[21]

These studies usually present the FHS as the result of the scientific progress and as an important touchstone for medical science in particular. However, they often ignore the social conditions for the existence of the study. In reality, the FHS and the emergence of risk factors or, as it was referred to in a seminal paper, 'factors of risk',[22] were only possible in a particular social and technical background. So, in order to understand the success of the Framingham Study and the current pervasiveness of risk factors, we need to look at the design and early stages of this scientific experiment. In other words, what were the conditions for the FHS to happen? What made the FHS such a successful experiment? We argue here that the FHS was made possible by the progressive overlapping and mutual influence of the political awareness about chronic diseases, and scientific and technical advances in the fields of epidemiology, statistics, computing and diagnostics.

The beginning of the FHS is frequently related to a growing interest on the issue of chronic diseases by the Public Health System (PHS) in the late 1940s. Although infectious diseases were still the highest priority, after the Second World War, the epidemiological transition and the emergence of chronic diseases began to receive some attention from the US government. One of the main concerns was assessing the distribution of these diseases and identifying better diagnosis and prevention techniques.[23] The idea of some sort of population-based study for understanding heart disease is usually attributed to Joseph Mountin, a public health policymaker assigned to the Bureau of States Services.[24] To a large extent, he was able to elaborate some of the guiding principles of this type of research, such as the need for screening and intervention at a local, community level.[25]

However, the main people responsible for what would become the FHS was a mid-level PHS employee called Gilcin Meadors and a small team that accompanied him. The team's first activity was to determine a site for conducting the epidemiological study envisioned by Mountin and commissioned by PHS. Among the possible locations for the study were several small communities that met the desired demographic and epidemiological criteria. Thus, the choice of the town of Framingham as the location for a large-scale study of heart disease did not occur by chance. Among the determining factors for the choice were the town's markedly industrial economy and its proximity to important universities and research centres (approximately 35 kilometres of distance from Boston), providing the skilled labour needed for a large-scale epidemiological study.

There was also the pivotal influence of David Rutstein from the Preventive Medicine Department at Harvard University and former medical director of the American Heart Association. Dr Rutstein was fundamental for convincing the local population and government officials about the importance and benefits of bringing the proposed research study to Framingham.[26] In 1947, Meadors and his team, with the support from Rutstein and a board of cardiologists from the New England Heart Association, started to devise the study's objectives and methods (Figure 6.1). At this point, an internal struggle emerged: Meadors and his team preferred a public health approach, seeking to understand the distribution of cardiovascular disease in a normal population of self-selected volunteers; Rutstein wanted to use the Framingham Study as a way to evaluate the efficacy of several diagnostic technologies such as X-ray, electrocardiogram and electrochemography – a fluoroscopy technique later abandoned by cardiologists.

Back then, a dieting ideology had already established itself in the American culture, but it wasn't directly motivated by the problem of chronic diseases. Low-fat approaches to diet were mostly focused on weight reduction and body mass instead of serum cholesterol levels and heart diseases.[27] In fact, Americans were traditionally a "meat-eater"[28] culture, and the post-war prosperity made the average American eat more fat than ever before. However, the relation between heart diseases and diet was mostly a scientific hypothesis restricted to some researchers and doctors. The passing of the National Heart Act by the US Congress in 1948 started to change this view and gave the study the official support and clear direction it needed. The act created the National Heart Institute (NHI) and granted a total sum of $500,000 for heart disease research all over the country. Also, the Framingham Study direction shifted from the PHS to the newly created NHI. With this change, the approach favoured by Meadors was reinforced by the concern with cardiovascular disease prevention sponsored by the federal government.[29]

Felix Moore, a sociologist and first NHI director, then helped Meadors to finally define the study's objectives and design. Under the influence of Moore, the proposed follow-up time was extended from 10 to 20 years. The selection of subjects was improved by the introduction of better sampling and randomization techniques. The variables of interest were also correctly defined. Nevertheless, this choice was not only conceptual but also practical – considering the ease of collection and reliability of the measurements, biomedical variables (like blood pressure and cholesterol levels) were favoured over behavioural ones (e.g. dietary habits). Delicate questions about income, class and even intimate topics such as the occurrence of sexual dysfunctions were excluded from the study design in order to ensure the participation of local volunteers. The standard procedures for the interviews and physical exams were consolidated in an operational manual to be strictly followed by the researchers.[30]

In 1950, physician Thomas Royle Dawber was appointed as director of the Framingham Study by Moore. A former PHS employee, Dawber had no previous experience in epidemiology. For him, epidemiology was 'clinical study at a community level'[31] and therefore should be of practical use to the medical community (what would explain the lack of interest in social variables throughout the study's early stages). Under Dawber, the objective of the FHS would be to correlate clinical and laboratory data with the individuals' medical histories, prior to the onset of the disease, in order to establish generalizations about predisposition or risk factors. Accordingly, the NHI proposed twenty-eight hypotheses relating environmental exposure or individual behaviour to cardiovascular diseases. These hypotheses served as guidelines for the initial exams with disease-free participants, conducted between 1949 and 1950, and the processes of data collection, tabulation and analysis.

After the initial round of examinations, participants were required to show up for a follow-up every 2 years. For each visit to the study, a medical history, physical exams, blood samples and other laboratory procedures were conducted and carefully recorded on paper files. All information was then reviewed by a panel of three medical doctors under the supervision of a statistician. Finally, the collected data were then codified and transferred to punched cards and, later, to magnetic tapes for the computational analysis. If a participant showed any signs of disease, he or she would be excluded from the disease-free group and accompanied with a different methodology. Hospital admissions were also recorded and deaths were reported from newspaper obituaries, personal physician communications or coroner reports.

This initial stage of the FHS was fraught with uncertainties, setbacks and technical difficulties often caused by the novelty of the research. On the one hand, because of the nature of the study, it took the researchers a long time before they were able to present solid results. Until the first half of the 1950s, only four papers were published by the FHS researchers and only 7 years after the study began, the researchers had accumulated sufficient data to prepare a preliminary report.[32] On the other hand, each new round of examinations introduced small methodological adjustments, either to accommodate the inclusion of new diagnostic tools or to test new hypotheses. Despite these setbacks, the study continued to produce important publications and results. In fact, it was during this period that the first papers and results focusing on risk factors were published.

The first results from the Framingham experiment were fundamental for a new understanding of heart disease (Figure 6.2). Nonetheless, the researchers could not find a unique causal relation between a marker or personal habit and disease, as in the case of smoking and cancer. Isolated, risk factors such as hypercholesterolemia, hypertension or smoking were not related to disease episodes in the Framingham cohort. Morbidity and mortality increases were observed only with individuals who presented these risk factors combined.

No evidence produced in Framingham at that time could directly relate diet and cardiovascular disease. In fact, questions about the participants' dietary habits have been included in the interviews sometime between the fifth and sixth examination rounds (1957 and 1960), but dropped from the study's design a little later.[33] Dietary intake was then seen as particularly hard to measure correctly and no promising results came from this research hypothesis.[34] Thus, only a few papers on diet and cardiovascular disease were published by the FHS team at that point.

A 1962 paper[35] summed up the approach Framingham's researchers had on diet. At that point, the regulation of the level of serum cholesterol and the development of coronary heart disease were statistically associated to the following risk factors: overall calorie balance, level of animal fat intake, level of vegetal fat intake, level of protein intake, level of cholesterol intake and iron intake and its relation to haematologic values.

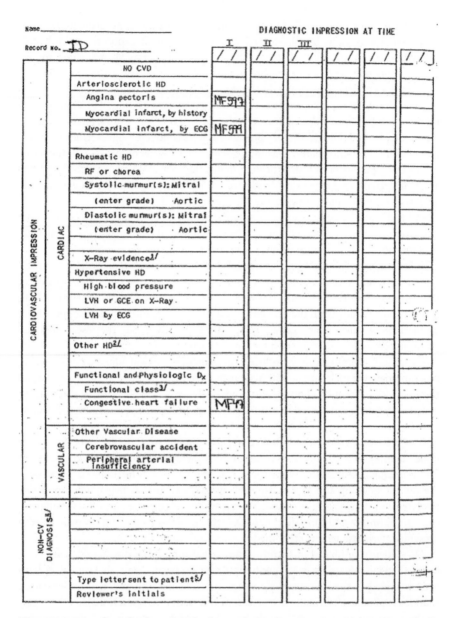

Figure 6.1 Exam form for the original cohort, *c.*1947. Courtesy: Framingham Heart Study Archives.

These 'dietary hypotheses' from Framingham were similar to Ancel Keys's premises from the Seven Countries Study[36] and previously published recommendations by the American Heart Association, suggesting that high-fat diets could be linked to heart diseases. Thus, it is possible to see how the diet-heart hypothesis and the risk factor

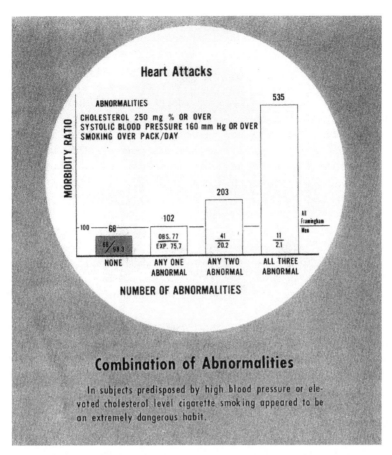

Figure 6.2 FHS results from a NHI report, 1961. Courtesy: Framingham Heart Study Archives.

approach did benefit each other: on the one hand, the Framingham researchers drawn from other studies in order to build their own research hypothesis; on the other hand, the supposed mathematical certainty of the risk factor approach helped to establish the overall credibility of dietary recommendations.

Trouble at Framingham and new beginnings

The second half of the 1960s represented a troubled time for the Framingham Study, initially because of a veiled conflict between the study's local researchers and NIH employees located in Bethesda, Maryland. Gradually the researchers at Framingham felt that decisions about the research and data analysis were being imposed by professionals far removed from the everyday reality of the study. In reality, a number of factors could be implicated in this controversy: first, the study was approaching the 20th-year mark – that is, the originally proposed deadline – and an NIH internal committee assessed that it had reached its objectives and therefore could be finished.[37,38] Second, at that time governmental research funding policy had shifted to developing laboratory and clinical tests, and particularly for researching diseases such as cancer, thus considerably reducing the political influence of FHS researchers.[39]

The uncertainty regarding the continuity of the Framingham Study can be explained by changes in the administration and research policies that took place at the NIH in 1965, which demanded a more bureaucratic and result-oriented administration. This could be related, on the one hand, to pressure from Congress (especially on the figure of Democratic congressman Lawrence H. Fountain) for greater transparency in relation to the funds allocated to the NIH. On the other hand, they are associated with an internal review process known as the Wooldridge Report. The report suggested a policy of constant revisions of NIH projects, especially in relation to its possible payoffs and possibilities of technical and scientific advancement.[40] The impossibility of establishing quantifiable goals and objectives for the FHS and the need for long-term follow-ups to produce results were the exact opposite of what was expected by policymakers and taxpayers, which could explain the recommendations for the closure of the study.

In any case, the direction of the study acted quickly. In 1966, realizing that support for the study was at stake, Dawber resigned from the Framingham Study and took a position in the Department of Preventive Medicine at Boston University. One of his pupils, William Kannel, was appointed as the new director. Dawber began a massive campaign to raise money to ensure continuity of the study in the case of effective cuts in government funding. In October 1969, after several internal disputes, the NIH ordered the discontinuation of the Framingham Study, effective in July 1970; after this date, the study would be reduced to a minimum staff of five (including another future director, William Castelli), who would be responsible for completing the examinations and for the final analysis of the data. Secretly, Dawber and a long-time FHS employee named Patricia McNamara began making copies of all the data stored since the beginning of the study – supposedly at a personal cost of $10,000 to Dawber himself.[41]

Since his departure, and with the help of Boston University, Dawber raised approximately $500,000 from private sources. From this total, approximately $40,000 were donations from more than a thousand Framingham residents who sent checks of up to $100, in a clear demonstration of the good relationship between the study and the community. The main donors, however, were insurance companies for which risk calculation methodologies were particularly useful. Thus, the continuity of the study was guaranteed, at least in the short term: the researchers would continue to be paid by the government, while the examinations and analysis of data would be maintained by the funds raised by Dawber. The public funding cut, however, did not go unnoticed – it was heavily criticized by the mainstream media and authorities, like Senator Ted Kennedy and the influential cardiologist Paul Dudley White.[42] Dawber had managed to mobilize important allies, which increased public pressure to continue the study.

To the pressure of public opinion and authorities was added an internal movement in the NHI, to direct funding for the FHS through research on the heredity of cardiovascular diseases (by then a blossoming area of knowledge). A research project was quickly designed and secured at the NHI. Once approved, this research was then managed by Boston University, under contract with the federal government for funding. In 1971, the Framingham Offspring Study was established, consisting of a second generation of participants. The second cohort involved the follow-up of 5,124 participants, mostly sons or daughters of the original participants who entered the study two decades earlier. Its main goal was establishing a genetics approach to the FHS. In addition, the exams and follow-ups of the previous cohort continued normally. In practical terms, federal funding for the study was only temporarily discontinued, to be reinstated under a new budget heading.

These innovations were a direct result of contextual and structural changes, which forced researchers to revise their practice and, in a certain way, to rebuild the study. In other words, the second phase of the Framingham Study was not a result of deliberate processes, or of previously elaborated strategies of its researchers, but much more of the adaptation of the study to the contingencies of the politics of research and the action of diverse social actors. Although the new arrangement initially represented less support from the federal government, it paved the way for expanding the scope and duration of the study and, consequently, for the continuity of its data production and visibility.[43] In particular, it meant the return of decision-making power to Dawber (then at Boston University), Kannel and his pupils (such as future director William Castelli).

In addition to this second-generation cohort, new groups of participants were included in the Framingham Study during the subsequent decades. In 1994, the Omni Cohort 1 project included minorities in order to face the country's demographic changes, to address the growing scientific interest on the issue of race and its relation with health and disease and particularly to correct a design flaw – for decades, the study focused mostly on risk factor for white Americans. Thus, 507 men and women – African Americans, Hispanics, Asians, Indians, Pacific Islanders and Native Americans – joined the study as regular participants. This cohort was expanded with the inclusion of new individuals considered as minorities between 2003 and 2005, totalling another 410 new participants.

More recently, the study has aligned itself to genomic research. Starting in 1991, participants in the Offspring cohort had their blood collected for the specific purpose of DNA mapping. In 2001, the selection for the third generation of participants (the Gen III cohort) started. These participants were submitted to both the original procedures and the sampling of genetic material. The original participants were not included in this stage because they represented a skewed sample – those with a higher propensity for cardiovascular disease had probably died and the survivors were largely healthy. To improve the statistical power of this genetic research, the New Offspring Spouse Cohort was also designed – if the spouse of an Offspring Study participant had never participated in the study and if at least two of their biological children were associated with Gen III, he or she would be invited to participate in the genetic screening, giving FHS researchers a more complete picture of hereditary elements related to cardiovascular disease risk factors.

From Framingham to the world

The influence of the FHS for our contemporary understanding of food, dietary habits and disease is often mentioned and celebrated, but not always substantiated or described. In order to elaborate a sociological description complementary to the historical narrative, we must emphasize the necessary conditions and the technical and political negotiations for the existence of the FHS. Based on the premise that the study is the result of a process of overlapping (and alignment) of a series of technical, scientific and political elements, it is possible to describe the conditions for the emergence and success of the FHS from a sociological point of view. Thus, we propose a sociotechnical model to describe and interpret the success of the FHS, based on four dimensions: epidemiological profile, institutions, science and technology and morality.[44]

The first condition for the emergence of the Framingham Study and other population-based epidemiological studies was the epidemiological transition, that is, the changes in distribution of diseases that affected populations during the twentieth century and, in particular, the emergence of new health problems. The comparison between the burden of diseases from the beginning of the last century and the 2010s shows it very clearly – instead of suffering from illnesses such as influenza, gastrointestinal infections, tuberculosis or malnutrition, contemporary Western societies have been mostly suffering from cardiovascular and cerebrovascular diseases, and different types of cancer.[45] The shift in epidemiological profile raised the public awareness and has put in motion actions like the National Heart Act, the creation of the NHI and, therefore, of the FHS. Thus, the problematization of the epidemiological transition was the first necessary condition for the existence of risk factors as a scientific problem.

The second condition was the intervention of institutions and government agencies. In modern Western societies and states, rationality and bureaucracy play a central role in managing diseases at a collective level. In particular, the FHS was directly subordinated to the governmental apparatus of the United States. Also, it was related (although indirectly) to professional organizations and universities. These institutions provided the study's researchers with financial resources and legitimacy, while at the same time directed the overall objectives and concepts of the study. Therefore, the relation between the study and institutions such as the National Institutes of Health and the American Heart Association ensured the legitimacy of the study's methods and goals; at the same time, it determined the roles of the different actors, limiting and conditioning the scope of the study according to their own interests.

In both cases, changes in dietary patterns were part of the expert's concerns and governmental responses. The rise in cardiovascular diseases was related, for example, to obesity; obesity, in its turn, was associated with post-war abundance, the availability of new food products and lifestyle changes. Dietary habits were perceived by experts to be at the problem's core and therefore became a central aspect of the governmental intervention through public health campaigns and official recommendations. Thus, risk factor statements served both scientists and policymakers concerned with heart disease.

The third condition is related to science and technology. If the study's institutional relations determined the problems to be addressed and the roles of those involved, science and technology provided the conceptual mechanisms and practical tools that made the study possible. A wide range of concepts, hypotheses, research methods and techniques for collecting and presenting scientific data previously created by other areas of knowledge were fundamental to the Framingham Study. Also, technologies such as the examination of serum cholesterol levels or the computational processing of the statistical data of the participants were fundamental to its success. By interconnecting these heterogeneous elements, the Framingham researchers created a functional, stabilized sociotechnical network that allowed the production of new scientific facts and then helped to shape risk factors statements that would become central for changes in individual and collective practices.

Finally, the Framingham Study was deeply influenced by a specific morality system. In this sense, the choice of certain hypotheses and the individualization of risk are directly influenced by the capitalist ethos and the socio-economic conditions of the American society of the time. Although never acknowledged directly by researchers and scientific articles produced by the FHS, the tension between individual responsibility (represented by an ideal of moderation as virtue) and abundant socio-economic conditions (economic prosperity, increased consumption, sedentary lifestyle, suburbanization) can be perceived in many of the study's premises, and particularly in the way risk statements are based on individual's habits and biomedical measurements (e.g. cholesterol levels and blood pressure). In other words, the FHS and the risk factor approach benefited from a favourable cultural environment for their acceptance.

The results from Framingham and the risk factor approach originate from the correct alignment by these different elements. In order to be recognized and accepted, the study researchers had to consider not only technical aspects but also social and institutional interests. The legitimacy and credibility of the study were the result of the persuasion of laymen and specialists, of institutions and individuals. That is, the FHS was designed and conducted to become a stable sociotechnical arrangement through the convergence of interests of different actors. The stability of the study helped the dissemination and adoption of its techniques and results in different social contexts. Throughout its history, the FHS was then able to establish itself as an 'obligatory passage point'[46] – a local network that allowed actors in the global network to accomplish their own objectives.

The inclusion of risk factors in official dietary guidelines is derived from this process. More precisely, the condemnation of saturated fats in official dietary recommendations coincides with the rise and widespread acceptance of the risk approach. This is because the methods and results from Framingham and other large-scale studies provided the policymakers the 'ready-made' statements needed to convince the public and to coordinate actions for public health. However, most of the criticisms directed at official dietary guidelines,[47,48] such as the Dietary Goals for the United States (issued by the US Senate Select Committee on Nutrition and Human Needs in 1977) or the Food Guide Pyramid (issued by the US Department of Agriculture in 1992), concern the misunderstanding or selective use of risk factors statements.

Dietary guidelines adopt a reductionist version of the idea of risk. They usually ignore or downplay the multivariate nature of risk statements, focusing mainly on a single causal relation, like the diet-heart hypothesis. Nevertheless, the proposed relation between high cholesterol levels and cardiovascular diseases, partially based on the data from Framingham, made its way into these official recommendations. Either by ignorance or political pressure, policymakers and experts came up with advices that had real consequences for dietary practices in the last century. This is especially significant for the case against saturated fats and the adoption of trans fat as a substitute, the so-called 'trans-fat fiasco' – sometime after the release of the first Dietary Guidelines and Food Pyramid in the United States, researchers found evidence that trans fat is actually bad for human health, because it increases LDL cholesterol and decreases HDL cholesterol. However, at that point, saturated fats were already vastly denounced in the United States and other countries. Risk factors became inseparable from our understanding of disease and diet.

Final remarks

During the twentieth century, food and diet came to be increasingly related to health and chronic diseases. This change in perception is largely based on risk factors and their perceived scientific qualities – rationality, neutrality, invariability and predictability. The risk factor approach was only made possible by the confluence of a series of social, political, scientific and technical circumstances and elements. This can be exemplified by the emergence of large-population epidemiological studies, especially since the Second World War. Through the combined use of knowledge and techniques from epidemiology, statistics, computing, nutrition and medical science, researchers in advanced countries were able to established risk statements that were later adopted by individuals, health practitioners and governmental organizations. These new ways of understanding disease also transformed the perception of food and diet, through the evaluation of the risk of fat consumption, dietary patterns and obesity.

The FHS was at the centre of this revolution. It represented both the government concern and the scientist's interest in unveiling the causes of heart disease and its relation to food and diet. Framingham was the birthplace of the very idea of risk factors, and its importance cannot be ignored. Public health policies such as dietary guidelines draw extensively from the notion of risk factors and the data from the study regarding, for example, the diet-heart hypothesis. If dietary fat intake is now seen as a danger to health, it is because the Framingham Study helped to disseminate the risk factor rationale and to provide scientific evidence for decision making.

Food and diet are now widely perceived as potential risks. This has dramatic effects on traditional practices, personal choices and the symbolic aspects of eating. In this sense, risk has contributed standardized food practices all around the world in the name of health and security. Yet, paradoxically, heart disease and obesity are still rising in most industrialized and developing countries, while consumers and even medical professionals are increasingly puzzled by conflicting scientific dietary recommendations. After all, risk has not fulfilled its promise to eradicate heart disease and new dangers appear every day. Therefore, a critical instance on the social and cultural effects of risk factors is paramount.

7

From John Yudkin to Jamie Oliver: A Short but Sweet History on the War against Sugar

Rachel Meach

In 2016, an anti-sugar campaign headed by celebrity chef Jamie Oliver was launched in the United Kingdom. Dubbed a 'crusade against sugar', Oliver's documentary *Sugar Rush* examined Britain's penchant for sweetness, exposing the health implications of excessive consumption and calling on the British government to tax sugary drinks in order to reduce obesity and diet-related diseases.[1] In the midst of the furore that ensued, the National Obesity Forum (NOF) and the Public Health Collaboration (PHC) published a report, which demanded a major overhaul of official dietary guidelines. The report condemned the dietary doctrine of 'low fat', which had dominated official dietary guidelines in the United Kingdom since 1983, alleging the advice was based on 'flawed science' which had failed to curb rates of obesity and type 2 diabetes.[2] Their call intensified the debate even further; while members of the PHC described low-fat guidelines as 'the biggest mistake in modern medical history', others warned that reversing the current guidelines may prove disastrous for public health.[3]

Central in this debate was the concern that by buying into the 'low-fat' ideology, people unknowingly increased their consumption of refined sugar as a result. As the food industry had replaced fat with sugar in many of its 'low-fat' products, nutritionists and the public alike began to question whether it was not fat after all, but sugar, fuelling the epidemic of chronic disease.[4] Consequently, a war of nutritional ideology between fat and sugar, first waged in the 1950s, has re-emerged in an attempt to solve the enigma of diet-related disease.

The idea that sugar consumption could be potentially detrimental to health is not a new one. Towards the end of the 1950s, heightened fears of coronary heart disease fuelled a search for the dietary components responsible for the dramatic rise in cardiovascular mortality and other diet-related diseases. During the surge in nutrition research that followed, nutritionists polarized into two distinct groups. One group followed American nutritionist Ancel Keys and believed that dietary fat was to blame; the other concurred with the views of British nutritionist John Yudkin that carbohydrates, primarily refined sugar, was responsible. In the decades that saw heart diseases accelerate, sugar consumption rose in parallel, increasing sevenfold since 1900.[5] Nevertheless, as evident in the dominance of 'low-fat' dietary recommendations that followed, Keys and his critique of fat won the debate and Yudkin's warnings about sugar lay dormant until recent years. This chapter explores the development of the diet-heart debate, analysing how ideas about diet and disease were disseminated to the public and the role they played in shaping official dietary guidelines and nutritional discourses in both Britain and the United States. The chapter begins with a historical overview of the link between sugar and disease before moving on to analyse the diet-heart debate in more detail, focusing in particular on the publications of John Yudkin, the late British nutritionist, renowned for his 'prophecy' on the dangers of sugar.[6] This section examines a range of Yudkin's works but specifically addresses his series of diet and weight loss books published during the 1950s to 1980s which sought to promote a low-carbohydrate diet before moving on to assess the impact Yudkin's warning had on twentieth-century dietary guidelines. The following chapter thus sheds light on the social, political and cultural factors that influence our notions of the ideal diet, reappraising the views of John Yudkin; it attempts to understand why his warnings about sugar were ultimately dismissed.

Sugar's place at the table

Sugar first made its way to England in the twelfth century and what little quantities arrived were typically reserved for the wealthy. Over the next five centuries, its availability increased slowly until around 1650 when the modernization and expansion of refineries allowed for greater production. According to historian Sidney Mintz, it was here that 'sugar began to change from a luxury and rarity to a commonplace necessity'.[7] Mass production and cheap labour lowered the price of sugar and it quickly found its place as a cheap source of energy within the diets of the working class. As a commodity only afforded by the rich, sugar was held in high esteem and its whiteness was seen to symbolize its purity, healthfulness and superiority over other sweeteners.[8] However, as the price of sugar declined, and thus became widely consumed, ideas about sugar and its nutritional status were challenged.

Both historians, the medical professionals and epidemiologists alike maintain that the link between sugar consumption and chronic disease has corresponded with its development and increased presence in Western diets. Denis Parson Burkitt, the late surgeon renowned for his work on cancer and nutrition, remarked of the association between refined carbohydrate and disease that the 'fear that sugar may be injurious is as old as the written history of this sweet food'.[9] Burkitt traced concerns surrounding sugar's nutritional value to India around 100 AD when soon after the cultivation and importation of sugar cane from New Guinea, Charake Samhita ascribed both obesity and diabetes to this 'new article of diet'.[10] In the twentieth century, American investigators Emerson and Larimore (1924), having traced the reported rise in diabetic mortality in New York since 1866, ascribed their findings to changes in dietary habits, especially the rise in sugar consumption. Emerson and Larimore were the first to draw a definite correlation between the influence of social and environmental factors such as diet and the incidental rise of diabetes.[11] Similarly in Britain, Stocks (1944), having studied the increase in diabetic mortality in England and Wales from 1861 to 1942, drew attention to the marked decline in diabetic mortality during the two world wars; this he believed was due to wartime rationing and reduced consumption of sugar. These findings, along with those of Himsworth (1949) were reassessed further by British surgeon Thomas Cleave in his book *The Saccharine Disease* (1974). A keen purveyor of the damaging health consequences of sugar consumption, Cleave drew a convincing link between the decline in sugar consumption during both world wars and the corresponding decline in diabetes mortality and the overconsumption of refined carbohydrates, notably sugar and flour, and the increase in many prevalent chronic diseases. Yet, despite this periodic connection between sugar consumption and disease, no other figure generated such controversy over sugar as the late British nutritionist John Yudkin. In a series of publications written during the 1950s to 1980s, Yudkin maintained that a host of chronic conditions, from diabetes, obesity and heart disease, to asthma, dermatitis and Crohn's disease, could be attributed to high consumption of sucrose. At the height of the diet-heart debate, Yudkin argued against the nutritional consensus of the time, stating that it was not fat, but sugar that was fuelling the post-war rise in cardiovascular mortality and many other chronic diseases.

A war of nutritional ideology

The emergence of the diet-heart debate at the end of the 1950s has been well documented.[12] Yet among these accounts, consideration of the context in which the debate emerged has often been overlooked. Beginning in the 1950s, as the manufactured-food industry expanded, refined sugar had found its place as a crucial ingredient in a range of new foods and was vital in creating the image, particularly in the United States, of a consumer paradise with an abundance of ready-made, convenience foods. Yet, as sugar was being added to an increasing range of foods, rates of diabetes, obesity and heart disease were quietly escalating. As a MetLife study published in the *New York Times* in 1951 revealed, body fat had become America's 'primary public health problem'.[13] This anxiety regarding the relationship between diet and disease was heightened further in 1952 when the US president Eisenhower suffered a heart attack, an event which thrust the issue into the public domain. By the end of the 1960s, a war of nutritional ideology was in full swing, symbolized by a polarized debate between two eminent nutrition scientists.

In 1958, nutrition scientist Ancel Keys launched his Seven Countries Study, a major survey of the potential risk factors of cardiovascular disease. Keys asserted that fat was to blame for the rise in heart disease and only a diet low in fat would lower cholesterol and reverse the intensifying trend fast becoming prevalent across most of the Western world.[14] Around the same time, British nutritionist John Yudkin found that sugar too appeared to correlate with heart disease in several countries and thus put forth his contending hypothesis that high sugar consumption was a key cause of heart disease. Initially, Yudkin seemed more agreeable to the idea that both fat *and* sugar were somehow implicated as mutually confounding variables, present in equally high levels in the diets of those he had observed. Writing in the *Lancet* in 1957 Yudkin claimed,

> A consideration of some of the more readily available data on the incidence of coronary deaths and on food consumption makes it difficult to support any theory which supposes *a single or major dietary cause* of coronary thrombosis.[15]

Unlike Yudkin, Keys was unwavering in his belief that the escalation of heart disease was being fuelled by a single nutrient: fat. Agitated by this, Yudkin took to the *Lancet* to accuse Keys and his colleagues of using 'awkward facts' and 'cherry-picking only the data which supported their view'.[16]

Despite his initial reluctance to support the idea of a single nutritional cause of heart disease, evident here in 1957, by the 1970s with the publication of the controversial (and later banned) *Pure, White and Deadly*, Yudkin too had subscribed to the idea of a single dietary cause of disease. Accordingly, Yudkin became persistent in his belief that a whole host of conditions, ranging from obesity, heart disease, cancer and diabetes to hyperactivity, eczema and arthritis, could all be traced back to sugar.[17] Absent in much of the literature on the diet-heart debate is a consideration of why fat *and* sugar could not both be feasible as mutual dietary explanations. The possible explanations for this are both personal, reflecting the professional ambitions of individual nutrition scientists, and political, shaped by changes in the formation of official dietary guidelines and the increasing influence of the food industry and government in their formation. Gyorgy Scrinis concept of 'nutritionism' is particularly useful for understanding the latter. According to Scrinis, beginning in the 1960s, there was an increasing tendency towards a reductive understanding of nutrients in which foods became distinguished as either 'good' or 'bad'. This Scrinis argues signalled the emergence of a new nutritional era, one which became wholly obsessed with fat and focusing attention on single nutrients rather than address the role of food production techniques, additives or the metabolic interaction of different nutrients.[18] Scrinis maintains that the narrow focus on fat, and later the different types of fat, served to focus the attention of the public and nutrition experts on the presence or absence of fat in foods, rather than on the processing techniques and other ingredients (i.e. refined sugar) used in production.[19] Within this context, whereby it became fashionable to differentiate between 'good' and 'bad' foods and focus upon single nutrient explanations of disease, overall attention unquestionably focused on fat. Correspondingly, the food industry, heavily influenced by the powerful sugar lobby, fuelled this significantly by translating the findings of Keys et al. into an enormous array of low-fat products.[20]

The tendency to focus on single nutrients thus reflected the wider context in which the diet-heart debate emerged, particularly changes occurring within the field of nutrition as the change in the language of dietary advice seen above. However, this explanation alone is insufficient to explain why one dietary theory (fat) should dominate and rival theories such as Yudkin's attracted only limited support. Both sugar and saturated fat were associated with the risk of heart disease, yet Keys and Yudkin's hypotheses were situated as competing single-nutrient explanations.[21] The possibility that both fat *and* sugar were mutually responsible for the rise in chronic disease was never seriously entertained, evident in the very public dismissal of Yudkin's ideas by most nutrition experts at the time and the deriding of his career by his contemporaries.[22] Thus, in addition to considering changes within nutrition and the wider context at the time of the debate, it is worthwhile to likewise consider Yudkin's particular impact on the debate – his professional ambitions and how he disseminated his ideas about sugar to the wider public.

The narrative of Yudkin's career is fascinating and provides a unique perspective of the diet-health debate so often overlooked. Yudkin began his research career towards the end of the 1930s, primarily interested in the effects of vitamins and vitamin deficiency in the diet upon health. However, alongside this research, Yudkin had greater ambitions. In an anonymous letter published in the *Times* in 1942, Yudkin called for a nationwide 'Nutrition Council' which would be responsible for setting nutritional goals and recommendations for the entire population.[23] Unnerved by the frank dismissal of this proposal, Yudkin persisted in his career in nutrition, becoming chair of physiology at Queen Elizabeth College, establishing a nutrition department and the first taught degree in nutrition in Britain. Yudkin's early academic publications from the 1940s to mid-1950s demonstrate a wide range of interests in nutrition, from vitamin deficiencies and nutrition quality to the psychology of food choice. Yet, by the 1960s, as the diet-heart debate intensified and attracted widespread publicity, Yudkin's interests narrowed, concentrating on the relationship between diet and the related conditions of obesity and heart disease, in particular connecting these with the consumption of sugar.[24]

The progression of Yudkin's career and the response to his ideas offers a window into the development of nutrition, in particular how nutritional debates can become caught up in corresponding cultural notions in an attempt to disseminate ideas regarding diet to the general public. An analysis of Yudkin's publications throughout his career demonstrates this to be the case, particularly reflecting popular ideas about gender and body weight. As his interest in the relationship between sugar and obesity augmented, Yudkin disseminated his warning against sugar widely in medical journals and newspapers but also, as discussed below, through a series of diet and weight loss books. In existing histories of the diet-heart debate, scholars have overlooked Yudkin's publications for a lay audience, choosing to focus on his scientific publications and academic papers instead. I argue here that Yudkin's diet and weight loss books are a crucial source for the historian that shed new light on the debate between dietary fat and sugar, elucidating why Yudkin's ideas were ultimately dismissed for decades and only revisited in recent years.

Sugar, slimming and the 'expert'

In 1958, Yudkin attended the scientific meeting of the British Medical Association (BMA) in Birmingham. Following a panel on obesity and exercise, Yudkin proposed that the BMA establish a panel of 'experts' to inspect slimming products, with which he claimed the public were being 'bombarded'.[25] Referring to advertisements for slimming products in the *British Medical Journal*, Yudkin held,

> I think we really ought not to have these advertisements in our journal. I should like to see the association setting up some sort of panel of people who know something about this and who would look at the products with which the public is being bombarded daily, and give some sort of seal to those which fulfil the well-recognised criteria of respectable slimming preparations.[26]

Meanwhile, the same year, and precisely a year after first publishing his critique of sugar in the *Lancet*, Yudkin entered into the diet industry himself, publishing his first book, *This Slimming Business*, in an attempt to disseminate his ideas to the wider public. The book proved to be a bestseller and brought Yudkin's attack on sugar and 'yo-yo dieting' to national prominence.[27] As the title of the book suggests, Yudkin's intention here was to branch out from scientific publications and reach a lay audience by tapping into the market of the expanding diet industry. Selling 200,000 copies in Britain alone, *This Slimming Business* was deemed a success and thus encouraged Yudkin to undertake further research into public attitudes towards health and nutrition.[28] In 1963, along with his colleagues at Queen Elizabeth College, London, Yudkin published the study 'Knowledge of Nutrition amongst Housewives in a London Suburb'.[29] In the study, housewives were provided with questionnaires and asked to answer a list of true or false statements relating to diet, revealing Yudkin's growing interest in the diet industry, in particular women's thoughts on slimming. In the study of London housewives, Yudkin notes,

> The housewives were asked what foods they would recommend to be cut out of the diet by a person who wanted to slim. It is interesting to see the high importance attached to foods containing carbohydrate, and the relatively low importance attached to foods rich in fats.[30]

Women's views on the foods to target are reflected in a number of questions; for example, when asked, 'If a friend wanted to slim what foods would you suggest they cut out of their diet?', the women ranked potatoes first, followed by bread and sugar while ranking fats firmly at the bottom.[31] While the study highlights the disparity between the anti-carbohydrate sentiments of British housewives and Keys low-fat ideology, perhaps the most interesting aspect is Yudkin's evident agenda in gathering popular ideas about slimming and weight loss. One of the most apparent themes in all of Yudkin's diet books published thereafter is the association between adopting this type of diet and 'a slim figure'.[32] Reflecting the context in which he was writing, when women, housewives in particular, were considered to represent the 'feminine ideal', it can be argued then that Yudkin began to focus his nutritional agenda on the appearance, rather than health of women, connecting his ideals of a low-sugar diet with the archetypal slim figure.

A year later Yudkin published his second diet book, *The Complete Slimmer*, later renamed *Lose Weight, Feel Great* for publication in the United States. Now positioning himself as the 'slimming expert', it became clear that appearance had become the primary benefit of a low-sugar diet, with improved health featuring merely as an additional bonus. Yudkin explains,

> The more you really understand and accept the logic of what I say, the more easily you will be able to accept the advice I give you. And the benefits are much more than simply a good figure. You may well achieve a degree of health that you may have forgot was possible.[33]

Clarifying his intended audience, Yudkin continues,

> Thirty of forty years ago, few people seemed to be worrying about whether they were too fat. Since that time, more and more people have been doing so. Mostly, these are young women whose excessive body shapes do not look the best in the current fashions. Of course, women's fashions change in what, to a man, seems an extraordinary and unpredictable way. But excessive bosoms, excessive hips, and an intermediate anatomy of similar dimensions, have been unpopular now for as long as women have discarded the many frills that were once considered feminine attire. Since that time, there has also been the cult of the seaside and sunbathing – the era of barest maximum. Women in fashion have, then, increasingly found it desirable to avoid inordinate curves and shapes and proturbances, which do not look well in the more revealing garments to which they have taken.[34]

A recurring message which appears in all of Yudkin's publications for popular audiences is that a low-carbohydrate diet is not only a means to good health, but is also essential to achieve and maintain a slim figure. It is clear that Yudkin, tapping into popular culture and advertising, viewed women as aspiring to emulate 'slim trim figures', or as he states in *Lose Weight, Feel Great*, 'being in fashion should not be confined to models'.[35] While Yudkin's interest in overweight and chronic disease undoubtedly stemmed from health concerns of consuming too many refined carbohydrates, the language used to communicate this idea to the public exploited cultural concerns regarding body weight and body image. Promoting what he describes as the aesthetic benefits of weight loss, Yudkin states, 'Let me hasten to say that I think the aesthetic incentive to avoiding overweight is commendable and quite important.'[36] In *The Slimmer's Cookbook* (1961), *The A to Z of Slimming* (1977) and his later *Eat Well, Slim Well* (1982), it can be seen, particularly from the front cover and illustrations inside the book, that women were the prime target audience of his nutritional agenda.

In conjunction with his diet books, Yudkin continued to publish widely in medical and scientific journals, challenging Keys fat hypothesis and decrying its growing popularity among nutrition scientists, the public and the food industry. Writing in the *Lancet* in 1964, Yudkin disparaged Keys 'Seven Countries Study', maintaining that heart disease could likewise be linked with high levels of sugar consumption.[37] In his own study of thirty-four countries, Yudkin had found the national consumption levels of fat and sugar to be almost exactly the same, thus leading him to conclude that it was as likely that sugar was responsible. Yudkin's article was met with great interest as a number of responses in the *Lancet* elucidate. One particular response came from an English physician, who, curious about Yudkin's links between sugar and heart disease, had carried out his own research into men and women's consumptions habits, yet remained unconvinced. The response pointed out that while women consumed more sugar and sweet foods than men, heart disease appeared to be a 'distinctly male disease'.[38] The physician further added,

> Professor Yudkin invites us to cut our sugar intake drastically, since 'we think it likely that we are dealing with a primary causal relationship between sugar intake and arterial disease'. Elsewhere in the same paper he treats this assumption as only as only a hypothesis at present. In other words, sugar – historically, the latest addition to the list of our nutrients – has become the newest fashionable villain of the affluent society. A difficulty arises however. Were there – as Professor Yudkin suggests – a causal relation between sugar intake and I.H.D, one would expect the highest prevalence of this disease among those who consume the biggest amounts of sugar, sweets, biscuits, chocolate, ice cream, and puddings. Tentative observations seem to contradict this. I am far from claiming scientific accuracy for a small poll which I carried out among my patients with coronary-artery disease, at local confectioners, and also by asking waiters about the dessert orders of customers of a few humbles snack-bars and West-End restaurants. But one thing emerged. Young adult women and the 'upper-middle-aged' women constitute the overwhelming majority of sweet buyers, and they do not hesitate to ask for a pastry or pudding as dessert instead of 'men's cheeses'. I questioned the healthy wives of my patients with I.H.D as to their husband's consumption of sugar, and it was not conspicuously higher than their own. As is well known, there is a distinct sex difference in the prevalence of I.H.D in favour of the female. Do oestrogens suppress the hypothetical action of sugar, and, if so, in what way?[39]

This response to Yudkin's premise highlights the peculiar way in which concerns about the relationship between diet and disease had emerged due to the increase of mortality from heart disease, which as this letter highlights, in both the United States and Britain was a distinctly male disease, particularly common among older, white, affluent men. Yet, the dietary advice produced in response to the diet-heart debate, as discussed above, targeted not this cohort of men, however, but rather young women.

Despite this peculiarity, a growing diet industry ensured Yudkin's diet and weight loss books sold well. According to historian Harvey Levenstein, Yudkin's 'fame, along with his quick wit and engaging personality' ensured wide coverage of his ideas and despite attempts by those who supported Keys to deride him in the media, he successfully sued for referring to his work as 'science fiction'.[40] Ultimately, however, Yudkin's personality was not enough to secure his popularity and professional status. Those who supported Keys used their influence with research-granting agencies to drain him of funding and by 1970 Yudkin found himself pushed into retirement from his professorship, leaving him unsalaried in a backroom office.

Yudkin could not be supressed, however, and during his retirement wrote his final indictment of sugar, the seminal *Pure, White and Deadly*, published in 1971. At the end of his career Yudkin found both himself and his theory marginalized and derided; yet, he remained resolute in his ideas:

> With many examples in mind of how information can be distorted or withheld, it becomes even more evident that people should not be left entirely to themselves to decide what they should or should not eat. Sooner or later, I feel, it will be necessary to introduce legislation that by some means or other prevents people from consuming so much sugar, and especially prevents parents, relatives and friends from ruining the health of babies and children.[41]

By the 1970s then, despite decades spent producing books targeting individual dieters, Yudkin believed the threat posed by sugar was not only more 'imminent and deadly', but that changing consumption habits could no longer be left to the individual and warranted state intervention.

Yudkin's work published at the height of the diet-heart debate thus demonstrate the development of Yudkin's career and the professionalization of the field of nutrition in addition to revealing much about the cultural context in which he was writing. That Yudkin, a renowned scientist, chose to enter the weight-loss industry to disseminate his ideas about sugar reveals the power of the diet industry and culture of slimming throughout the 1960s to 1980s. Despite the fact that the debate had arisen out of concerns about heart disease, which seemed to occur mainly in men, by the 1960s onwards it was women who had become the main targets of dietary advice on either side of the debate. According to Joan Brumberg, one explanation behind this can be found in the rapid change during this period in dieting and bodily ideals; 'After a brief flirtation with full-breasted, curvaceous female figures in the politically conservative post-war recovery of the 1950s, our collective taste returned to an ideal of extreme thinness and an androgynous, if not childlike figure'; as a result, she argues, our cultural tolerance for body fat diminished and women became the target of 'experts' to strive for a lean body.[42]

How conscious Yudkin was in his decision to tailor his advice towards women is uncertain. La Berge asserts how a century-long preference for slim bodies and losing weight using low-calorie diets was well entrenched as the diet-heart debate arose. Slimming and weight reduction, she argues, was a widespread social and cultural phenomenon among women from as early as the nineteenth century, waxing and waning in response to changing social, cultural, economic and political conditions.[43] Thus, in both Britain and the United States, the diet-heart debate emerged within a context in which a diet culture was already firmly entrenched, of which the incentive had long been both aesthetic and medical.[44]

Yudkin's books sold well initially, and despite lacking the nutritional consensus of his colleagues, as the debate gathered momentum several key developments unfolded which seemed to add weight to his case. For the first time, nutritionists began to distinguish among different types of sugar along nutritional grounds. Until the 1960s, white and brown sugar, honey, syrup and molasses had been treated as a discrete category; however, in the late 1960s both nutritionists and non-experts alike began to rank these in a hierarchical order positioning white refined sugar, once known for its purity and healthfulness, firmly at the bottom.[45] Additionally, the American counterculture provided a weighty critique of the American diet, questioning the healthfulness of the food supply and drawing attention to the over use of artificial additives, both chemical and 'natural' such as sugar, in modern foods.[46] By the 1970s then, fears over 'hidden sugars' had mounted and the idea that additives could even be linked to childhood disorders like hyperactivity, an idea popularized by allergist Benjamin F. Feingold, gave increasing cause for concern.[47]

Dietary goals and guidelines

In 1973, the US Senate Select Committee on Nutrition and Human Needs was established to focus attention on the 'overnourished' and what to do about the rising rates of chronic disease. The committee spent the next 4 years looking into aspects of the American diet that had been linked to the leading killer diseases and concluded that too much fat, sugar, cholesterol, salt and alcohol were linked to cancer, cardiovascular disease, diabetes, coronary heart disease and cirrhosis of the liver. While both fat and sugar were listed as contributing to these diseases, the panel's final set of dietary goals, issued in December 1977, 'Dietary Goals for the United States', also referred to as the McGovern Report, manifested these findings into low-fat, high-carbohydrate recommendations.[48] In addition to warning the public about obesity, the guidelines advocated increasing carbohydrate consumption to 55 to 60 per cent of total daily intake while reducing fat from 40 to 30 per cent.[49] Not only did the new recommendations apply to the general population, but also to those with chronic, diet-related disease such as diabetes. In breaking with decades of low-carbohydrate recommendations for diabetes, the American Diabetic Association (ADA), Canadian Diabetic Association (CDA) and the British Diabetic Association (BDA), in line with the changes made following the McGovern Report, increased the carbohydrate allowance for diabetics. Moving towards a diet similar to that of the general population, diabetics were now recommended to consume a high-carbohydrate diet. The BDA's 'Dietary Recommendations' for the 1980s stated,

> The traditional view that restriction of carbohydrate is an essential part of the dietary management of diabetics can no longer be regarded as correct. Provided that the energy content of the prescribed diet does not exceed individual requirement, the proportion of energy consumed as carbohydrate is immaterial to diabetic control.[50]

Accordingly, the new guidelines for diabetics recommended a maximum of 35 per cent of dietary energy from fat and 55 per cent from carbohydrate, representing a significant reversal from former guidelines and years of research on nutrition and diets for diabetics.[51]

The publication of *Dietary Goals* reflected the federal government's official support of the low-fat approach. While the guidelines recommended that fat, sugar, salt and alcohol all be consumed less, it was the reduction of fat in particular which was emphasized continuously thereafter. Between 1978 and 1979, the American Society of Clinical Nutritionists, the American Heart Association and the National Cancer Institute all fell in line and produced their own low-fat recommendations and by 1980 a scientific consensus was emerging which promoted a low-fat diet as the appropriate diet not only as a preventable measure for those at risk of heart disease and cancer, but the entire population.[52]

The saccharine saga

While it appeared that Yudkin's warning about sugar had failed to achieve the same level of recognition as Keys's warning about fat, one subsequent event suggests that on some level, his ideas about sugar took hold. The debate surrounding the banning of artificial sweeteners, particularly cyclamate and saccharin, and the protest against the ban, suggests that there was substantial demand for a low-sugar alternative. In 1977, the same year as the McGovern Report had been published and low-fat became the dominant nutritional consensus, contention arose over the use of artificial sweeteners in foods following the results of a study in 1970 by the Canadian government which found saccharin as a potential cause of bladder cancer in rats.[53] In response to the study, the FDA considered labelling saccharin as a drug, making it only obtainable in pharmacies. This suggestion was met with considerable protest from food manufacturers, consumers and lobbyists alike.[54] The diabetic community in particular, both patients and their diabetic associations, while naturally wary, disapproved of the suggestion which would ultimately mean a diet completely devoid of the sweetness they had become accustomed to with the availability of special diabetic foods (see Figures 7.1 and 7.2). The ADA commented on the FDA's decision, warning that the unavailability of sugar substitutes could have 'very grave' effects for the 10 million Americans with diabetes, 'making it more difficult for these individuals to control their condition by dietary means'.[55]

In 1977, the *New York Times* reported how the FDA's 2-day public hearings into its proposal to limit the use of saccharin were met with 'a mass outpouring of protest' as 'eight witnesses representing organisations of diabetics testified that the FDA proposal would undermine the efforts of 10 million diabetic Americans to stick to their sugar-free diets'.[56] With mounting pressure from the public, diabetic associations and lobbyists, coupled with the fact cyclamate had already been banned the decade prior and there were no 'no-sugar' alternatives, the FDA eventually reversed its decision, settling on warning labels on food packaging instead. Ultimately then this event suggests that while Yudkin's concerns about sugar may have failed to manifest as the dominant recommendation within nutritional advice, he nevertheless influenced the

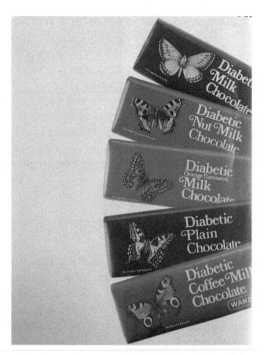

Figure 7.1 'Wander's Diabetic Chocolate'. Advertisement featured in supplement of the Chemist and Druggist (1979). Courtesy of the Wellcome Library, London.

public's ideas about sugar consumption, in particular its association with obesity and henceforth the reluctance to give up artificial sweeteners as a substitute to its sweetness.

Conclusion

By examining the publications of the late British nutritionist John Yudkin, both his academic publications and those produced for a lay audience, this chapter has considered how mid-century warnings about sugar were disseminated to the public, how these were shaped by the wider social and cultural context and the impact of these upon the diet-heart debate as it unfolded in Britain and the United States. Amidst a rapidly changing food environment and expanding food industry that increasingly used sugar in food production, alarming rates of coronary heart disease and obesity spurred nutritionists, the media and the public to consider the connection between diet and disease and the role of single nutritional components in fuelling the emerging epidemic.

In subscribing to the trend which emerged in the 1960s of explaining the epidemic rise of chronic disease in a reductive, single-nutrient manner, Yudkin, through the use of diet books, sought to generate greater interest in his nutritional advice about sugar by appealing to women's health concerns, primarily that of being overweight. While

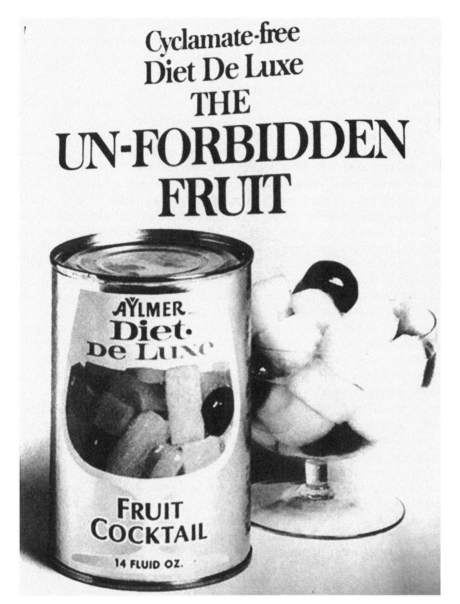

Figure 7.2 'Diet de Luxe Fruit Cocktail'. Advertisement featured in quarterly newsletter of the Canadian Diabetic Association, Vol. 20, No. 1 (1979). Courtesy of the Joslin Archive, Joslin Diabetes Centre, Boston, MA.

the main objective of his books was undoubtedly to disseminate his beliefs concerning the link between sugar and disease, he did so while simultaneously endorsing the cultural ideal of the slim body to his readership. Left derided at the end of his career, Yudkin's warnings ultimately fell on deaf ears. However, what can be assumed by his publications is his recognition of women as a prime target audience as he sought out professional merit. This was not because they were more susceptible to heart disease, but rather, because of their presumed penchant for sweetness.

The latest war against sugar, led by public figures such as Robert Lustig in the United States and celebrity figures like Jamie Oliver in Britain, has witnessed a resurgence of interest of Yudkin's otherwise dormant ideas. Reprinted in 2012, *Pure, White and Deadly* has been hailed a 'prophecy' which foretold the consequences of our increasing consumption of sugar long before the scientific evidence was available. While this has drawn due attention to the growing amount of sugar in our modern diet, these new debates have tended towards the same narrow focus on the ideological war between Keys and Yudkin, or fat or sugar, rather than the production and processing of foods, the interaction of combinations of different nutrients or overconsumption of food generally. Recent research suggests that both Yudkin and Keys could have been right – that neither sugar or fat alone can lead to heart disease but a combination of them together as 'sweet fat' in packaged foods. Nevertheless, a narrow preoccupation with single nutrients has avoided, or at least stalled, research investigating this in a more systematic manner.

Ultimately, that Yudkin chose to disseminate his ideas about nutrition and health in this way not only reveals much about social and cultural atmosphere in which he was writing, ideas pertaining to gender, health and expert knowledge, but also demonstrates that by the 1960s, nutrition scientists were now finding themselves transcending the realms of the research laboratory and the scientific journal and becoming popular and commercial figures. By entering into the diet industry and with significant coverage in both the popular press and public health media, the debate penetrated the public sphere and influenced ideas about diet and health much greater than any previous nutritional debate. Accordingly, this attention afforded the debate much greater scope to influence official dietary guidelines and nutritional recommendations, for both the general public and those with diet-related diseases. The result has been decades of nutritionally reductive, nutricentric guidelines and food aisles in abundance of low-fat products, which have ultimately failed to curb rates of diet-related disease.

Part Three

The Politics of Dietary Change

8

The Popularization of a New Nutritional Concept: The Calorie in Belgium, 1914–1918

Peter Scholliers

The history of the calorie is known, but that of its dissemination into wide layers of society remains enigmatic.[1] Who introduced this concept to the general public, when, through which means, with which arguments and aims? How was 'calorie' received within current, general views on eating? Was 'calorie' readily associated with doctors, physical condition or overweight, and did it emerge within views on feeding babies, vulnerable children, pregnant women and ill people? Did disinterest, suspicion, curiosity or enthusiasm prevail? Questions like these may help interpret the way the general public conceives of health recommendations at large, which is essential for interpreting their reception and application. Studying dissemination of nutritional information is not new, though. Various channels have been studied in diverse places and times, including cookbooks,[2] exhibition reports,[3] official campaigns,[4] manuals of domestic education,[5] recommendations by dietary societies,[6] advertisements[7] and public radio broadcasts.[8] Focusing on gender, disease, public intervention or commercial interest, these studies have revealed huge variations of diffusion regarding form, content, aim and audience. The present chapter analyses the way a nutritional concept has been popularized in a precise context, which offers new insights into mediators and their messages.

The contours of this investigation

The way 'calorie' appeared in Belgian newspapers during the Great War presents a relevant case for assessing how the general public may have come across new notions about healthy food. This claim needs justification. 'Kilocalorie' (or Calorie[9]) has been applied to human nutrition since the 1840s, used for assessing the energy intake and the optimal diet. 'Calorie' became familiar among dieticians since the late 1880s. By 1900, 'calorie' had found its way into doctors' practices,[10] and today it is part of the 'nutri-quantification' of food and familiar to most people.[11] Rather than 'carbohydrate', 'albumin' or 'healthy diet', I chose 'calorie' because of its innovative trait in a period when dietetics entered a new phase.[12] Worldwide, the Great War played a catalysing role in the spreading of 'calorie'.[13] For instance, 'calorie' was not used in manuals of Belgian household schools prior to 1914, to emerge in the early 1920s, while hands-on dietary brochures appeared during the war referring to 'calorie', which was not the case before 1914.[14] With the German invasion of Belgium on 4 August 1914, food import and distribution were abruptly disrupted and, for 52 months, all issues related to food became highly sensitive and visible.[15] Occupied Belgium had a (German) government that did not care about the food shortages, thus leaving food concerns to private ingenuity. 'Popularization', lastly, is the way to present scientific notions in a widely understandable form.[16] Mass media capture readily how these notions spread throughout society.[17] During the war, newspapers continued to be published for an eager public in need of information, although censorship was established, material problems accumulated and news sources became restricted. Some newspapers disappeared, others were launched and clandestine press grew but very haphazardly. The average number of copies of censored newspapers reached 500,000, that of clandestine press 20,000, showing the ongoing importance of periodicals as the information source.[18]

Two databanks are used: one that contains *all* periodicals pertaining to Belgium, published between January 1914 and December 1918,[19] and the Royal Library's collection of newspapers published prior to 1914.[20] I selected 'calorie', 'calories', 'calorieën' and 'kalorie(s)', which yielded 948 hits. After reducing to articles that relate to food, I obtained 125 articles between 1890 and 1913 and 142 articles between 1914 and 1918. The years 1892–1898 yielded 3 articles (out of a total of 267, i.e. 1.1 per cent), 1899–1903: 18 articles (6.7 per cent), 1904–1908: 56 (20.9 per cent), 1909–1913: 48 (17.9 per cent) and 1914–1918: 142 (53.1 per cent) (Graph 8.1).

During the war, the 142 articles were published in 42 newsprints of very diverse nature (general newspapers alongside workers' weeklies and family magazines; most under German control). Some dailies stand out with regard to the attention paid to 'calorie' – most pieces appeared in censored *Vooruit* (10.5 per cent of the total), followed by *La Belgique* (censored), *L'Echo belge* (clandestine, published in Amsterdam) and *L'Indépendance belge* (clandestine, published in Paris and then London) (each with 7 per cent). Assuming that the word *alimentation* reflects adequately the interest of the periodicals for all matters of food, the following ratio *calorie/alimentation* emerges: 1914 – 2.9 per cent, 1915 – 7.3 per cent, 1916 – 3.3 per cent, 1917 – 14.9 per cent and 1918 – 12.0 per cent. Despite the increase in both proportional and absolute numbers, the interest in 'calorie' was not overwhelming. To put this finding in perspective, I count the frequency of 'calorie' in relation to food in Dutch and French newspapers between 1890 and 1918.[21] Attention in Belgium and the Netherlands, comparable countries with regard to size and number of inhabitants, ran quite similarly, and the influence of the Great War is undeniable (Graph 1). The latter also clearly shows in France, although interest emerged earlier, which may be explained by the active role of French nutritionists in caloric research since the 1840s.[22]

In Belgium, the first reference to 'calorie' in relation to food appeared in *Journal de Bruxelles* (3 July 1892, 6), the second in *Le Peuple* (28 September 1895, 1). The first was unsigned, and the second was signed by a physician. Prior to 1914, articles had titles as 'Force motrice humaine' (*L'Avenir du Luxembourg*, 7 October 1905), 'Mangeons des calories' (La Meuse, 22 June 1909) or 'L'homme est un poêle' (*Dernière Heure*, 26 July

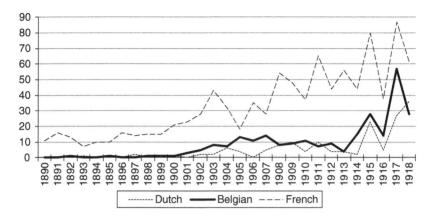

Graph 8.1 Mention of food-related use of 'calorie' in Belgian, Dutch and French newspapers, 1890–1918.

Sources: Notes 20, 21 and 22

1913). The novelty of 'calorie' appeared tellingly in an article of *Le XXe Siècle* of 14 January 1910, writing, 'However, our ignorance was, until now, excusable, because the calorie wasn't familiar to us.'

Mention of 'calorie' during the war did not develop linearly. 'Calorie' appeared most in 1917 (38.7 per cent of the total of 1914–1918), followed by 1915 and 1918 (both 20.4 per cent), 1914 (10.5 per cent) and 1916 (9.8 per cent). The growing interest in 1914 and 1915 was undoubtedly linked to food supply difficulties, and the high number of 1917 may be explained by the start of the German U-boat attacks, leading to severe food shortages, skyrocketing prices and vast health problems. The low number of mentions in 1916 (also occurring in France and the Netherlands) may be explained by relatively steady food supply. The 142 articles are tackled by asking 15 questions that translate into quantifiable answers. Some questions are easily answered by 'yes' or 'no', but others need interpretation. This quantitative approach points at particular issues, which are further addressed by close reading of the articles. I start the investigation by considering the author and the form of the pieces, then the language of the articles will be analysed to conclude with the investigation of their content.

Authors with a mission

A newspaper article signed by a doctor may have got more attention and authority than an unsigned one. Yet, unsigned pieces are telling about the way 'calorie' was used by non-expert authors, which matters greatly when considering media usage of nutritional notions. In 1914, 1915 and 1918, articles were equally divided between signed and unsigned, but in 1916 and 1917, the number of unsigned pieces surpassed

Table 8.1 Authorship of articles, 1914 to 1918 (in %)

	Unsigned	Signed	Signed by doctor
1914	47	6	47
1915	45	17	38
1916	65	14	21
1917	72	14	14
1918	52	24	24

the signed ones (Table 8.1). The deteriorating food supply can explain the increase of unsigned articles in 1916 and 1917, reflecting the growing worry of general observers.

Prior to 1914, it was not unusual that doctors published in newspapers. In 1914, doctors signed almost half of the articles, but in 1917 this was only 14 per cent, to rise again to 24 per cent in 1918 (Table 8.1). In absolute figures, doctors provided about ten articles each year. Some doctors had a regular column, but others appeared only once. An example of a weekly publication is provided by Ghent-based social-democrat *Vooruit* and middle-class *Gazette van Gent* (both under German control) in December 1914 and January 1915, authored by Dr A. Van de Velde.[23] The name of Dr Delattre popped up a couple of times,[24] alongside fifteen names of other doctors who contributed at least one article that included 'calorie'. Assuredly, doctors gave more food advice in newspapers during these years, but without using 'calorie'. Non-doctors signed by their name, such as French journalist L. Baudry de Saunier,[25] who paid large attention to food in the chic, France-based weekly *L'Illustration* (e.g. 11 May 1918, 21). A few authors signed with their initials or penname, for instance, Tante Colinette in her habitual 'Coin des ménagères' of censored middle-class *La Belgique* (6 May 1917, 1). The latter suggests that 'calorie' has entered the sphere of the housewife.

Formal aspects like the size, the place of the article in the newspaper and the use of tables and figures inform about the weight of each article. Generally, signed pieces were larger than unsigned ones (Table 8.2). Yet, now and then, unsigned articles had a considerable length, such as the one appearing in patriotic, London-based *Stem uit België* (9 February 1917) of 3,590 words, considering the question whether international food aid of Belgium profited to the German war effort. Conversely, signed pieces, even by doctors, sometimes were very short, such as Dr Durand's sixty-five-word article in patriotic, Amsterdam-based daily *L'Echo Belge* (29 September 1918, 4), in which he reassured the Belgians about sufficient caloric supply after the war.

Would signed pieces appear on highly visible spots in the newspapers, that is, pages 1 or 2, with catching titles in capitals or bold? This varied according to the sort of publication, the total number of pages and the layout. Some, like *L'illustration* having about forty pages, always put an image on page 1, very general contemplations on page 2 and solid pieces further in the magazine, but most newspapers had no more than four pages (broadsheet format), where relevant news appeared on pages 1 or 2. Taking both unsigned and signed articles together, pieces bearing 'calorie' obtained quite some visibility in 1914 (86 per cent of the total were published on pages 1 or 2), but this fell radically afterwards (Table 8.2). In 1915 and 1916, articles referring to calories were

Table 8.2 Signed and unsigned articles broken down by size, page in the newspaper and use of statistics (in %, to be read horizontally by category)

	Size				Page			Stats	
	<300	300–600	600–1,000	>1000	1	2	Elsewhere	No	Yes
1914									
Unsigned	14	28	58	0	57	29	14	86	14
Signed	0	12	63	25	37	51	12	50	50
1915									
Unsigned	31	39	15	15	38	15	47	77	23
Signed	0	0	31	69	19	37	44	31	69
1916									
Unsigned	33	45	0	22	11	56	33	78	22
Signed	0	0	40	60	40	20	40	60	40
1917									
Unsigned	44	15	26	15	23	31	46	74	26
Signed	6	6	6	82	31	12	57	31	69
1918									
Unsigned	47	20	13	20	47	33	20	73	27
Signed	14	7	28	51	29	7	64	64	36

increasingly published 'elsewhere'. In 1917 and 1918, the signed pieces appeared far less on pages 1 and 2 than the unsigned ones. Thus, 'calorie' had been appropriated not only by doctors but also by all authors, putting 'calorie' on eye-catching pages.

Inserting a table tells about acquaintance with 'calorie' and may have created a sense of expertise, although it also may have intimidated the reader. Statistics surely caught the eye. Clear differences appear between unsigned and signed articles regarding their use. Throughout the war, unsigned pieces made lesser use of statistics than signed articles, the former using figures in about 25 per cent of the cases (Table 8.2). Signed articles largely had statistics, although not systematically. In 1914, half of the signed articles used figures, rising to almost 70 per cent in 1915 and 1917, but dropping to 40 per cent in 1916 and to only 36 per cent in 1918. Some of these offered very exhaustive information about calorie values and intake. For instance, the censored, popular Christian-Democratic *Het Volk* (8 November 1917, 1) published a large table with the quantity of protein, carbohydrates, fat and calories of fifteen foodstuffs (Figure 8.1).

The direct cause for publishing a piece on food and health including 'calorie' differed throughout the war. In 1914, most authors referred to general circumstances of food supply ('Event' in Table 8.3), which remained a reason to publish a piece throughout the war. Yet, this diminished in favour of other occasions. Authors replied to an article in another newspaper or a brochure, particularly in 1915, 1916 and 1917. Equally, a specific action or policy ('Achievement' in Table 8.3) could lead to a newspaper article, particularly toward the end of the war. A lecture or an exhibition

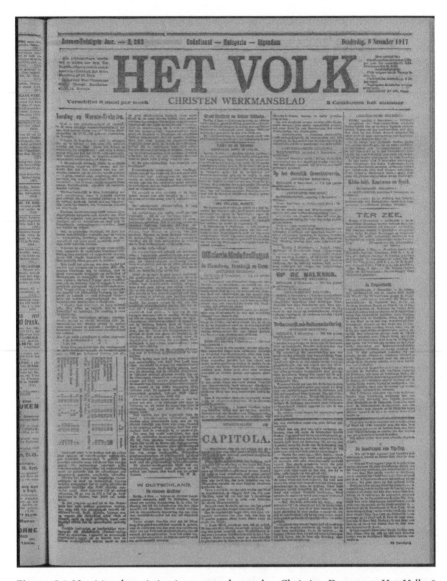

Figure 8.1 Nutritional statistics in censored popular Christian-Democrat *Het Volk*, 8 November 1917, page 1, signed by Dr F. D., 'Voeding en warmte-eenheden' (*The diet and warmth-units*), c.1,400 words. The article defines calorie, explains the way food is absorbed by the body (making the analogy with a stove), mentions the daily necessary supply of 3,000 calories and provides a table of the content of proteins, carbohydrates, fat and calories of vegetable and animal foodstuffs.

Source: https://hetarchief.be/nl/media/het-volk-christen-werkmansblad/W2bUldUkGaGKVWhqUUS WuowQ

Table 8.3 Direct cause for publishing an article with the mention of 'calorie' (in %)

	Exhibition	Publication	Lecture	Event	Achievement	None
1914	0	13	0	87	0	0
1915	0	56	3	34	0	7
1916	0	44	7	28	7	14
1917	4	47	7	9	22	11
1918	3	24	3	56	14	0

also led to referring to 'calorie'. For instance, *La Belgique* (29 June 1917, 2) reported that the Brussels municipality had organized an exhibition in which various dishes were shown alongside their "rendement en calories" in relation to a healthy, affordable diet.

All sorts of authors, thus, used the notion of calorie in newspapers and magazines, and, in general, doctors wrote long, well-informed pieces. The crucial point, here, is that not only doctors published about 'calorie' – next to them, many anonymous authors used this concept readily. This leads to the following section of this chapter, which investigates the language and tone by which 'calorie' appeared in newspapers and magazines.

Convincing rhetoric

Overall, the 142 articles envisioned 'calorie' in a neutral way – it appeared as a down-to-earth, accustomed notion. Yet, this distant, impartial approach gained importance during the war, growing from 67 per cent in 1914 to 72 in 1916 and to 83 in 1918. 'Calorie', thus, was not surrounded by enthusiastic adjectives or praising language but was increasingly considered a familiar acquaintance.

Positive appreciations appeared in 1914 and 1915 (26 and 17 per cent of the total), when 'calorie' was framed as scientific progress. Dr Van de Velde, for example, wrote, 'Thanks to this computation, one can calculate or, better, translate, each foodstuff [into caloric value]' (*Vooruit*, 25 April 1915, 1). Negative and even hostile pieces were also published, especially in 1916 and 1917 (21 and 13 per cent of the total). In *L'Etoile belge* (8 June 1914, 1), Constantinus ridiculed the analogy of the human body with a machine that both would need combustibles expressed in calories and depicted the physician as an *empêcheur de manger* ('eating preventer'). Some authors used inverted commas to show scepticism (e.g. censored Catholic *Le Siècle*, 24 June 1916, 2), and now and then, 'calorie' was disapprovingly linked to science of the German aggressor (e.g. clandestine *L'Echo belge*, 19 July 1917, 3), one of the rare cases of clear difference between the censored and the free press related to 'calorie'. A Dr Durand mocked the overpowering statistics about caloric content of foodstuffs, which required 'at his side a chemist, a mathematician, a physicist and a couple of members of the Academy of Sciences' (*L'Echo belge*, 13 July 1918, 1).

Dr Van de Velde gave an example of a critical but pragmatic approach of 'calorie': 'In general, and though the method of food units is more scientific than that of calories,[26] the value of food is commonly expressed in calories. This is easier to explain because human nutrition is simply comparable to combustion' (censored Comité National-weekly *Landbouwleven*, 4 January 1917, 9). The doctor referred to the Dutch dietician A. J. C. Snijders,[27] who questioned the accuracy of calories to measure nutritional values – calories supplied by meat differ from those supplied by margarine, whereas food was not only used to convert into labour but also to maintain healthy bodily functions, which required protein, sugar and fat. Van de Velde, thus, was quite pragmatic when using 'calorie' in his newspaper articles. A more hostile stance appeared in a note by E. Van Sweden in *Vooruit* (18 June 1917, 2). The author accused the *Comité National*, among other things, to use 'calorie' in establishing rations, which had become irrelevant by 1917. Moreover, he goes on, 'The theory that a given amount of calories is required to nourish the human body, is incomplete.' A very critical view on the use of 'calorie' was written by Dr Francis Heckel (*L'Illustration*, 10 November 1917, 18–19).[28] He admits that wheaten bread contains more calories than wholemeal bread but argues that the latter comprises vitamins and was better for digestion. He deplored the increasing use of 'calorie' – 'The introduction of calorimetry was soon followed by the creed that all nutritional value of foodstuffs could be captured by caloric values.' Alcohol, he continues, expressed in calories, would induce no one to solely ingesting alcoholic beverages. Van de Velde, Van Sweden and Heckel, thus, introduced a scientific debate into the popular press, expressing caveats about 'calorie'.

Some authors eagerly applied name-dropping to forge authority, but most articles did not refer to scientists or science(s). Only in 1915 and 1917, names of scientists appeared in the newspapers somewhat more than in other years (Table 8.4). Breaking down the articles by signed and unsigned, it appears that the unsigned included slightly more names of scientists. Did authors thus expect to increase their authority? When names are referred to, commonly more than one scientist was mentioned. For example, the anonymous author of *Le coin de la ménagère* referred to Frémy, Voit and Ballaud (*La Belgique*, 19 December 1915, 5) and a Dr Van Caneghem referred to Atwater, Tigerstedt, Voit, Hermans, Seiffert and Müller (censored business paper *La Métropole*, 29 August 1917, 2).

Even though names of experts and reference to sciences are absent in about 70 per cent of newspaper pieces that use 'calorie', the fact that names were actually used reveals the sources of expertise. About 150 references to names of experts

Table 8.4 References to experts and science, and context (in %)

	Expert(s)*	Science*	Context				
			Health	Hunger	Supply	Cost	Other
1914	26	33	40	20	0	13	27
1915	42	24	21	62	0	7	10
1916	29	28	21	14	58	0	7
1917	36	35	24	16	53	0	7
1918	21	24	10	7	73	3	7

*The remaining percentage signifies no reference (e.g. 1914; in 74% of the articles, there is no reference to experts and in 67 per cent no reference to science[s]).

appeared in the newspapers throughout the war. Rubner, von Voit and Snijder were mentioned the most (seven times each); Atwater, Gautier, Labbé, Slosse, König and Müller appeared somewhat less (between two and five times); while a long list of chemists, physicians and sociologists were mentioned only once. Some of these had gained international reputation, while others had local recognition. Now and then, newspaper authors introduced them respectfully as 'professor' or the 'eminent scholar', sometimes adding the name of a town or university. However, a certain P. V. created a professor Schweissfuss (France-based *Courrier de l'armée*, 20 July 1916, 1), making fun of *Ersatz* foodstuffs that were launched by German chemists. Rubner was mentioned alongside his colleague Schweissfuss ('Sweat foot'), who would have published *Über Selbernährung durch eigenes Fett* ('auto-feeding by own fat'), that is, catching one's own sweat to turn into nutritive calories.

Claiming authority and relevance also occurred via reference to big issues, such as diseases, the cost of living or hunger, which would underline the weight of an article (Table 8.4). Most articles using 'calorie' were written within such broader context, and only a minority had 'calorie' as distinct subject. Particularly, articles about hunger and diseases led to mentioning 'calorie' in 1914 and 1915, whereas pieces on food supply used 'calorie' in 1916 and 1917. Probably, 'hunger' addressed mainly the working classes, while 'supply' included everybody, which may explain the shift of interest in 1916. Yet, 'health' would incorporate everybody, although the importance of this theme, related to 'calorie', diminished after 1914. Rising food prices, an issue that caused great anxiety, hardly led to references to 'calorie'.

Yet another means to assess the forging of authority or attracting of interest consisted of referring to other nutritional concepts. In 1914 and 1915, 'calorie' appeared quite often together with other nutritional concepts, such as 'carbohydrate', 'fat' or 'protein'. The mentioning of 'calorie' with only 'carbohydrate' or 'protein' was rare. Yet, throughout the war, 'calorie' appeared increasingly solely in the set of articles (27 per cent in 1914 but 70 per cent in 1918), as if the usage of this concept alone sufficed to seize food necessities. Other nutritional concepts (fat, iron and, very marginally, vitamin) hardly appeared.[29]

A final technique to induce readers consisted of addressing them in a particular way. Throughout the war, readers were directly addressed (e.g. 'You, my reader'; 'My friend'; 'Between you and me'; 'My amiable readers') in a positive way about 'calorie', but this approach weakened (87 per cent in 1914 but 52 per cent in 1918). A more neutral or distant solicitation applied since 1915, merely notifying readers, without wishing to convince them. This, again, may be interpreted as increasing familiarity with the notion of calorie.

Definitions and recommendations

In the 1900s and early 1910s, 'calorie' was a concept that needed to be explained. Was this need felt throughout the war? And if so, how was 'calorie' defined and framed? In 1914, 47 per cent of the articles offered some sort of definition or periphrasis, but this number fell quickly to a poor 7 per cent in 1918 (17 per cent in 1915, 14 per cent in

1916 and 13 per cent in 1917). Apparently, after the first year of war, authors did not feel the urge anymore to explain 'calorie'. It had become familiar during the austere war years because of frequent messages not only in the media, but probably also during lectures, doctor's visits, exhibitions and even daily conversations.

Most explanations of 'calorie' in pre-1914 newspapers were quite short, leaving much to the imagination of the reader, unless they engaged in woolly treatises on food ingestion. The phrase 'A calorie is the heat needed to warm 1 litre of water by 1°C' was often used,[30] but the link between heating of water and healthy human digestion was rarely clarified. The more frequent reference to 'calorie' in Belgian newspapers during the war slightly changed this. Three types of descriptions emerged: the plain, the equivocal and the scientific. The latter may be illustrated by a sizable piece, 'Notes on food' (*Vooruit*, 17 December 1914, 2) in which Dr Van de Velde swiftly mixed physics with physiology and combined nutritional values with food advice and retail prices. He listed the most common foodstuffs that were particularly rich in fat, carbohydrate or protein, providing the link between these and the supply of calories and their cost.

Plain language was used when defining 'calorie' in censored middle-class *Journal de Gand* (10 June 1917, 1), 'The calorie is the unit of measurement of the energetic value of food', and no further explanation was given. However, most definitions were rather complex, enigmatic and blurred presentations of 'burning calories' in the body. An unsigned article of the clandestine Christian metalworkers' fraternity *Journal des métallurgistes belges à Bonnières* (1 May 1918, 7) provides an example. After having referred to albumin, fat, minerals and carbohydrate; explained which foods provide which nutrients; and pointed at the fact that all foodstuffs produce energy under various forms, 'calorie' is put forward to indicate input and output of energy. A list of calories by foodstuff and according to work effort is given, leading to this cheerful conclusion: 'With these data, it becomes easy to propose rational menus that supply the body with the exact stuffs.' The metaphor of a stove appeared regularly, but a candle and fire were also used. *Het Volk* (8 November 1917, 1), for instance, wrote, '[Human] life is like a lamp or fire, that according the degree of intensity, may be lowered or enhanced, but needs to be kept burning and, thus, needs constant alimentation [. . .]. The more it burns, the more fuel is required.'

Equally relevant are the articles that do not explain or present 'calorie'. For example, the censored middle-class *Le Bruxellois* (2 July 1915, 3) announced the publication of a brochure,[31] 'It includes lots of new data about food, cooking, and the quantity of calories that our fragile body needs.' This approach intensified after 1915. 'Calorie' seemed to have become part of daily language, as seen in *La Belgique* (6 December 1916, 2), announcing with regard to public soup distribution that each portion should have a quantity that is 'non inférieure à 300 calories', without any clarification of this value. Moreover, 'calorie' appeared in articles with a political bent, stating that workers were not sufficiently fed – metallurgists obtained a maximum of 800 calories per day, whereas nutritionists claim that they need at least 2,300 calories for light work (patriotic Le Havre-based *Informations belges*, 19 May 1917, 1). Thus, 'calorie' has entered industrial relations. The programme of voluntary labour of Belgians in Germany promised workers and their family extra calories (*La Métropole*, 2 October 1917, 2). Increasingly, 'calorie' replaced 'food'.

'Calorie' was also used in a rather light and even playful way, as seen in *La Métropole* (27 June 1916), when it wrote that Berlin housewives queued for 4 hours to obtain a little butter, which cost them the amount of calories that the butter would provide. Perhaps the best indication to state the widespread and evident use of 'calorie' during the war appeared in 'Pour les chiens' (*Echo de la Sambre et Meuse*, 4 June 1918, 2), calculating a dog's meal in calories. Equally, a piece on canaries' food mentioned higher need of calories during winter (*La Belgique*, 26 July 1916, 3). By and large, 'calorie' seemed to have been taken for granted since most authors did not deem it necessary to explain the notion. This can be seen as a successful further penetration in popular media of a new scientific notion.

An irregular but significant number of articles did not target a particular audience ('None' in Table 8.5, moving between 13 and 41 per cent). In 1914, articles that contained 'calorie' particularly concerned the working classes ('Social status' in Table 8.5), but this attention diminished during the war to the benefit of the *average* consumer ('Mix' in Table 8.5). 'La machine humaine' or 'le citoyen' replaced increasingly 'l'ouvrier'. Yet, other particular groups obtained the newspapers' attention. Exceptional was the mentioning of sportsmen and their caloric needs (*Journal de Gand*, 3 January 1915, 4). In 1915 and 1916, the diet and health of Belgian internees in German prisons became a big concern. For example, Paris-based *L'indépendance belge* (29 June 1915, 4) wrote, 'Each prisoner of war will obtain 2,700 calories', doubting whether this amount will be provided. In 1916, concern emerged about the health of children. In *La Belgique* (6 December 1916, 2), for example, the caloric intake of schoolchildren and pregnant women is considered.

Housewives got some attention throughout the war. Already in August 1914, Dr Delattre called upon the *ménagère* to supply nourishing food (*La Dernière Heure*, 15 August 1914, 1). Housewives' talents appeared elsewhere too – *la bonne ménagère* would undoubtedly provide sufficient calories at low cost, when serving bread, pulses, potatoes, sugar, milk and fats (*Le Bruxellois*, 29 April 1915, 2). An unsigned piece gave another, more critical role to the housewife, when writing, 'The physician, using scientific knowledge, taught [housewives] about caloric value of food; but the housewives, far less clever but more realistic, convert these values in money' (*Le Bruxellois*, 10 May 1917, 3). This article opposed daily practices and, particularly, the cost of calories to theoretic advice for calorie intake.

Table 8.5 Implied audiences and recommendations (in %)

	Implied audience						Recommendations		
	None	Age	Prisoners	Social status	Housewife	Mix	None	Diet	Calorie
1914	13	0	0	40	7	40	33	40	27
1915	24	0	20	14	3	39	72	14	14
1916	37	14	21	0	7	21	65	21	14
1917	20	4	4	14	7	51	69	0	31
1918	41	0	7	10	8	34	55	0	45

The latter opposition between science and common wisdom occurred a couple of times. A clear example is the unsigned article in *La Belgique* (14 January 1917, 3), in which the author makes fun of the *ingénieux chimistes* who would prescribe a precise quantity of calories per day, although, 'We only had for his sorts of calculations the training of a preacher, having always been favoured by a stomach that knows by itself what it wants.' *La Métropole* emphasized that the human body needs more than just calories (1 June 1918, 3). Right after the war, this scepticism about 'calorie' emerged again: 'The food supply will reach 3,500 calories per day and per head. 3,500 calories! We will certainly fatten. Nonetheless, the housewives aren't very enthusiastic: 3,500 calories or 35 million, who cares!' (*Le Matin*, 13 December 1918, 1).

Now and then, dietary recommendations were given in which calories were essential. Tante Colinette in her 'Coin de la ménagère' (*La Belgique*, 6 May 1917, 8) pleaded for using more eggs instead of meat, although both were very expensive. Nevertheless, she wrote, 'Regarding the production of heat, we know that 1 g of albumin supplies 4 calories, 1 g of fat 9 calories. The white of the egg provides about 18 calories and the yolk 62, and in total we obtain 80 calories per egg. Moreover, eggs digest easily.' In the same vein, a Dr Henseval advised not to use saccharine instead of sugar, because the former had no nutritive value (censored Catholic *Le XXe Siècle*, 24 March 1918, 7).

Yet, as shown in Table 8.5, during the war dietary advice was given irregularly, with few recommendations in 1915, 1916 and 1917 (in about one-third of the articles), somewhat more in 1918 (45 per cent) and much more in 1914 (67 per cent). I divided the articles between those with general food recommendations and those where calories played the dominant role.[32] The latter exceeded the former in 1917 and 1918. An example of this already appeared in December 1914, when Dr Toulouse moulded his food advice entirely according to caloric requirements. In clandestine *Le Belge* (16 December 1914, 1), he instructed what to eat if the food supply would deteriorate. The norm of 3,000 kilocalories was the quantity to attain, and he proposed a daily menu with bread (pasta or rice – 1,300 calories), pulses (500 calories), fats (400 calories) and sugar (400 calories), to which meat, eggs or milk should be added. The same outline was followed in various pieces that appeared in 1917 and 1918. An unsigned article in censored Brussels-based *L'Echo régional hebdomadaire* (29 April 1917, 1), for example, established first the caloric requirement and then proposed a couple of nourishing menus with caloric quantities according to the price of foodstuffs. Guidelines for equilibrating the daily menu also use calories (i.e. about one-third calories of animal origin). The presence of 'calorie' in these recommendations may be interpreted as the achievement of caloric hegemony in matters of food advice at the end of the war.

Food advice was directed to everyday cooks, but 'calorie' also appeared when all sorts of authorities were addressed. In the absence of a government in Belgium and because the German invader neglected food provisioning, 'authorities' included the *Comité National*, the French government, local aid organizations and administrations and, towards the end of the war, international organizations. Calling upon these authorities was nigh absent in 1914 (7 per cent of the articles), but rose in 1917 and 1918 to respectively 53 and 45 per cent (1915 – 31 per cent, 1916 – 36 per cent). Local authorities were asked to intensify quality control (e.g. *L'Echo régional hebdomadaire*, 29 April 1917, 1). *Les Petites Abeilles*, the Brussels aid organization for little children, was congratulated for providing more than sufficient calories (*Le Bruxellois*, 7 April 1916, 2). From late 1916 onwards, the caloric content of the *soupe populaire*, provided by regional bureaus of the *Comité National*, was largely discussed, which regularly led to calling upon public authorities to improve food import, increase rations or use intensively local farmers' products. 'Calorie' was prominent in the debate, as Dr Thibaut illustrated (censored *Le Peuple Wallon*, 26 May 1918, 1), when writing, 'The nutritious value merits huge attention, and more than ever I plead for a soup that contains 500 calories, which represent about one fifth of the daily ration.'

By the summer of 1917, the dietary and health situation of all Belgians had highly deteriorated, to which medical reports from Charleroi, Bruges, Mons, Ghent and other towns testified in the press. 'Calories' played a central part in the reports for measuring the degree of starvation. *La Métropole* (3 October 1917, 2) published the report written by the administrator of the local bureau of the Comité National of Mons (Hainault), explaining that 1,130 calories per day could not keep alive a man. Clandestine Le Hague-based *Vrij België* (17 August 1917, 3) published a piece by Dr Van Caneghem about the atrocious food condition in Bruges, which ended by saying that, in the absence of a clear public authority, he was desperate. 'Anonymous' authorities also emerged elsewhere, as in *Le Bruxellois* (11 November 1916, 2), calling upon *les pouvoirs compétents*. This, however, changed when the press started to report about plans for international aid. Foreign food aid for occupied Belgium existed since October 1914, but in late 1917 new initiatives were taken. Tellingly, the norm of this aid was expressed in calories.[33] Thus, *Le XXe Siècle* (6 December 1917, 1) reported on the international conference of the allied armies on food supply of the occupied countries,[34] where it was decided that a minimum would be provided of 2,000 calories during the war and of 3,000 once the war is over. Censored *Le Bruxellois* (31 December 1917, 1) labelled these quantities as pure fiction. This, however, could not prevent that the *Comité National* and the overseas aid were praised, which shows in the piece 'Hoover, ami de la nation belge' (*Le XXe Siècle*, 18 August 1918, 1) – despite the fact that the norm of 2,000 calories per day and person was rarely obtained, the efforts had been immense.

Conclusions

Between 1 January 1914 and 31 December 1918, the word 'calorie' in connection to nutrition appeared in 142 articles spread over 42 Belgian newspapers and magazines of diverse kind. This cannot be considered an overwhelming success. Yet, wide-read newspapers mentioned 'calorie' in various contexts much more than before the war, and articles were often substantial, written by physicians and laymen. The 142 articles did not deem it necessary to repeat definitions, assuming that readers increasingly knew about 'calorie'. A clear sign of 'calorie' becoming customary was the fact that food recommendations were modelled according to caloric needs, which was unseen prior to 1914. Perhaps an adequate evaluation of the use of 'calorie' during the war is given by journalist Baudry de Saunier when expressing his optimism about the possibility of *methodically* studying the diet, which would highly benefit the housewife (*L'Illustration*, 28 September 1918, 23).

Yet, the newspapers and magazines did not denote 'calorie' with eagerness, which may be explained by the fact that this concept was used since the early 1890s and that, moreover, even fervent users of 'calorie' were somewhat sceptical. Furthermore, 'calorie' was now and then considered with apprehension because of the awareness that energy requirements were only one part of human nutrition, and that own, habitual experience (the housewife's wisdom or 'my stomach') had its say. On top of that, 'calorie' was part of the conflict between censored and free press.

The role of the war was crucial for the popularization of 'calorie' in Belgium. Food supply and the daily, healthy diet worried an ever-growing number of people and institutions. Gradually, the size of needs, hunger and food aid was measured by calories, which was handy for international and local organizations. Via one figure (the mythical 3,000 calories), goals, success and failure could be assessed. The case of Belgium is pertinent because of the absence of a government that could inform people about the optimal diet under warfare. Semi-public (the *Comité National*), local and international bodies and, perhaps predominantly, the media, took over the state's role in popularizing the 'calorie'.

9

Nutritional Reform and Public Feeding in Britain, 1917–1919

Bryce Evans

In the popular British memory of the world wars, food rationing has come to obscure the major *public feeding schemes* undertaken by the state. In Britain during the Second World War, there existed a vast network of over 2,000 state-subsidized 'British restaurants', the inspiration for which came from their First World War predecessor – 'national kitchens'. National kitchens were large canteens where hundreds and sometimes thousands of people at a time would sit on long benches to eat cheap yet nutritious food together. These state-supported feeding experiments were also witnessed in other European nations during the war. Indeed as the First World War intensified in mid-1916, seriously threatening food supplies for the civilian population, the British press reported admiringly on the great communal feeding schemes in the enemy's capital, Berlin, and other German cities.[1] And yet the international historiography surrounding wartime public feeding schemes remains underdeveloped.[2] In Britain, national kitchens were locally run, yet part of a major nationwide government-sponsored programme to alleviate food poverty and its effects. They grew out of grass-roots projects within working-class communities to combat wartime supply disruption and price inflation and were first sponsored by the British government in May 1917. By mid-1918, there were over 1,000 national kitchens in Britain.[3] In general, national kitchens remain an under-documented phenomenon in modern British social and economic history,[4] and in particular the role of nutritional reformers in shaping British state-sponsored public feeding in the First World War is unknown. This article addresses this gap in knowledge by detailing the colourful debate surrounding nutritional reform and feeding policy in First World War Britain.

Origins: Recruiting the food reformers

The cost of living and instances of food shortage had increased in Britain since July 1914,[5] but for the first 2 years of war such trends tended to be localized.[6] Food shortages were combated by locally run communal feeding schemes. In Britain's big cities, voluntary groups provided cookery and food economy classes for working-class women, either at communal venues or at women's homes.[7] Other voluntary initiatives aimed at providing nutritious food to the urban poor during wartime, for example, London's 'invalid kitchens', which were patronized by the humanitarian Muriel Paget and were predominately female-run. But with the intensification of war came the transition from Prime Minister Herbert Henry Asquith's 'Wait and See' administration to his successor David Lloyd George's 'Push and Go' ministry in December 1916. Faced with the heightened U-boat campaign of spring 1917, a commission of enquiry linked labour unrest to food price inflation and recommended the opening of industrial canteens.[8] In May 1917, the newly appointed food controller Lord Rhondda (millionaire Welsh businessman D. A. Thomas) publicly advocated the state taking on responsibility for communal feeding for all. With food rationing still many months away, the government's priority was to ensure a basic standard of physical well-being for its populace deriving from an improved national diet.

Rhondda wanted a blueprint for the scheme and tasked an understudy at the Ministry of Food named Kennedy Jones with searching for a tangible example of successful communal dining which could be used as a template by local authorities who might want to take the idea on. Kennedy Jones was a former journalist and Unionist politician who had contested the 1916 Wimbledon election on the radical right-wing ticket of the 'Do-it-Now party' and was a 'man of action' with a reputation, appropriately enough, for 'getting things done'.[9] As mentioned, the real inspiration for communal dining had come from the voluntary efforts of women in Britain's inner cities. Yet in looking for consultants for the brave new world of the national kitchen, Jones instead turned to a group of prominent male middle-class food reformers – R. Hippisley Cox, H. J. Bradley and Eustace Miles – to spearhead the new state-backed 'Kitchens for All'.

Eustace Miles, the most famous of this triumvirate, was a vegetarian who ran a well-known health-food shop and restaurant in Charing Cross, London. Born in 1868, Miles's extraordinary contribution to the culture of the day was his fusion of physical manliness and vegetarianism. A graduate of King's College, Cambridge, he was a handsome and athletic man who combined brains and brawn. A champion on the tennis court, he published widely off it, writing works not only on diet, exercise and self-help, but also on the classics. In 1908, just shy of 40, he won the Olympic silver medal for real tennis in the London Olympics; this was no mean feat since many of his opponents – including the gold medallist – were 20 years younger than him. He was also a successful businessman; the pricey but popular Eustace Miles Restaurant Company Ltd opened in 1906. Partly due to his relentless self-publicity, Miles seemed to embody the masculinist confidence of the British Empire in its Edwardian twilight. Miles's favourite theory was that the meaty, heavy Edwardian diet was deleterious to health and explained various health problems from poor physical fitness to mental problems to disease.[10]

Miles's muscular, manly and outdoorsy image would do much to counter the prevailing stereotype of the vegetarian man as sandal-wearing, wrong-headed and politically suspect.[11] The intellectual set may have patronized his restaurants (George Bernard Shaw was a shareholder), he may have indulged in non-mainstream beliefs such as reincarnation and he may have backed the suffragette movement; but Miles was simultaneously a national treasure when it came to health as a patriotic virtue, a former real tennis champion of England and the world, an Olympic medallist, a philanthropic champion of free food for the poor, virile, active, a popular man of commerce and an all-round good chap. Whereas the first Vegetarian Society (founded in Manchester in 1847) advocated 'a many-sided liberalism', by contrast later vegetarian projects – such as the London Vegetarian Society (1888) – emphasized the health benefits of a non-carnivorous diet on the individual body.[12] Miles was not only influenced by the latter movement, by the outbreak of the First World War he was pretty firmly established as its poster boy. The new *Public Kitchens Handbook* (1917) written by Miles and his collaborators Cox and Bradley was published in time for the opening of Britain's first government-backed national kitchen on London's Westminster Bridge on 21 May 1917. The involvement of Miles, in particular, lent the whole venture a celebrity air, one heightened by the ministry's choice of Queen Mary to open the first site. By the end of the year, national kitchens were popping up in almost every British high street.

Eustace Miles the 'nutter': The brave new world of egalitarian eating

Probably at some future time it will be difficult to believe that each household in the country did its own separate marketing, buying small amounts of food from retail dealers a hundred per cent above cost price, that every hundred houses in a street had each its own fire for cooking, and that at least a hundred human beings were engaged in serving meals that could have been prepared by half a dozen trained assistants.

This was the verdict of Cox, Bradley and Miles in their *Public Kitchens* handbook. There was an upbeat and distinctly futuristic air to the handbook, which claimed that national kitchens were destined to become the new 'centres of civilisation'.[13] Some within the ministry fretted anxiously at the socialism implied by all this and the name itself – 'national kitchen' – sought to reassure that this was a firmly patriotic venture. However, the model that emerged was certainly different to established restaurant dining. These were large canteens where one received a ticket upon entering and then exchanged it for cheap meals at the counter. At the flagship 'Kitchen for All' on Westminster Bridge, a small staff – two cooks, two kitchen maids, a superintendent and a cashier – proved sufficient to cater for between 1,200 and 2,000 people at a time.[14] For speed, customers purchased coupons from a cashier upon entering the premises rather than handing over money after eating. Contact with 'shippers and important dealers in the great markets' meant that meat was procured at 25 per cent of retail price – savings which were in turn passed on to customers.[15] Most national kitchens opened at lunch and dinner time (from 11.30 am to 2 pm and between 5 pm and 8 pm). Fish was the predominant dish for the evening meal. The ministry only provided funding (including 'national kitchen' branding and the fitting of canteens with the latest kitchen equipment) on the basis that certain conditions be met, the most important of which was that prices were kept affordably low and within a set pricing structure to ensure that food was available to all, regardless of class and income.

Another aspect crucial in differentiating national kitchens from charitable soup kitchens was the need to keep up appearances. The Ministry of Food, taking inspiration from the food reformers' wish that national kitchens become 'centres of civilisation', instructed that each outlet 'must not resemble a soup kitchen for the poorest sections of society', but rather a place in which 'ordinary people in ordinary circumstances' could purchase an attractive yet cheap meal.[16] Staff had to be well dressed, the cooks had to demonstrate experience and the décor could not be chintzy. Gramophones and pianos were recommended to add to the ambience.[17] A report in the *Scarborough Post* on Hull's central national kitchen encapsulated this:

> The Hull people do not go into a back street. They avail of commanding premises in a good and busy thoroughfare, they fit their premises on modern lines, and there is no suspicion of shabby genteelness to be observed. On the contrary, were it not for the artistically painted signs you would never dream it was a National Kitchen. The place has the appearance of being a prosperous confectionary and café business. It is dainty and pleasing to the eye and the goods delivered are in appetising form. The business done is enormous. So far fourteen kitchens have been started in Hull.[18]

But for all the modernism and ambitious scale of these ventures, the food reformers who played a role in shaping them were also conscious of traditional prejudices. Free Trade was a popular pre-war policy in Britain, and the cheap white loaf it delivered was a symbol of national pride. Somewhat paradoxically, this nationalistic pride in the cheap white loaf simultaneously celebrated foreign production within a global market system while scorning alien cultures of consumption.[19] The *Public Kitchens Handbook* displayed an awareness of these popular British Edwardian preconceptions. Its authors advised that to ensure long-term popularity national kitchens should 'bow to prejudice' by serving established British meat-based dishes. The guidebook criticized the 'appalling ignorance' of the British people when it came to preparing attractive food. This situation, which the handbook's authors termed a 'national disgrace', had led to the neglect of many different cuisines, most notably those of the 'pleasant land of France – the shrine of all true chefs'. Yet, foreign cuisines and the greater use of vegetables should be introduced only gradually, they instructed. Gravies should be prepared in the 'British way' – from the juices of their own meats – and not, 'as in many restaurants where foreigners rule', from a mixed meat gravy.[20]

As mentioned, the *Public Kitchens Handbook* was spearheaded by Eustace Miles, very much the celebrity food reformer of the day. But Miles's fame did not save him from being lampooned. Take, for example, 'The Mutton Chop', a popular ditty of the time:

> Let Eustace Miles find muscular force
> In carrot cutlets with Plasmon sauce
> Or other equally messy slop
> But give me my old fashioned mutton chop[21]

'Plasmon' was one of Miles's health food products. Another was 'Emprote', a nut-based energy bar marketed to cyclists and walkers. That great traditionalist curmudgeon of the era, the writer G. K. Chesterton, rubbished what he saw as faddish consumerism masquerading as rugged authenticity. In a put-down aimed at Miles, he deliberately misremembered the name of his non-meat substitute as 'nutter'.[22] Chesterton, unsurprisingly, was no fan of national kitchens either, writing elsewhere that a 'communal kitchen' was not 'a real kitchen'.[23] Miles, though, was aware of such popular prejudice against him and the vegetarian image in general. He himself disliked the term 'vegetarian' because of its cultural connotations. 'It stands for cranks and bewhiskered gentlemen and other undesirable people', he once told a reporter, 'my slogan is a "balanced meatless diet". I eat vegetables, eggs and cheese like yourself and others, in their right proportion.'[24] Miles's awareness of a popular 'common-sense' disdain for vegetarian food was borne out in the *Public Kitchens Handbook*. If the desire among proponents of national kitchens to transcend the Victorian philanthropy of the soup kitchen was palpable, so too was the worry that national kitchens would be seen by the public as lofty avant-garde projects pushing trends like vegetarianism. Accordingly, the *Public Kitchens Handbook* noted guardedly the public 'suspicion' that soup kitchens only served bland 'bean-based dishes'.[25]

Nutritional impact and national character

On the other hand, the wartime imperative not to waste food allowed Miles and his fellow food reformers to reiterate their favourite warnings about the negative nutritional effect of peeling and boiling vegetables. 'The peel, tops and outside leaves contain valuable salts which are lost when poured down the sink and boiling alters the composition of the salts.'[26] Instead, simmering, stewing, frying or braising vegetables was recommended. Flavour, the handbook told its readers, was paramount, stimulating the digestive fluids and helping to extract the full food value whereas 'dull cooking' left the digestive fluids 'inert'.[27] These concerns about 'proper cooking' dovetailed with the health-giving benefits of vegetarianism, which Miles was keen to stress. In the years leading up to the First World War, the number of vegetarian cookbooks published in Britain and America increased, with three prominent volumes published in the first year of the war alone.[28] Communal dining, a feature of the early vegetarian movement on both sides of the Atlantic, was viewed as a way to promote the healthiness of the vegetarian diet through social interaction.[29]

The latest research on diet change during the war, which challenges some of the upbeat conclusions of the The Working Class Cost of Living (Sumner) committee of 1918, points to a reduction in the consumption of sugar, cheese, butter, butcher's meat, fruit and vegetables, and the increased consumption of bacon, sausages and margarine. This resulted in an overall reduction in vitamins A and B12 for skilled and unskilled workers and reductions in vitamins C, D and riboflavin for skilled workers.[30] Such revelations would have disappointed the authors of the handbook who, in attempting to strike a balance between healthy eating and popular consumption, envisaged that the meat consumed in national kitchens would compensate for potential shortages of foodstuffs which were not considered key. Therefore, although the handbook was co-written by Miles, a committed vegetarian, it devoted considerable time to explaining how to ensure meat was cooked attractively. Even cheap cuts of meat should not be merely boiled 'for there is an unexplained repugnance to a grey hash'. Instead, all meats should be 'lightly fried, then cooked slowly with a little stock and vegetables'. Deep frying was recommended as the most economical means of cooking meat.[31] There was also a desire to improve the national character through improving diet and reducing waste. The poor physical standard of British recruits to the Anglo-Boer war of 1899–1902 had resulted in a national anxiety about how poor nutrition negatively impacted national fitness.[32] The *Handbook* therefore combined patriotism, food culture and diet, its authors hoping that national kitchens would 'avoid the tendency of all large kitchens to provide "factory food" and would instead be "centres of civilisation" fostering the "art and skill" of good food rather than its "manufacture"'.[33] Gas was favoured for cooking over electricity because 'few persons familiar with its use were available' and the price too high; the latest technology, such as roasting ovens, steamers and water jackets, was to be used only where available.[34] It instructed that 'odds and ends must be used' – peelings, stalks, outside leaves and tops of vegetables, to say nothing of bone and gristle'.[35]

Ultimately, the final draft of the ministry's official *National Kitchens Handbook* was edited heavily by civil servants, who deleted some of the food reformers' social wishes. For instance, the favourable social consequences anticipated by food reformers like Miles as a corollary of the movement, such as the power of communal dining to quell popular demand for alcohol, did not make it into the final draft.[36] What nonetheless remains striking is Miles and company's awareness of the need for a balance between nutritional good practice and popular national cultures of consumption. Inspired by food reformers like Miles, it seems that national kitchens managed to achieve this equilibrium. This was certainly the opinion of the famed author Arnold Bennett. Bennett's comments on national kitchens, published in the *Daily News* in mid-1918, are significant because of the author's relationship with modernism and literary modernism in particular. There was something distinctly futuristic about the universalism of communal dining, something which chimed with the ethos of high modernism of the 1910s and 1920s and its impulse towards a radical break with the past.[37] Well-fed and middle-aged when he composed his opinions on national kitchens (one of his legacies was an omelette named after him by chefs at London's Savoy Grill), Bennett – who liked to think he knew a thing or two about gastronomy – went on to echo some of the sniffier verdicts of the *Public Kitchens Handbook*, claiming that the average British person 'does not understand either cooking or diet' and that French restaurants far surpassed their British equivalents. On the other hand, Bennett has also been represented as a champion of the expanding British working class, in contrast to his modernist literary contemporaries, many of whom held the ever-expanding masses in little more than contempt. A popular author and journalist who was open about the fact that he wrote for money, Bennett aimed his writing at a mass audience and aspired to be more in touch with 'the people' than his detractors of the intellectual avant-garde.[38] This aspect, too, is in evidence in Bennett's remarks on national kitchens where, although critical of the term 'communal', he characterized resistance to the scheme as 'reactionary', identifying middle-class snobbery as the enemy.

> I do not know how many national or municipal kitchens there are today. Probably not more than five hundred. There ought to be perhaps twenty thousand [. . .] municipal authorities ought to lead instead of waiting to be pushed. Innumerable towns are extremely sluggish [. . .] The impetus for them should and must come from the middle class. The lower class, for obvious reasons, is notoriously the class with the most adamantine prejudices about food. It has never had the chance to educate itself in diet and cooking. It is wants a huge, unmistakeable example, and that example it ought to have.[39]

That 'unmistakeable example', wrote Bennett, was the national kitchens. They were eliminating waste, achieving economies of scale in buying and serving food cheaper, guarding against disease and offering ordinary people a greater variety of dishes than would otherwise be available. Anticipating the universalism and purchasing power of supermarkets, he saw national kitchens as the way to overcome the small shopkeeper's refrain, 'That is what I have to sell. You can take it or leave it.' What's more, Bennett (who, ironically enough, was to die of typhoid after defying the advice of a waiter not to drink water from the tap at a Parisian restaurant) identified expert nutritional advice as key to national kitchens' success. Identifying the 'expert scientific management of their cooking processes' as favourable to the efforts of 'any single family – no matter how ingenious or up-to-date', he claimed,

> A large proportion of the nation still has a secret contempt, and even hatred, of scientific methods and exact knowledge. Speak to it of calories and [. . .] it will shy. Mention the theory of a scientific dietary and it will at once suspect that you intend either to starve it or to render the meal-table a purgatory. Say that the open fire and the saucepan are not the last word of culinary apparatus, and it will praise the cooking of its grandmother, who had nothing but the open fire and the saucepan. This reactionary spirit has got to be faced in the open and defeated by the force of proved facts.[40]

Some of these thoughts toed the official line, of course, and Bennett, who was at the time performing his war service as director of propaganda for France at the Ministry of Information, heaped the customary praise on Minister of Food Control Lord Rhondda. Yet Bennett's enthusiasm for the national kitchen was clear; insisting that national kitchens 'ought to be encouraged and patronised and cried aloud for', he recommended that they continue after the war and not be written off as an extraordinary war measure.

However, as discussed later, the coming of peace in 1918 would complicate the term 'national' and what exactly it signified. Many would urge a return to the pre-war mantra of free trade as an essentially British value, something contrary to state-supported social eating whether it was dubbed 'national' or not. Moreover, the introduction of ration books issued to individuals and families from early 1918 had already started to damage national kitchens. Bennett remarked on this, citing an instance in Salford where customers had criticized the quality of the meat served in the national kitchen, claiming that their ration book coupons entitled them to better-quality meat than that on offer. Bennett blamed this on the managers of the Salford national kitchen, giving examples – notably – from municipal kitchens in Hamburg, where the ration value of a coupon could instead be spread over several days (and several meals). What he failed to appreciate was that the damage had already been done. With people adjusting to consumption via the rationing system, press coverage of incidents like this confirmed for some that the national kitchen, as Bennett characterized prejudice against it, was a 'quasi-paternal' institution meant only for the very poor.

The role of domestic science colleges

Bennett's call for more scientific experts when it came to food and diet was shared by the Ministry of Food. Hippisley Cox, Bradley and Miles were not the only high-profile food reformers recruited by the Ministry of Food to assist in the national kitchens movement. Three prominent women – Maud Pember Reeves, Constance Peel and Kate Manley – were recruited by the Ministry of Food to head a women's department, which became the national kitchens advisory committee. Reeves was a suffragist and Fabian socialist, who in 1913 published *Round about a Pound a Week*, an influential survey of poverty in Lambeth which pointed to the structural causes of poverty rather than maternal negligence.[41] Her co-director Peel was familiar to the fashionable classes as editor of *The Queen*, a regular contributor to *The Lady* and, from 1918, editor of the women's page in the *Daily Mail*. Manley was an inspector of domestic subjects for the Board of Education.[42] Since Reeves' 1913 report had called for free school meals, Manley provided an important link between social reformers like Reeves and Peel and the educational authorities. Reeves' role was interrupted by the bereavement of her son in June 1917 but Peel travelled nationwide on behalf of the ministry, delivering almost 200 addresses promoting the economical use of food.[43]

Nutritional instruction, then, was a key part of the national kitchens message. Reacting to the mounting food supply difficulties of late 1917, domestic scientists issued advice informed by contemporary beliefs. The conference of teachers of domestic science produced a pamphlet in May 1917 which not only contained the blunt instruction that people must 'eat less food' but also advocated Fletcherizing – 'well masticated, or in other words, well chewed food, yields more nourishment to the body than food which is eaten quickly and is not properly chewed'.[44] Elizabeth Waldie, head teacher at the Glasgow and West of Scotland College of Domestic Science, the largest of the three great Scottish cookery training schools, published her bestselling *Economical Recipes Suitable for War Cookery* in 1917. Cooking must respond to 'the greatest struggle of nations the world has ever known' by supplying energy for war work and achieving fuel economy, she wrote. Waldie broke wartime nutrition into four food groups. 'Flesh Formers' – scarce sources of protein such as meat, eggs and milk – which could be replaced by cheaper meats, nuts, beans and dried fruit; 'Heat and Energy Producers' – fats which were in short supply – could also be obtained from suet, nuts, seeds and fish; 'Sugars and Starches' – for which Waldie recommended replacing jam with syrup and treacle; and 'Blood Purifiers and Bone Formers' – to be found in mineral salts and vegetable acids and now largely to be gotten from green vegetables, she instructed. Waldie's book of *War Cookery* also provided a number of substitute recipes. These included 'Poor Man's Goose' (made from pig liver), 'Brains on Toast' (made from sheep's brains) and 'Very Economical Plum Pudding'.[45]

Unsurprisingly, the Ministry of Food's national kitchens division was keen to harness the expertise of individuals like Waldie as well as using Britain's colleges of domestic science to its advantage. Cookery schools had been increasingly forced to adapt to the wartime ethic of egalitarian eating in instruction as well as recommendation. Waldie had redesigned her college's entire syllabus in the summer of 1917 in order to ensure that every course adhered to the imperative of cookery instruction 'of the greatest nutritive value at the least possible cost'. As part of the national Food Economy Campaign, the college dropped its Special Certificate in High Class Cookery in favour of free cookery courses to large audiences on topics such as 'meatless cooking'.[46] In general, Britain's schools of domestic science 'did their bit' by publishing leaflets on wartime cookery, running cookery classes for widows and even carrying out experiments into 'fatless dishes' and other nutritional innovations.[47] To the Ministry of Food, collaboration with these domestic economy experts was an enticing prospect.

The feeling, though, was not mutual. Whereas the Edinburgh School of Cookery resolved, in April 1917, to establish 'one or more communal kitchens', its Glasgow equivalent worried that the autonomy of cookery training schools was threatened by the emergence of national kitchens.[48] The Liverpool school, for its part, sent a board member to inspect London's national kitchens; after hearing her report, the board agonized over the 'very great expenses' for 'equipment and upkeep' and hoped they would not end up being incorporated into the project and thus end up footing the bill.[49] These fears were confirmed and the movement towards a more statist political economy of food further underlined when, in May 1918, cookery colleges received instruction from the Ministry of Food that all new national kitchens 'in large population centres' were to be located near to cookery training schools. Training schools were to educate future national kitchen staff. In assisting the formation of national kitchens, college principals were instructed to liaise with their local education authority and food control committee.[50] In April 1918, the Ministry of Food took over the restaurant and training kitchens of London's National Training School of Cookery. The ministry hoped that availing of the 'really first-class cooking' of the training school would reinforce the point that national kitchens were not merely cheap and cheerful.[51] Meanwhile, the schools bemoaned their loss of autonomy.

Steadily, leading teachers of domestic science were poached by the Ministry of Food, which bettered the salaries of the best teachers if they agreed to leave their posts to become national kitchen supervisors.[52] In May 1918, Scotland's war cookery guru, Elizabeth Waldie, was headhunted by the ministry and made supervisor for national kitchens in the south-west of Scotland.[53] Such tactics revealed that the alliance between colleges of domestic science and national kitchens was always an uneasy one. The Ministry of Food was, on the one hand, keen to recruit the principals of domestic science colleges onto consultative committees but, on the other, increasingly reluctant to release food to their institutions for educational purposes.[54] Domestic science colleges, in turn, felt squeezed; it was not long, however, before national kitchens raised the ire of another, more influential, commercial lobby.

Resistance grows and national kitchens decline

In August 1918, Glasgow Corporation's special committee on national kitchens was approached by a six-man deputation from the Glasgow District Restaurateurs' and Hotel Keepers' Association. The restaurateurs had gotten wind that the corporation was to buy a large restaurant in the city centre and run it as a national kitchen. This central location, they claimed, would be hugely detrimental to the restaurant trade in the city. What annoyed the Glasgow restaurateurs most was the location – the new restaurant would operate not in the city's slums but on the bustling Argyle Road.[55] Naturally, the resistance to public feeding from the catering trade recurred throughout the country. This was not a matter of the trade trying to profiteer at a time of scarcity, maintained restaurant owners; rather, the very principle of state-subsidized restaurants was immoral since it offended that quintessential British value – the notion of 'fair play'. Similarly, a letter to the ministry from London caterer John Pearce claimed that national restaurants, thanks to 'preferential treatment' from the state, had simply failed to 'play the game'. Writing in late 1918, he claimed that the Ministry of Food could have fulfilled its duty by establishing national kitchens during dock strikes and hunger marches, but had preferred to concentrate on competing with private retailers.[56] This communique encapsulated another staple of popular pre-war free trade culture – the democratic ethic of the neutral state.[57] With the post-war return to normal trading conditions, proponents of 'fair play' like Pearce found the whiff of the big state increasingly malodorous.

The armistice of November 1918 was to provide another blow to the broad ethic of collectivism. It was followed by the post-war winding down of the Ministry of Food and, with it, the forward march of the national kitchen was steadily brought to a halt. Cost-cutting now became the priority for the Ministry of Food, and national kitchens found themselves squarely in the firing line. To save money, national kitchen supervisors were no longer to be trained by the leading British domestic science colleges but were to receive their entire training at headquarters in London.[58] Elizabeth Waldie, who had been so enthusiastic about taking up her post as supervisor of national kitchens that she had turned down a substantial pay rise from her former employers in favour of the job, left her post shortly thereafter, taking up a new job as inspector of the Scottish Education Department.[59] With the lease on the flagship national kitchen at London's New Bridge Street set to expire in May 1919, the national kitchens advisory committee declared that its closure would be 'disastrous' and the 'moral effect' of closure 'very bad'.[60] But the ministry was by this stage busy selling on its national kitchens elsewhere to private food retailers like London's Spiers and Ponds.[61] Councils were obliged to inform the ministry of plans for the closure of locally run kitchens. The committee frequently protested against the closure of local premises, citing social need, but was powerless to force borough or district councils to keep their kitchens open without central financial support.[62] At the signing of the armistice in November

1918, the number of officially registered national kitchens in Britain had dwindled to 363; 6 months later, there were 120 less.[63]

By early 1919, the national kitchens division had taken over catering in royal parks – a further sign of the kitchens' journey from popular and cheap communal ventures to established institutions. Sure enough, these catering units were soon charging more than affordable restaurants like Lyons. Soon the national kitchens division was doing handsomely from its running of refreshments in parks, reporting that £700 had been taken from four sites during the Easter holidays in 1919. The national kitchens advisory committee urged that 'arrangements for poor children' be made through a special discount children's lunch[64] but it was clear that national kitchens, by this point under Kennedy Jones' stewardship, were evolving from cut-price communal ventures into highly profitable and expensive park cafes. Jones claimed that catering in royal parks had provided food at 'reasonable prices'.[65] The advisory committee's Maud Pember Reeves countered that prices were 'excessive' and that they were unable to service large numbers of people.[66] Certainly, the sites at Kensington Gardens, Kew Gardens, Hyde Park, Regent's Park and Primrose Hill had turned over an impressive £4,000 in 3 months.[67]

For all the committee's social concern, it was clear to all concerned that national kitchens had morphed into something quite distinct from their original purpose, now serving tea and cakes rather than hearty vegetable-based meals. By late 1919, national kitchens had closed their doors for good. The national kitchens division was wound up, its advisory committee disbanded. While some kitchens persisted as non-affiliated ventures, the last instance of mass feeding carried out under the national kitchens division's auspices was feeding hot cooked food to the thousands of police and lorry drivers called into London to take up the transport duties of striking railway workers.[68] In just 2 years, the national kitchens movement had performed a 180-degree turn, resembling something quite different from the communal vision imagined by the food reformers first recruited to advise on them.

Conclusion

The British 'national kitchen' of the First World War was part of a wartime movement across Western Europe towards state-supported communal dining, a model of social eating quite different to the food bank model prevailing in Britain and elsewhere at the time of writing. In providing affordable yet nutritious food to the masses, the British government was determined that these new venues transcend social class and be attractive social spaces 'for all'. The goal (to improve dietary standards *en masse*) was, of course, underlined by an unspoken and more cynical motive – to ensure fit fighting and working bodies to support the continuing slaughter of war, a British priority which had first been flagged by the notoriously poor physical standard of recruits to the Boer War at the turn of the century. The real 'blueprint' for the scheme came from organic voluntary efforts started by working-class women but, in keeping with the masculinist standards of the age, this was soon forgotten as the wartime priority of male potency interjected. The very name of the venture reflected conservative anxieties about the subversive potential of socialism, and indeed vegetarianism.

Yet, at the same time, the British national kitchen movement was infused with a genuinely progressive élan and many who were involved with the project thought themselves part of a long-term nutritional and social effort to improve national character and eliminate disease through diet. Food reformers recruited to advise on the project, like Eustace Miles, were certainly typical of this forward-looking spirit, if at the same time wary of the ridicule they had previously attracted for their beliefs. The government's recruitment of staff from the nation's domestic science colleges further reinforced the move towards scientifically informed social progress through dietary innovation. As such, the national kitchen is symbolic of a broader shift in Britain from pre-war imperial free trade towards a form of war socialism. As with other wartime measures, this would prove short-lived once the guns had fallen silent, but the national kitchen was to re-emerge in the Second World War 20 years later, this time rebranded 'British Restaurant'. Then, the same old conservative anxieties about large numbers of people congregating to dine cheaply were to re-emerge. These anxieties, though, were tempered by greater nutritional understanding and advice – social and nutritional – which echoed many of the observations of the First World War food reformers, perhaps proving that Eustace Miles and his ilk were not such 'nutters' after all.

10

The Sin of Eating Meat: Fascism, Nazism and the Construction of Sacred Vegetarianism

Francesco Buscemi

This chapter analyses the negative perception of meat-eating and the positive sense of meat abstention shown by the propagandas of three ferocious European dictatorships: the Italian Regency of Fiume, Italian fascism and Nazism. In relation to the topic of this book, what is interesting is that the disease linked to dietary change, here, is not physical illness. Rather, it is a moral form of disease. In fact, these propagandas related eating meat to their enemies, especially in the Fiume and in the Nazi cases. In the languages of these propagandas, eating meat meant impurity, inability to reach the highest level of knowledge and wisdom and, finally, how all dictatorships refer to their enemies, which is, inferiority. That is why I have termed this kind of vegetarianism as 'sacred', because, in the intention of the propaganda, it conferred a label of 'sacrality' on those who professed it, in contrast with those who did not.

To better understand this, it is important to underline what vegetarianism was in those years outside these dictatorships. More specifically, it would be really reductive to talk about a single vegetarianism. Rather, in those years, many forms of this food practice were already present, even though involving a minority of people, compared to what happens today. However, vegetarianisms existed and spanned science and nostalgia, politics and religion. For example, science was certainly central to the experience of Dr John Harvey Kellogg and to his attempt to prepare cereals in new ways. However, Dr Kellogg was also a member of the Seventh-day Adventist Church, a religious group that banned meat from their diet. For Kellogg, thus, being vegetarian improved both physical health and inner spirit.[1]

In Europe, often vegetarianism related to nostalgia for a golden age extraneous to modernity. Germany was at the forefront, as the many social groups and cults gathering under the big umbrella of *Lebensreform* (life reform) demonstrate. Lebensreform was a German movement that originated around 1880 involving many social and religious movements fighting modern life and industrial development, and supporting vegetarianism and rurality. It split into many components in the Nazi years.[2] Its links to the Nazi ideology are developed below.

In Italy, vegetarianism was late. While in Britain the first vegetarian society was founded in 1847, the fist Italian vegetarian association originated in 1952. Until then, vegetarianism was considered as a sort of illness relating to odd people. In this chapter, I demonstrate that Asian and religious references were necessary to fascism in order to turn this unusual food practice into ideology.[3] The constructive nature of vegetarianism under these dictatorships is confirmed by the fact that fascism and Nazism only liked vegetarianism on an intellectual and sometimes dietary level[4] and that politically the three tyrannies were in contrast with the vegetarian associations.[5]

Many studies have investigated the propagandistic apparatuses of fascism and Nazism, focusing in turn on a broad historical approach,[6] strategies,[7] everyday lives,[8] and the media.[9] Only a few, however, have centred on food and more specifically on meat and vegetarianism. Sax[10] has brilliantly analysed Nazi policies towards animals, and his account of the Nazi construction of animal protection has been really useful for this current study. Alexander Nützenadel[11] investigated the fascist food (and meat) policies, which fought undernutrition drawing on neo-Malthusian theories, aimed to guarantee self-sufficiency to the Italians, but failed because of the economic crisis. I have focused on the demonization of the enemy through meat,[12] and Bernhard Forchtner and Ana Tominc have looked at a vegan neo-Nazi group on YouTube and its recipes.[13]

All of this concerns Italian fascism and German Nazism. Literature on the Italian Regency of Fiume is instead much less developed and is almost exclusively in Italian. Due to this absence from the international debate, in the next section, I explain what this dictatorship was, also drawing on the few studies about it.

The Italian Regency of Fiume

The Italian Regency of Fiume and of Carnaro (the gulf of Fiume) occurred from September 1919 to December 1920. In contrast with the Italian government, a group of Italian citizens (the *arditi*) invaded the region and took power of it. They were led by the Italian poet Gabriele D'Annunzio, whose point was that Fiume and Carnaro naturally belonged to Italy, but that the Italian government was too weak to conquer it. D'Annunzio was the head of the regency for the entire period. In December 1920, the Italian army entered the city and easily defeated the *arditi*, putting an end to the regency. However, for many historians, that experience was one of the bases of the later fascist dictatorship in Italy.[14]

There are two different historical perspectives of the Italian Regency of Fiume. The first one centres on its progressive policies,[15] such as women's right to vote and equality between all the religions. Renzo De Felice defines the regency as a modern regime stemming from a combination of the various radical tendencies occurring in Italy and Europe at that time.[16] Related to this, article 2 of the constitution of the regency established that all people are equal without any differentiation of gender, religion, race or class.[17] Moreover, the left-wing intellectual Antonio Gramsci supported D'Annunzio.[18] In the end, some see Fiume as a combination of the worker movement and of an idealized worship of God Pan and Nature.[19] Linking to it, other historians see the regency as an anticipation of the hippie movement of the 1960s.[20] In fact, it supported a natural way of living and an ideally pure Nature. Many *arditi* publicly followed alternative (for those times) lifestyles, such as homosexuality and nudity, which at that time and later were banned in both dictatorial and democratic contexts.[21]

The second historical perspective of the regency highlights that D'Annunzio's regime was a kind of rehearsal of fascism. *Il Comandante*, as the *arditi* and the propaganda used to call him, was one of the main supporters of Benito Mussolini,[22] and certainly the regency anticipated many fascist elements, such as the cult of personality and the resort to violence to impose dominion and power, even against the will of the majority of people.[23]

It was to reach these aims that the Italian regency developed a strong propagandistic apparatus, which, apart from traditional weapons such as journals and fliers, also adopted less frequent forms of communication, for example, letters and books, which I analyse below. In fact, many of the *arditi* were actually intellectuals and novelists, such as Giovanni Comisso and Guido Keller. Analysing this propaganda is necessary to understand what meat meant in Fiume during the regency.

The majority of Fiume propaganda centred on D'Annunzio, who is seen as a sort of spiritual figure, even involving omnipotence and deity. Just as already demonstrated with Nazi propaganda,[24] even Fiume propaganda split the world between purity and impurity. D'Annunzio perfectly embodied purity in each of his representations. The *arditi* were represented as pure as well, but on a lower level than D'Annunzio, seen as unattainable. However, legionnaires were always represented as courageous and violent, the slim and athletic men risking their lives to defend the *Italianness* of Fiume.

Another protagonist of Fiume propaganda, and Fiume regency in general, was Guido Keller. Keller was one of the principal collaborators of D'Annunzio's, and an important official in Fiume's hierarchy. He was an aviator, and for the fascist propagandist Pozzi, flying was for him a way of freeing his spirit.[25] Keller was a nature lover and vegetarian who used to sleep on trees, talk to animals and go around totally naked. He loved to contemplate natural landscapes and studied birds and their way of flying.[26] 'We are flowers with our secrets of vastness', he used to say.[27] Overtly homosexual as other *arditi*, in Fiume Keller promoted and practiced free love.

Keller was the sole man among the *arditi* who was on familiar speaking terms with D'Annunzio.[28] Leeden considers him a hippie about 50 years in advance of the time,[29] even for his interest in Hindu and Buddhist philosophies. He believed that Oriental races were superior to the Western ones, and that the Western world only overwhelmed Oriental civilizations thanks to its superiority in violence.[30]

As a result of these intellectual interests, Keller discovered the swastika symbol, which was a Hindu and Buddhist element relating to Nature's equilibrium and harmony. Keller adopted the swastika as the symbol of the group of writers and intellectuals that he led in Fiume, called Yoga. This name, for Giovanni Comisso, had no links to the Indian discipline.[31] Interestingly, Keller chose the swastika in 1920, the same year that this symbol was adopted as the logo of the Nazi Party in Germany. Apart from the temporal coincidence, there is no evidence of contact between the two groups.

A great part of Fiume propaganda centred on pushing the Italian state to recognize Fiume as a part of Italy, but the Italian government always refused to intervene. This is why the Italian government is often represented by Fiume's propaganda as the worst enemy of the regency, and the Prime Minister Francesco Saverio Nitti is continually ridiculed. If D'Annunzio and the *arditi* are continually depicted as the quintessence of purity, Nitti and his allies are often represented as impure. As in the case of Nazi propaganda, purity and impurity were also often expressed in Fiume through food in general and meat in particular.

The Italian historian Giordano Bruno Guerri[32] explains the relationship between D'Annunzio and food through the story of D'Annunzio's turtle, who died because it ate too many roses in the garden. From that day onwards, D'Annunzio put the dead animal on the table of his house, in order to remind his guests of eating moderately. Guerri adds that *Il Comandante* loved simple food and fruit.

This inclination to extoll the moderation of food also affected Fiume propaganda. The *arditi* are always represented as slim and light. The airy, slim man in many of D'Annunzio and Keller's writings was the same fast and active man extolled by Futurism.[33] Lightness became a mental, moral and existential category, which was opposed to gravity. This brought about the myth of the slim, rebel man, in contrast with the heavy man who is slow and conservative.[34]

This view is in many of D'Annunzio's propagandistic messages against Nitti. Here, food is key to the construction of the negative image of the prime minister. On the 11 September 1919, the day before entering in Fiume, D'Annunzio addresses his speech *Italia o Morte* (either Italy or death).[35] First, he attacks the resignation of Italian people in considering Fiume a non-Italian city. To underline the passivity of the Italians, D'Annunzio says that they are only satisfied with digesting their daily meal, and only concerned about their food in future days. Second, he focuses on Nitti's passivity, saying that the prime minister wants his and Italians' souls to be filled with 'adipe e grassezza' (fat and stoutness). Third, to underline Nitti's passivity again, D'Annunzio says that every day the prime minister shifts one length more in his belt loop, as he is becoming fatter and fatter.

In a propagandistic text written by Keller, Nitti is seen as a traitor who eats and drinks as long as it is possible, while in other propagandistic texts the *arditi* are always slim, like their knives.[36] Finally, one of the historical personalities who inspired D'Annunzio and the *arditi* is Giuseppe Garibaldi, the hero of Italian Risorgimento, who, not by chance, is represented as having a big soul and a small body.[37]

Meat has often been analysed as the food through which men extoll their masculinity.[38] Many studies have underlined how, through meat, men come in contact with blood, sex and death.[39] Even in everyday life, meat production, preparation and consumption have always been seen as a male activity.[40]

While the masculine role of meat has been frequently acknowledged, it is interesting to note that this did not happen in Nazi propaganda, where meat was frequently associated with the Jews, and Kosher slaughter and the Jewish butcher were further opportunities to stereotype and attack an entire race.[41] In the end, for the Nazis, meat was impure, then belonging to the enemy, while purity was frequently represented by old myths in which eating meat was forbidden, or by Hitler's vegetarianism, which was subsequently seen as a propagandistic construction rather than a real inclination.[42]

In this scenario, it is interesting to find out how Fiume propaganda represented meat. Even though the Fiume regime acknowledged a woman's basic right to vote, it was certainly a male-led regime. Analysing meat in its propaganda is thus useful in order to understand its adherence either to the more widespread interpretation of meat as a masculine food or as an anticipation of the demonization of meat put forward by Nazi propaganda.

The group Yoga aimed to achieve uncorrupted lives and mirrored Oriental philosophies, and the same members defined it as 'a union of free spirits who tend to be perfect'.[43] Keller's vegetarianism pervaded the whole group. In his book *Le Mie Stagioni*,[44] Giovanni Comisso describes the relationship to food of the members of the group in detail. Comisso writes that Keller persuaded the others to reject meat and eat vegetables and honey, sometimes together. Eating was considered a fastidious necessity, and they almost managed to get rid of this obligation. The members rented some fruit fields around Fiume and used to climb the trees to eat fruit as a complete meal. Apart from fruit and vegetables, the members of the Yoga used to eat cheese and milk, and Keller also used to eat rose petals, because he considered them well fed by the sun. In the end, for the members, this was the way to also eat landscape, sun, wood and, above all, thoughts, adventure and love.[45]

So far, this interesting way of constructing food during the Italian Regency of Fiume has been seen as a strange caprice of bizarre intellectuals or an anticipation of the Futurist cuisine.[46] Instead, I argue that, as is clear in this part of Comisso's book, the vegetarianism of the members of the Yoga was a means to get in contact with Nature and with a higher level of knowledge. Meat leads to heaviness and passivity, and Keller's vegetarian recipes, rather than anticipating Futurism, paved the way to a higher kind of life and to purity. Vegetarianism in Fiume was a way of cleansing the body and soul from the intoxications of daily life, and was also suggested by the old Oriental myths followed by many *arditi*.

This is even more evident in another of Comisso's books, *Il Porto dell'Amore*,[47] when it is said that heavy food brings sleep, and if we get rid of it we would double our available time. Sleeping is the most immediate expression of passivity, the evil in the propaganda of the regime. As highlighted in point number 44 of the constitution of the regency, the perfect *ardito* must be light, in order to run, fight, ride, swim, but also play music and sing.[48] Meat is not the right food to achieve this level of active participation or purity. Impurity may be found in banks, beards and prejudices, which are killing Fiume, which is instead a pure, idealized place.[49]

To achieve purity, four members of the group went to live in a small house around Fiume. Keller, Comisso, Henty Furst and Léon Kochnitzsky experienced a simple, vegetarian and healthy life. Comisso, in one of the letters to his family,[50] explained that in that house they only ate honey, fruit, milk and butter. The gained lightness permitted them to go to the forest in the night and sleep beneath the trees. Comisso defines it as an unimpaired life that he had never hoped to realize for his body. Again, body and soul may go hand in hand thanks to abstention from meat.

Apart from vegetarianism as a food habit leading to purity, Fiume propaganda also dealt with the symbolic meaning of meat highlighted by Nick Fiddes.[51] In two letters[52] that they exchanged during the regency, D'Annunzio and Keller tell of an episode that occurred some days earlier. D'Annunzio was at home, suffering from high fever, and Keller brought him grapes. When the *Comandante* asked Keller why he brought grapes, the vegetarian *ardito* answered that a grape is the symbol of blood and military. D'Annunzio agreed and wrote that grapes are the purest fruit generated by Italian blood. The fascist propagandist Sandro Pozzi added that the *Comandante* knew that all the youth of the 14,000 Italians who died in conquering Fiume was present in that grape.

These letters show a very interesting symbolic replacement. What D'Annunzio and Keller, and later Pozzi, are talking about is blood, the blood of the soldiers dead for the *Italianness* of Fiume. Usually, when blood is represented by food, it is represented through meat. In this case, conversely, it is grapes that represent blood. Finally, grapes are also the medicine that heals the *comandante*.

Meat, conversely, is often represented in order to symbolize impurity and, above all, the enemy. A document from the *Ufficio Stampa e Propaganda* (press and propaganda office)[53] states that the honour of the nation has been bartering with three different objects each linked to three different enemies: the smile of a French prostitute, a rise at the London stock exchange and a quintal of American meat. Therefore, in this idealized perception of Italy, meat is represented as corrupting Italian purity and as impure as prostitution and money.

Nazi propaganda

All of this becomes clearer if we analyse the way in which another criminal dictatorship, Nazism, represented meat. Much literature has analysed Hitler's vegetarianism. Philosophically, it seems that Adolf Hitler became a vegetarian due to the great admiration he had for the composer Richard Wagner, who believed that meat-eating had contaminated human beings and shortened their lives. Obsessed with the risk of cancer, Hitler decided to give up eating meat to improve his health.[54] James Cross Giblin points out that Hitler's acknowledged problem of excessive gas was even worsened by his vegetarian diet.[55]

But it is the constructed nature of Hitler's vegetarianism that is important here. Robert Proctor has advanced that Hitler was represented as a vegetarian by the Nazi propaganda even before 1933, in order to underline his ascetic approach to politics and life.[56] Sax analyses how vegetarianism also spread over many Nazi officials and how this conferred a character of higher status on them.[57] Importantly, Carol Adams has demonstrated that Hitler's vegetarianism was disputable (sometimes he used to eat ham) but socially constructed by the propaganda to add sacrality to the image of the leader.[58]

This ascetic and sacred character of vegetarianism is fundamental to understand how a dietary choice became a political weapon. In fact, more recently, I have analysed the negative representation of meat-eating constructed by Nazi propaganda in order to vilify the Jews.[59] Zygmunt Bauman[60] has explained that Nazism may only be comprised fully through the dichotomy purity/impurity, and even the other two analysed dictatorships strove to construct their 'sacred' nature and the aspiration to a spiritual existence. Thus, to Nazi propaganda, meat was a symbol of impurity, highlighted by the cruelty of kosher slaughter, the stinginess of the Jewish animal traders and the dirt and blood of the Jewish butchers. Interestingly, Fiume propaganda newspapers also identified the enemy in the butcher, when they attacked Croatian butchers because in Fiume they mistreated Italian customers.[61]

If Nazi propaganda represented meat to signify impurity and the enemy, it also created a bright side to all of this, that is, meat abstention.[62] Hitler and other Nazi officials often showed off their vegetarianism, as opposed to the Jews' passion for meat, even, in the criminal Nazi construction, for the human one, when they drew the Jews as cannibals.

However, the Nazi construction of vegetarianism was really complex and also involved faith and worship. Nicholas Goodrich-Clarke[63] has already explained the close relationships between vegetarianism, old myths and religions which fascinated the Nazis. In particular, one of the key names to understand this is Friedrich Eckstein, a member of Lebenreform who created a group of theosophists who drew on German and Spanish mysticism, freemasons, oriental religions and the Templars. Another German intellectual who overtly influenced the Nazis was Karl Heise, one of the leaders of the vegetarian Mazdaznan cult, a neo-Zoroastrian group.

It is important to underline that neither Eckstein and Lebensreform, nor Heise and the Mazdaznan groups had to do with Nazism directly. Lebensreform was a social movement also involving the philosopher Rudolph Steiner which also influenced the hippy movement thanks to its supporting natural life; similarly, the Mazdaznan cult principally asked for a return to the past.[64] The vegetarianism of these movements was only a food practice encouraging a more natural and healthy lifestyle. However, their further developments and some interpretations of their values led to Nazi ideology.

Later, in fact, a part of the Lebensreform movement shifted towards a more nationalist approach and gathered around Richard Ungewitter, who in his best-selling book *Nudity and Culture* wrote that the natural and vegetarian lifestyle would regenerate the German race and defeated the diabolical Jewish one.[65] In 1923, this strand of Lebensreform created the Artaman League, a rural movement that turned vegetarianism and naturism into a nationalist ideology. The movement drew the attention of Heinrich Himmler and Rudolph Hess, and became a part of the Nazi party in 1934.[66] A part of the members of the Artaman League created the Blood and Soil movement, in which German ruralism was opposed to Jewish nomadism. One of its leaders was Walther Darré, who became minister of food and agriculture as the Nazis took power in 1933, and was later an official of the Schutzstaffel, the defence squadron also named the 'SS'.[67]

The Mazdaznan cult, instead, already had racist perspectives. While wanting to turn Earth into a garden again, in fact, the movement also considered the Aryan race more able to do it than the others. Vegetarianism was key to all of this, as in some Mazdanan theories it allowed people to reach a higher level of regeneration. The movement was critical of Nazism and was banned in 1935, as the regime considered it as a group of subversives.[68] However, it certainly anticipated many racial perspectives of the Third Reich and the involvement of vegetarianism in them. What for Mazdanan theories was regeneration, in Nazi ideology became supremacy, a sort of higher level of purification, which in any case implied hierarchy between different races.

Similarly, in Fiume, D'Annunzio used to associate Nitti's heaviness and the voracity of the Jews.[69] In Fiume, 'elected', strong men reject meat, in order to be able to connect to higher entities and the coveted state of purity. Relevantly, in the first manifesto of the Yoga movement,[70] an article accuses the enemy of wanting to destroy the sky to give more importance to the Earth. Lightness is an essential characteristic to achieve this ascension. This is why in the same manifesto the movement states that Yoga wants to kidnap heavy people who hamper the velocity of those who have taken Fiume. Similarly, Comisso says that Yoga must wipe away heavy people from D'Annunzio's entourage.[71]

Moreover, and similar to Nazism, which created a strict animal protection law, Fiume also showed concern for animal safety. For example, Fiume fought the practice of dynamite fishing, as it results in a massive killing of animals apart from damaging fishermen and consumers.[72] Similarly, in Yoga, the poem *H2O = Forza + Amore*, by Ottaviano Targioni Tozzetti, extolls the role of animals in Nature.[73]

Sacred fascism

Italian fascism is the third dictatorship analysed here in relation to meat. Fascism took power in Italy in 1922, when the Fascist Party won the election. Once in charge of the country, the party briefly transformed the fragile Italian democracy into a dictatorship, which would find its natural ally in Nazism. Italian fascism was made up of various components, really different from each other. Each of these components had a precise idea of the dichotomy Nature/Culture. For example, there was a *strapaese* (ultra-local) and a *stracittà* (ultra-urban) fascism: the first was a combination of Catholicism, ruralism, classicism, realism, hierarchy and authority; in contrast, *stracittà* relied on modernity, technology and innovation. Thus, while the first component was much more based on Nature, the second one mostly drew on Culture.[74] In a recent study, Alberto Capatti[75] finds the roots of Italian vegetarianism in the attention of the fascists to uncorrupted Nature and spiritualism, thus in the first strand.

In this debate, Giacomo Boni and the so-called sacred fascism played a relevant role. Before fascism, Boni was one of the most important Italian architects and intellectuals, and the one responsible for the archaeological site in Rome. Ideologically, he tried to retrieve the old Roman religion and some pagan rituals. As Mussolini took power, he believed that the new dictator was the perfect leader, able to give Italy an international credibility, and that fascism originated directly from the ancient Rome.[76] By thinking so, he totally agreed with Mussolini's idea that fascism was a sort of continuation of the Roman Empire.

A strict vegetarian, Boni planted spelt in Rome, on the Palatine hill, saying that the Roman law was conceived by brains fed with spelt.[77] Thus, even the law of the fascists, who he defined as Roman's heirs, should have been fed the same way. Personally supported by Mussolini, who appointed him senator, Boni projected a ceremony to celebrate the first anniversary of the rise of fascism. He died in 1925, sharing only a few years with fascism. However, he was buried on the Palatine hill, and the regime organized an extraordinary funeral to pay homage to him.

Sacred fascism continued after Boni's death and was a mixture of esotericism, tradition, nostalgia and vegetarianism. As with the Yoga movement in Fiume, and as

Boni repeatedly did, Sacred Fascism also showed admiration for India, arguing that the European peoples originated from the Indian one.[78] India was considered as a guiding light and, as in Fiume, vegetarianism linked to the sacred levels of existence and led to the glorious past made up of purity. Apart from Boni, also Giuseppe Tucci, another vegetarian, played a relevant role in supporting sacred vegetarianism. Tucci has not been studied enough by the historians of fascism, and a few studies only partially analyse how decisive he was in bringing spiritualism to Italian fascism and in covering the regime with apparent purity. Tucci was an Orientalist specializing in religions and an explorer who served the regime without any second thought. On the one hand, Mussolini understood his importance and turned him into a sort of intellectual ambassador of fascism in Asia, detaching him from the University of Rome and appointing him supervisor of the Italian schools abroad at the Ministry of Foreign Affairs; on the other hand, his theories on the purity of Oriental religions became a consistent part of fascist ideology, vegetarianism included.[79]

The fact that this spiritual vegetarianism was only a superficial and exterior myth is clear when we see that vegetarianism was also used by propaganda to connote Mussolini's enemies. In a recent study,[80] I have analysed how vegetarianism has been represented in *La Stampa*, the oldest Italian newspaper, from 1870 to the present. It has emerged that in the fascist years, vegetarianism was represented in two opposite ways: as a food practice of the enemies and as a spiritual habit of the pure people.

The most evident example of the first way regards two Anglo-Saxon personalities, the Irish writer George Bernard Shaw and the American actor Gary Cooper. Both are referred to as vegetarians and represented as strange people. In an article,[81] George Bernard Shaw is considered as a false rebel whose anarchic and vegetarian humanitarianism is destined to fail. In another article,[82] the Italian dramatist Luigi Pirandello, who supported fascism, says that he links the fact that George Bernard Shaw only eats dull spinach and carrot to the fact that he spends much time in dull English hotels, living, in the end, a sad life. Finally, in a third article concerning everyday life,[83] vegetarianism is seen as a food habit helpful for ill people, while for women meat is recommended, as it does not threaten their beauty.

However, for fascist propaganda meat rejection also connoted people in search of spirituality and purity. This idealized version of vegetarianism, linking vegetarianism and a higher level of existence, is evident in an article[84] which celebrates the enthusiasm of the young Indian university students educated according to the values of Mahatma Gandhi and Rabindranath Tagore. Discipline, spiritualism and the wish to improve are the main characteristics of these youngsters, represented as clean from any nuisance of everyday life. One of the keys to reaching their distance from ordinary inconvenience, in order to concentrate on spirituality, is vegetarianism. Abstaining from meat, in fact, allows these youngsters to cleanse their lives and to make them 'pure' and disciplined.

Certainly, this kind of vegetarianism was not a systematic element of the fascist propagandistic machine, as it was in Fiume, and never reached the level on which it was represented by Nazi propaganda. Similarly, even though in the first period of fascism Mussolini was reported to eat only yogurt, milk, fruit and vegetables and no meat at all,[85] the Italian dictator's diet cannot be compared to Hitler's one and his already studied vegetarianism. However, also fascism saw vegetarianism as an instrument to pursue perfection and purity.[86] In the end, the fact that all these three dictatorships drew on this type of vegetarianism in order to represent themselves as 'pure' is of great relevance to understanding their real nature.

Conclusion: Class and religious roots in sacred vegetarianism

What has been said so far demands a higher level of interpretation, to discover what this approach to meat-eating and meat abstention means. The first reason may be identified in social class, at least for Italy. Certainly, meat has always been an expensive food often not affordable for the lower classes. Thus, the demonization of this item of food undoubtedly served the purpose of increasing the already abundant doses of rabble-rousing under these dictatorships. Hasia Diner[87] found the Italian diet of the pre-fascist period deeply divided in terms of class, with the poor having no access to meat. Miriam Mafai[88] points out that during the Second World War, the diet of the working class was even poorer. Between the two periods, there was fascism, and it is easy to imagine that the dictatorship strove to increase consensus. Nazi Germany and Fiume under the regency also had the problem of attracting people's favour. The demonization of meat put forward by the three dictatorships, thus, may be seen as an attempt to gain more support from the poor, that is, the majority of people.

To continue in this line concerning the need of these dictatorships to entice ordinary people, we may rather look at religion. Many studies have pointed out that the dictatorships of the twentieth century have drawn people's consensus even resorting to mystical discourse, and representing themselves as religions and their leaders as 'worldly' gods. The older generations of historians termed all of this as *political religion*, a fortunate definition created in 1938 by the American-German historian Eric Voegelin,[89] and also put forward by Michael Burleigh.[90] For these historians, the religious auto-representation of Nazism (and of other dictatorships) had to be explained within the crisis of the monotheistic religions and of spirituality in general. In short, Nazism and communism filled the religious void affecting many European peoples in the first part of the twentieth century and succeeded in representing themselves as religions.

Some younger historians[91] have found this view quite conservative and have proposed the term *religious politics*, rather than *political religion*. They equally underline the importance of sacred rituals and religious auto-representations of Nazism, but have advanced that they were not linked to the crisis of the true religions, and that the old definition risked depoliticizing Nazism. Rather than a secular and neopagan religion, for them, Nazism was a constructed faith that tried to smooth the differences among the true religions, in order to be accepted by anyone. In Italy, Emilio Gentile[92] says something similar in regard to fascism, also mentioning Herbert Schneider's idea that fascism realized a deification of Mussolini.[93]

It is in this light that we may read the approach of these dictatorships to meat, what I call 'sacred vegetarianism'. Certainly, the vegetarian cults that I have analysed in this chapter, apart from a few exceptions, never allowed principles such as racial superiority or violence. However, some of them linked meat abstention to a higher level of physical and, importantly, spiritual wellness and purity. It was this 'spiritual plus' that attracted fascist and Nazi propagandists, and that allowed them to turn a simple food practice into the ideology of 'sacred vegetarianism'.

Rather than creating a new religion, sacred vegetarianism was thus the attempt to highlight a trait that was common to more worships. As in Richard Steigmann-Gall,[94] by attenuating the differences among the existing religions, Nazism, through meat abstention, tried to create a ritual that could be acceptable for everyone. Those who disagreed were impure. In this sense, and referring to the topic of this book, the illness constructed by these propagandas for those who eat meat is sin, the moral illness that many religions often apply to those not belonging to them. Moreover, meat rejection was not only linked to monotheistic religions, it also had links to many ancient myths, on which the Nazis based their ideology, as repeatedly found throughout this chapter.[95]

The fact that rejecting or cutting down meat was already part of many existing worships makes me agree with the second group of scholars, those theorizing religious politics. In fact, linking to various religions, Nazism tried to simplify and unify what the existing religions said in order to draw people's faith and trust. The deification of D'Annunzio, Mussolini and Hitler also seems to support this second thesis. In fact, the three men never wanted to replace the existing God of Christianity, who was really popular in their respective countries. In 1929, Mussolini even signed a fundamental agreement with the Vatican state, the *Patti Lateranensi* (Lateran Pacts), which regulated the relationships between Italy and Vatican. On the one hand, the Italian state gained at least little religious independence; on the other hand, the Vatican state benefited from many financial exemptions in the Italian territory.[96] Thus, Mussolini acknowledged the importance of the Catholic religion and never tried to overwhelm it. His being represented as divine never collided with other divine entities.

Religious politics, and with it meat perspectives, served the purpose of considering these dictators as divine and helped their sacralization and the legitimization of their absolute power. Through meat, they could gratuitously invent false categories of purity and impurity, and separate the supposed pure people (the sacred themselves and their followers) from the equally supposed impure ones (the sinful enemies). This, for example, is at the base of the Nazi condemnation of Kosher slaughter or of the idealization of vegetarianism in Fiume.

Unfortunately for these dictators, the falsity of their taking care of animals and Nature was soon uncovered. What confirms that this approach to meat-eating was only propaganda and political construction was the fact that, while constructing sacred vegetarianism, these dictatorships were significantly in contrast with the real vegetarian associations in their countries.[97] This ambivalent behaviour also explains the two different representations of vegetarianism in the Italian newspaper *La Stampa*. In conclusion, for fascism and Nazism, meat-eating was a comfortable sin to attach to their enemies, a socially constructed sin that contributed to classifying humans into pure and impure, friends and enemies, us and them.

11

'Milk Is Life': Nutritional Interventions and Child Welfare: The Italian Case and Post-War International Aid

Silvia Inaudi

Several studies have shown the steady increase in the popularity of milk in the twentieth century as the ideal form of nourishment, notably in relation to the promotion of maternal and child health. In the interwar period, the spread of nutrition research on the significance of proteins and vitamins to physical health was instrumental to introduce this assumption.[1] In-school distribution played a relevant role in fostering milk consumption, and national subsidized school milk programmes in Western Europe were already implemented in the 1930s (e.g. in Britain and the Netherlands[2]). The expansion and consolidation of state-promoted school milk schemes, in replacement of local and private ones, took place in the post-war period. Furthermore, in the aftermath of the war, when the concerns for the consequences of shortages and malnutrition on child health moved to an international level, the interventions and the propagandistic action of UNICEF played a key role in the distributions of the product through schools.[3]

Several researches have questioned the promotion of massive milk consumption and shown how the implementation of school milk programmes was in many cases more connected with the interests of farmers and dairy lobbies than with the well-being of children, targeted as prospective consumers.[4] Although the interaction of material and ideal interest varies within states, this factor cannot be neglected, particularly for the post-war period, when several countries of Western Europe, thanks to their agricultural and technological progress, had to face a massive increase in milk production, which led to the expansion of milk-drinking campaigns. In Britain, in 1944, the school milk provision became a statutory duty and in 1946 free of charge for the parents; in France, the Mendès plan, launched in 1954, granted free milk to all the children attending public and private elementary schools.[5] In the case of the Federal Republic of Germany, the pressure exerted by the lobbies has been identified as a significant factor related to the replacement, in 1950, of the school meals by the distribution of subsidized milk.[6]

In Italy too, after the Second World War, milk rapidly became a symbol of social intervention, despite its modest spread among Italian households and the backwardness of the dairy sector. It was also crucial in the cultural construction of an educational paradigm able to shape the health and eating habits of the Italian families, especially of those belonging to the medium-to-low economic classes. School lunches aided the spread of milk among children, which was strictly connected to the international aid long provided to Italy as a result of food shortages, in particular in the southern parts of the country. This chapter analyses the aims, the potentialities and the limits of the programmes implemented from the post-war years to the beginning of the 1960s, with a particular focus on international influences, so as to put the Italian experience in a wider context.

International aid and food assistance
to children in post-war Italy

In September 1944, the United Nations Relief and Rehabilitation Administration (UNRRA), established in November 1943 to help the countries ravaged by the Second World War, included Italy among the recipients of its subsidies.[7] Following the signature of the official agreement in March 1945, the delegation of the Italian government for relations with UNRRA was established in April 1945 to cooperate in the fulfilment of the tasks required by the programmes. The delegation was chaired by Lodovico Montini, brother of future Pope Paul VI and a member of the Christian Democratic Party (DC), who was very close to Alcide De Gasperi.[8] Due to its former enemy status, Italy was initially the recipient of relief interventions aimed only at the most vulnerable categories, followed by a series of wider and more articulated programmes from 1946 onwards. The first food programme implemented was, therefore, targeted at deprived mothers, mothers-to-be and children aged 0 to 15. It was based on the distribution of free supplementary food rations for values that ranged from 501 calories for infants up to 866 for children aged 9 to 15.[9] At its peak, the programme covered about 2 million people, including 1.7 million children (according to estimates by the UNRRA Italian Mission, amounting to 10 per cent of the most deprived children[10]). The distribution of supplies in Italy took place mainly through school canteens, kindergartens and public and private collective institutions; during the summer, it was continued through summer camps. Despite the miserable social and economic situation, the programme provided those who could get access to it with a significant public health tool. Notwithstanding the relative imbalance in rations, due to Italy's dependence on the types of food provided by international aid, essential products were at least accessible. From a quantitative point of view, milk (powdered, evaporated and – to a lesser extent – condensed) was preceded only by flour.[11] Its distribution was of the utmost importance for mothers-to-be and children and provided help in fighting against the sky-high child mortality rate.

At the end of the UNRRA Mission, the Italian delegation was replaced in September 1947 by the *Amministrazione per gli Aiuti Internazionali* (AAI – Administration for International Aid[12]), placed under the supervision of the Italian Presidency of the

Council of Ministers and Montini's chairmanship. Throughout its long life (it was dismantled in 1977), the AAI represented an example of social administration which tried to develop a subsidiarity-based concept of welfare, and where the Catholic tradition of social engagement united with the Anglo-Saxon culture of self-help.[13] The AAI played an important role in both childhood welfare and food safety.

The AAI was instrumental in the continuation of the food assistance programme for children. The fulfilment of the programme in the 1940s was made possible by the allocation of part of UNRRA Lire Fund and other international aid, notably the Aid from the United States of America (AUSA, 1947). A prominent role was played by the newly established UNICEF, with which the Italian government signed an agreement in November 1947 under the supervision of the AAI.[14] This cooperation had a relevant impact on the solidity of the food programme in the years that followed, as the Interim Aid (1948) programme, marginally managed by the AAI, was deprived of any welfare aim. The establishment of the Marshall Plan and the evolution of political and socio-economic goals eventually led to the exclusion of the AAI from the management of the American aid.[15] Therefore, UNICEF remained AAI's main international interlocutor for the childhood assistance.

Why milk?

Milk epitomized UNICEF's welfare action and represented its most significant product in terms of distribution, at least until the end of the 1950s. This was related to the alleged economic influence of the United States – at that time the global leader in the production of powdered milk – and to the establishment of a Western scientific model aimed at presenting milk as the 'perfect food'. UNICEF's focus on milk was largely criticized, even more with the expansion of its initiatives outside of Europe.[16] Certainly, UNICEF played a significant role in the promotion of milk in child nutrition in post-war Italy, a country characterized by dramatic socio-economic unbalances in terms of spending power and access to food. UNICEF's influence was also strengthened by the growing prominence of the scientific debate on the principles of nutrition and the importance of the policies on safety and food education, which had been deeply altered by the objectives of the fascist regime.[17] Finally, several other political and socio-economic factors brought milk to the forefront of the whole childhood nutrition debate.

Milk – which, according to Thorvald Madsen, head of UNICEF's Mission in Italy, was 'a sort of obsession' for Chairman Ludwik Rajchman[18] – was undoubtedly one of the most relevant issues in the talks between UNICEF and the AAI. The negotiations for the allocation of milk supplies were constantly connected to the monitoring of policies implemented by the Italian government aimed at the recovery and expansion of the dairy sector. From 1949, production in Italy returned to pre-war levels. However, it was heavily unbalanced, as more than 80 per cent of dairy production and most of the plants were concentrated in the northern part of the country, for historical and economic reasons.[19] This problem could only have been solved by implementing a long-term investment policy focused on the agricultural and zootechnical sectors. The inclusion of Italy in the project known as Milk Conservation Programme (MCP) for the promotion of independent milk processing plants[20] – notwithstanding the emphasis placed by the Italian government on the vital need of food supplies – responded to production and health needs. In the experts' view, the spread and upgrading of pasteurization plants was a priority, and several studies had shown how instrumental dairy processing plants were in dramatically reducing the impact of infections related to poor or non-existing hygienic conditions (e.g. typhus).[21] In addition to this, milk was one of the products most likely to be subjected to food fraud. In the 1950s, investments in pasteurization plants increased significantly, even if they were not equally spread and were largely concentrated in northern Italy.

The MCP provided machinery not available in Italy as well as technical assistance for a certain number of plants, whose location was chosen by UNICEF and the Food and Agriculture Organization (FAO) in cooperation with the AAI and the Ministry of Agriculture. UNICEF's programme peculiarly combined food safety and welfare goals, which led to the free distribution of fixed quantities of milk to the children aided by the AAI across a 7- to 10-year period, so as to cover the paying off of the machinery. The programme consisted of two phases. The first phase, from 1949 to 1952, was aimed at the establishment and/or upgrading of central dairies in important Italian cities (Turin, Florence, Rome, Bari). The second phase, completed at the end of the 1950s, was mostly aimed at the central and southern parts of Italy, with the establishment of about ten processing plants.[22] This initiative was not only instrumental in boosting consumption levels, but also in meeting imperative hygienic and sanitary needs, given that as late as 1958 the percentage of hygienically compliant milk in central and southern Italy ranged from 50 per cent in Campania to a mere 5.4 per cent in other southern regions (e.g. Calabria).[23] The plants established in southern Italy under the MCP, however, were fewer than those initially planned, mainly due to the lack of agreement with local authorities and producers. Occasionally, the welfare goal represented an obstacle, as in the case of the failed upgrading of the Naples central dairy, because the municipal authorities did not agree on the transfer clause related to percentages of milk to be distributed.[24]

The focus on milk did not stem only from the analysis of the economic, structural and sanitary problems of the dairy sector, but also from several studies undertaken on the food and consumption habits of Italian families. According to a FAO survey on the daily calorie intake between 1948 and 1949, Italy – with an average of 2,343 daily calories – ranked among the worst countries in the Western world in terms of both total calorie and dairy product intake (the latter accounting for about 4 per cent).[25] At the beginning of the 1950s, Italy was among the worst countries in terms of consumption per head, with an average of 48 kilograms per year, a figure which dramatically decreased in the central and southern parts of the country. According to nutritional studies carried out at the beginning of the 1950s, the Italian diet did not meet the average need of animal proteins and calcium by 17 per cent and by 50 per cent, respectively, with the protein deficit peaking at 70 per cent in central Italy, 84 per cent in southern Italy and 85 per cent in the islands.[26] The problem of malnutrition came to the fore of the political debate following the dramatic results of the Parliamentary Committee of Inquiry on Poverty in Italy (1951–1953), whose appointed vice chairman was Montini. According to the survey, 11.8 per cent of the Italian families (6,200,000 million people) lived in extreme poverty and another 11.6 per cent (5,900,000 million people) endured severe hardship. The diet of the poor classes was based almost entirely on low-cost products, such as farinaceous foods, accounting for more than 60 per cent of their income. The consumption of animal source foods (meat, fish, dairy products, eggs) was inadequate or very low.[27] The consumption of milk in poor families was lower than 19.2 per cent compared to the national average; however, the consumption among these families in southern Italy was 64–66 per cent lower than the national average.[28] Strong differences existed among professional categories, with the agricultural sector showing the lowest level of consumption. The diet in southern Italy was therefore theoretically very high in calories (due to the large quantities of carbohydrates consumed), but qualitatively poor, especially in terms of protein intake.[29]

Several studies carried out in those years highlighted the consequences of malnutrition and nutritional deficiencies on children. A significant survey conducted in 1949–1950 by Gino Frontali and his team on behalf of the National Research Council (CNR) showed that the dietary regimen for children in the worse-off classes was often inadequate in terms of calorie intake and almost always in terms of protein, calcium and vitamin intake. An adequate animal protein intake was observed only among babies (however, not in southern Italy and in the islands), mostly in connection to a milk-based diet. All children across all social groups showed a deficiency of calcium.[30] Several studies conducted in the first half in the 1950s associated the limited consumption of dairy products with delayed growth, brittle bones, reduced resistance to tuberculosis and the indirect tendency to rickets.[31] Still in the mid-1950s, some surveys carried out by the National Institute of Nutrition (INN) showed the excruciating presence of rickets in southern Italy's depressed areas, such as the province of Salerno, where 25 per cent of the children suffered from rickets despite their abundant exposure to sunshine. According to the study, the disease was linked to the inadequate intake of milk and consequent calcium deficiency.[32]

These studies and the comparison with other analysis conducted at the international level led to a greater public campaigns action in favour of milk, whose inadequate consumption was mainly due, in the view of doctors and specialists, to scant knowledge of the intrinsic qualities of this product. Both the High Commissariat for Food (ACA) and the High Commissariat for Hygiene and Public Health (ACIS), mostly on the basis of international surveys, largely drew attention to the importance of milk as a key nutritional component to make up the deficit deriving from a cereal-based diet.[33] Milk consumption was almost mandatory in the case of children and adolescents, as the proteins of milk were considered not only excellent but also not comparable to those of meat and eggs in terms of biological value. This was mostly due to two factors: on the one hand, the quantities of milk needed to balance the proteins of meat and eggs were smaller and cheaper; on the other hand, the calcium/phosphor ratio was higher.[34] In consequence of its quality/price ratio, milk was therefore propagandized as a panacea, notably among the poorest social classes. This was despite its extremely high cost relative to the average salary level in Italy.[35] Moreover, the price of milk varied greatly from region to region and was higher especially in the areas with lower levels of consumption because of its reduced availability and the logistical problems linked to its production and distribution.

In the wake of the medical and scientific debate, the increasing attention given to school lunches – together with the adhesion to the MCP programme – was instrumental in AAI's more prominent role in the spread of milk consumption. This was due not only to the influence of UNRRA's experience (warmly recommended by its experts[36]) but also to Montini's vision of the new role of schools in the global education of children within the Catholic tradition of people's canteens.[37] The AAI played a key role in the popularization of this service that, however, was mainly a welfare programme aimed at the children in need, at least until the school and welfare reforms of the 1970s. From the beginning of the 1950s, school canteens were hailed on several occasions as the most effective way to spread milk consumption. Its distribution, notably in kindergartens and elementary schools, following the example of various European countries and the United States, was seen as a measure of civility, as well as a 'crucial method' to boost consumption (see Figure 11.1).[38]

A boost to the consumption of milk, and of dairy products in general, came from the strong bond between the most influential medical and nutritional experts and the interests of the dairy and agricultural sectors. In autumn 1950, the *Comitato Nazionale di Coordinamento Studi per il Latte e i suoi Derivati* (National Committee for the Studies on Milk and Its Derivatives) was created; it gathered the most important national organizations on behalf of the companies producing, processing and distributing dairy products.[39] In 1952, Sabato Visco, the director of the INN, was appointed president

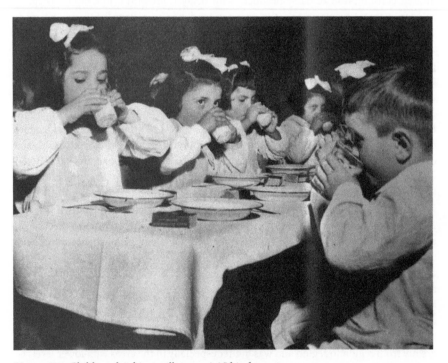

Figure 11.1 Children drinking milk in an AAI kindergarten.

Source: AAI magazine *Vie Assistenziali*, no. 11 (1959)

of the committee. He also represented Italy at the board of the International Dairy Federation in 1953.[40] The committee promoted several important events, such as the International Study Days on Drinking Milk held in Amalfi in 1954 and the 14th International Congress on Dairy Produce organized in Rome in 1956, both under the auspices of FAO.[41] Under Visco's presidency (1952–1959), the committee acted as a major *trait d'union* among the scientific community, dairy producers and the Italian government.[42] In 1955, the Ministry of Agriculture delegated Visco to draw an organic plan of initiatives aimed at increasing the consumption of milk[43] and allocated a grand total of 1 billion liras for publicity activities in 1956.[44]

Milk had an almost iconic role within the framework of the AAI food programme, thanks to the relations with the INN (the two bodies which had been closely cooperating since the outset of the programme); relations between Montini and the fringes in the DC that were more committed to the integration of productive development and the instances of social Catholicism – notably, Amintore Fanfani, who was the Minister of Agriculture between July 1951 and July 1953; and to the combined action of UNICEF and the FAO. After all, milk was a symbol of social struggle in the name of childhood, regardless of political hue. In 1951, the *Unione Donne Italiane* (Union of Italian Women), the Italian Communist Party's women's organization, created the slogan 'All Italian children in need should be given at least a wool shirt and a cup of milk a day!'. This led to the allocation of funds aimed at tens of thousands of children in some Italian cities, such as Naples, thanks in part to the involvement of prominent political personalities, such as the member of parliament Luciana Viviani.[45]

The AAI milk programme

In its first contact with UNICEF, the AAI initially tried to secure enough funds to maintain the food programme at the same level as UNRRA's. Montini's long-term plan was aimed at granting rations a more balanced and appropriate provision of food in terms of effective needs throughout the whole Italian territory. This programme could not be completed because of Italy's dependence on international aid and the financial, structural and labour situation of the network of schools and welfare institutions involved in the project. The relations with UNICEF were undermined by practical and bureaucratic problems, as the Fund did not fully understand the different food habits in Italy, and milk was the main element of debate and misunderstanding.

Between 1947 and 1951, UNICEF allocated about $15 million in food supplies to Italy, with powdered milk totalling 62,774,000 lbs, followed by fats (13,038,000 lbs), meat (11,127,000 lbs) and fish (8,073,000 lbs).[46] UNICEF's intervention was initially restricted to foundling hospitals, orphanages, maternal refectories and nurseries (and to children's camps in the summer). In 1949, however, it was extended to preschool and school canteens in central and southern Italy and gave assistance to almost 1 million people.[47] This decision was possibly determined by the UNICEF's concerns about the serious impact of milk consumption in schools with the reduction of international aid. A particularly worrying scenario involved the prospective exclusion of milk from school canteens, as it was rarely drunk during meals and was therefore difficult to space out its consumption, in particular in central and southern Italy where a considerable part of the welfare initiatives were based.[48] The poor quality and taste of the milk available played a negative role in its spread among children, as the type of milk distributed was mainly of the poorly soluble Roller skimmed type, often rejected by children because of its nauseating taste. Whole milk powder was of much better quality, but it was distributed exclusively to children up to the age of 1 due to its high price. The AAI, whose aim was the distribution of whole milk at least to children up to the age of 3, was granted derogations only in the case of foundling hospitals, where children potentially exposed to the highest risks of malnutrition and illness were sheltered. The difficulties in the distribution of this milk, caused also by the lengthy process of reconstruction of nurseries, caused a paradoxical increase of the stocks available.[49] The requests for the supply of other types of milk other than Roller were long rejected and various alternatives were explored to make it more appealing (e.g. with the addition of cocoa, when available).[50] Because of its unpalatability, some welfare institutions illegally traded milk with other foods that were more agreeable to the children, thus fostering a flourishing black market.

The AAI was only able to start its first distribution programmes of pasteurized fresh milk in 1952. The shared vision of Mayor La Pira, Montini and Fanfani made Florence the ideal 'pilot' city for a broad-spectrum experiment. In fact, free milk was distributed to all primary-school students, regardless of their families' income.[51] In 1953, an agreement between the AAI and the Ministry of Agriculture gave birth to a project later known as the Milk Programme. Thanks to the ministry's intervention, the distribution of milk from MCP plants was supplemented by the purchase of fresh milk in needy areas with central dairies or pasteurization centres. This initiative, however, involved only some tens of thousands of children and the distribution of powdered milk declined at the end of the UNICEF Mission in Italy (1952). Despite the allocation of yearly financial aids by the Italian government, the AAI food programme had to face significant quantitative and qualitative cuts for some years.[52] International aid was, once again, instrumental in revitalizing the food programme and the distribution of milk. Italy was included among the beneficiaries of the Agricultural Trade Development and Assistance Act (better known as Public Law 480), issued by the US government in 1954 for the clearance of the internal agricultural surplus. In the wake of the emotional impact of the Inquiry on Poverty, the AAI restlessly worked to obtain all the internal and external political support needed to redirect these aids to the development and the improvement of its programme. The first agreement between the US and Italian governments (over a 3-year period) was ratified on 30 June 1955 and followed by four more agreements until 1962. The AAI's project, mainly aimed at improving and developing school lunches in kindergartens and primary schools, was based on the distribution of supplies whose nutritional value varied – depending on the level – from 750 calories to 1,000 (1,800 in the case of the summer camps, where a large number of children with serious health and nutritional problems were accommodated) and was particularly focused on the increase of animal protein intake (see Figure 11.2). In its heyday, the programme provided aid to almost 1,800,000 children.[53]

L'alimentazione italiana, the magazine on food education published by the *Istituto di Tecnica e Propaganda Agraria*, commented on the US agreement by highlighting

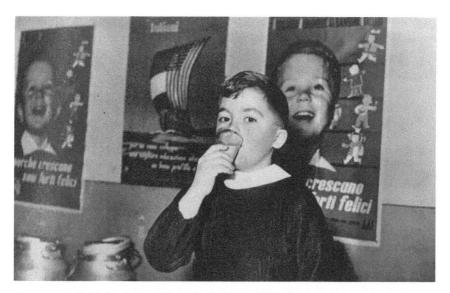

Figure 11.2 Child drinking milk. In the background, AAI food programme advertising posters.

Source: AAI magazine *Vie Assistenziali*, no. 2 (1958)

how 'the extension of the distribution of milk to all the recipients was particularly valuable' for the physiological and economic reasons mentioned before.[54] However, the milk drunk by children in Italy was not the fresh full-cream milk distributed in those years in other European countries and in the United States themselves, which started a special school milk programme in 1954.[55] Due to Italy's dependence on US surpluses, powdered skimmed milk was once again the main type distributed to Italian citizens. According to the analysis carried out by the INN, the American milk was of better quality compared to that of UNICEF, because of its perfect state of conservation and solubility. The potential controversy on the type of milk distributed was diffused by a series of considerations regarding AAI's school lunches – developed by INN and FAO experts and based on the recommended dietary allowances – in which high-fat butter and cheese were distributed, especially in the areas most subjected to the risk of malnutrition. According to Visco, these dairy products 'largely make for – even too much, I daresay – the very few grams of fat that have been skimmed from milk for technical reasons'.[56] In his opinion, no contribution of vitamin C or B1 should have been 'ridiculously' expected, or even a contribution able to cover the energy requirements of the body. The ration would provide 'a certain quantity of calcium and proteins having a high biological value'.[57] All these elements could be found in powdered skimmed milk and in sterilized low-fat milk – the former being the object of a heated debate, as in the case of the pasteurization process in the interwar period[58] – distributed by the AAI in some areas also thanks to the creation, via MCP, of two sterilization plants in Ragusa and Gioia del Colle. The choice of the type of milk to be administered relied on economic, transportation and hygienic factors.[59] Therefore,

Visco was not the only one hoping for the introduction of low-fat milk in the diet of malnourished people until the technological and economic gap between the northern and the central/southern parts of Italy was bridged.[60] Although, by law, pasteurized milk should contain not less than 3 per cent fat, the AAI was allowed by ACIS on several occasions to receive and distribute semi-skimmed milk, so as to cut costs in view of a wider distribution of fresh milk without having to wait for a reform of the legislation (which dated back to 1929 and was completed in 1963).[61] At the peak of its programme in 1961, around 1,400,000 children were still fed on powdered milk, while approximately 400,000 children were given pasteurized or sterilized milk. On average, distribution lasted 120 days, with a dosage equal or equivalent to 200 grams of milk for at least 5 days a week.[62] According to the INN, this time lapse was enough to observe significant height and weight progress.[63] The INN also promoted the distribution of biscuits with a 20 per cent content of powdered milk to be eaten with milk, so as to make snack time more appealing and to avoid the excessive intake at one time of a product which was still unknown to most children.[64] The distribution of biscuits first took place in the province of Salerno, within the framework of a pilot project to fight malnutrition in depressed areas, and was later endorsed by the AAI in the form of special distribution of milk with sugar and/or chocolate in northern, central and southern Italy, in isolated areas without the structures needed to provide regular meals and where the hygienic reconstitution of powdered milk was impossible and potentially harmful.[65] The AAI developed some original solutions, as in the case of the Sassi of Matera, with the creation of dispensers, known as 'milk bars', which provided access to small bottles of sterilized milk with straws.[66]

Combining social welfare and market needs: The role of milk

The extension of AAI's food programme through the distribution of the US agricultural surpluses fostered a heated debate in Italy, especially in the dairy sector. Between 1949 and 1958, the annual rate of production of Italian milk for feeding and industrial purposes increased fourfold compared to the years 1911–1940.[67] It was largely believed that the increase in consumption among the Italian population as a whole, through a clever, organic and articulated publicity campaign, could and should provide an adequate solution. A substantial purchase of supplies in view of their free distribution among the population, as in the case of the agreement between the AAI and the Ministry of Agriculture, was seen as a helping hand for the dairy sector. On several occasions, the Ministry of Agriculture seemed to be willing to arrange a massive distribution of fresh milk among primary school children. However, the huge investments needed, the political and structural difficulties as well as conflicting economic interests hindered its realization.[68] In a report drafted in 1955, Visco estimated that the costs of 200 grams of milk a day, for about 180 days, to all the students aged 6 to 14 (approximately 6,500,000 children), would have topped 10 billion liras per year, distribution costs excluded.

The extension of this programme to the whole infantile population aged 0 to 14 (around 11,650,000 people) would not have been affordable. As Visco stated, 'Such a policy cannot be implemented rapidly and on a large scale.'[69] From a theoretical point of view, the distribution of fresh milk in school canteens was largely seen as necessary and commendable. However, at least in the 1950s, this initiative could only be implemented on a small scale, given the productive unbalances in terms of distribution and storage, which would be tackled only from the 1960s with the introduction of Tetra Pack and UHT milk.

The distribution of US surplus dairy products, especially of powdered milk (which was not subjected to the import ban existing in the Italian legislation), was seen as a prospective danger because of the depression of the domestic market. The AAI reacted by advancing the future purchase of milk and its derivatives, under the agreement with the US government, at that time financially unaffordable for the organization. American aid was conceived as a gradually decreasing financial contribution, balanced against the increase of the funds allocated by the Italian government to maintain the results achieved.[70] A steady increase in the use of fresh milk was anticipated, based on the agreement with the Ministry of Agriculture. However, purchases on the market were always minimal, notably for powdered milk (all the more so because the AAI owned a production plant in Frosinone, the Solac, built with the contribution of the MCP), whereas a slight increase was observed for fresh milk. More generally, the observance of compensatory economic terms laid down in the agreements with the United States was largely disregarded or even lower than what was assumed by the AAI. When American aid came to an end, the food programme headed towards a slow decline. This was ascribable mainly to the political changes connected to the rise of the centre-left coalition, rather than to the economic boom and its positive effects (in fact, several analysis showed that, until the mid-1970s, a high percentage of children in southern Italy was still malnourished, despite the almost total elimination of disparities in food consumption in that decade[71]). The planned welfare and school reforms within the framework of a wider economic planning (even though they were only partially carried out) involved the rethinking of social-welfare policies, which had an impact on budget allocations.[72]

According to Montini, the distribution of milk was to be seen not only in the light of its obvious socio-medical value, but also as a prospective investment which would accustom the new generations to 'eating rationally' and would gradually generate 'a spontaneous demand for the product beyond and in addition to the mandatory welfare channel'.[73] Montini's vision was common to that of many reformers of that time and implied great trust in science and in the educational drive towards popular consumption. Teaching Italian families living on a low budget to eat better and consume a diet varied and rich in nutrients was not just possible but mandatory. The free distribution of food to children, notably milk, in the light of its importance from a medical and nutritional point of view, epitomized a political action which combined welfare and food education.[74] In fact, from the mid-1950s, the AAI launched educational courses and initiatives for caretakers, teachers and children alike, which would play a pivotal role in raising awareness on those subjects among Italian families.

Conclusion

As elsewhere, in Italy milk played a highly relevant and symbolic role within the debate on the ties between nutrition and child health which ran from the end of the Second World War to the 1960s. This was the consequence of a combination of scientific beliefs, economic interests and political goals. International influences, primarily UNICEF, were of crucial importance, whereas the analysis of the relations among dairy lobbies, experts and governments remains more complex, as they were extremely tight but not as pervasive as in other countries. Due to the limited economic investment of the Italian government, the food programme as a whole was therefore dependent on international aid, thus preventing the AAI, within the framework of the campaign to promote milk consumption, not only to achieve its mid-term objectives, namely the total replacement of powdered milk with fresh milk produced in Italy, but most of all to contribute to ensure the free distribution of milk to all children in school.[75] The latter was part of the AAI's prospective evolution of school lunches into a wider public service with educational purposes, as well as nutritional and health aims. The distribution of milk to children (much as the food programme in its entirety) continued to be targeted at the most needy categories.

The evaluation of the specific effects of milk distribution remains complex, as it was integrated, as much as possible, into the school lunches. At the general level, the food programme was certainly popular and in general supported by local bodies; in spite of its limitations, it was free and represented the only possibility for many poor children to have access to foods which otherwise could have never become part of their diet. Notwithstanding the efforts of the AAI, milk did not become popular among all the children assisted by the programme (probably because of the above-mentioned reasons). The effects of the milk programme on the expansion of consumptions remain uncertain, even if the analysis carried out on sales, particularly in the southern areas where the MPC plants were located, and - in this case, in public holidays - in the depressed area monitored by the INN, produced encouraging results. However, at the beginning of the 1970s, the statistics showed a high consumption of milk only among children until the age of 5, as well as the persistence of a large consumption gap between southern Italy and the rest of the country.[76]

12

Like Oil and Water: Food Additives and America's Food Identity Standards in the Mid-Twentieth Century

Clare Gordon Bettencourt

The need of the immaterial is the most deeply rooted of all needs. One must have bread; but before bread, one must have the ideal.

Victor Hugo
The Memoirs of Victor Hugo, 1899

According to Victor Hugo, nutritional fulfilment is completely separate from spiritual or intellectual fulfilment, but is it really that simple? Hugo puts forth the model of bread versus the ideal, but what about ideal bread? At the time Hugo wrote his memoirs, America and Europe were grappling with the impact of industrialization on food production.[1] Consumers faced a marketplace laden with unsafe adulterated foods that were often tainted with disease and harmful additives. Watered-down milk, diseased meat and lead dyes all posed serious health risks during the late nineteenth century. Bread specifically was commonly adulterated with alum, which was linked to gastrointestinal problems. Throughout Europe and in the United States, regional and nationwide measures were taken to regulate food purity and safety. While it seems that Hugo may be taking bread for granted, it is likely that consumers at the time were not just searching for bread, but a healthy, wholesome, ideal bread.

Humans have produced bread since transitioning from hunting and gathering to agricultural cultivation during the Neolithic period.[2] Bread has been produced by professional bakers since the second century BC, when the first baker's guild was formed in Rome.[3] Despite the long history of bread production, changes did not end with the addition of alum. The introduction of chemical food additives in the first half of the twentieth century, and their widespread implementation in the middle of century, transformed the entire American way of eating. Using chemical emulsifiers in bread as a case study, this chapter will assess the proliferation of food additives in the American marketplace to consider the policy response to additives through the food identity standards provision of the Food, Drug, and Cosmetic Act of 1938, the health implications of these ingredients and the cultural significance of processed convenience foods.

This research is in conversation with the historiography of food adulteration, pure food legislation, consumer history and the history of medicine. The existing historiography of pure food legislation in the United States has focused largely on the passage, implementation and function of the Pure Food and Drug Act of 1906. Work by Lorraine Swainston Goodwin, James Harvey Young and Marc T. Law have proven essential to understanding this landmark legislation.[4] A handful of scholars, many of them writing in the discipline of law rather than history, have analysed the passage and function of the Food, Drug, and Cosmetic Act of 1938.[5] Food regulation is deeply bound up with the history of food adulteration. Bee Wilson has written the most helpful and comprehensive text on food adulteration in Europe and America.[6] Historians of medicine, especially Matthew Smith, have shown the connection between food additives and health concerns.[7] The work of historians of consumption, Lizbeth Cohen and Tracey Deutsch, has chronicled how women have purchased food and reacted to food regulation and marketing.[8] Finally, Aaron Bobrow-Strain's work on the history of American bread outlines how commercialization and industrialization impacted bread production and consumption in the United States.[9]

With the historiography of these areas of history in mind, this chapter investigates a legislative proposal to permit chemical emulsifiers in the bread standard of identity during the 1940s as a case study in the wider use of additives in the post-war period. This chapter will argue that the increasing power of large food manufacturers, emergence of new convenience foods and shifting gender roles of the mid-twentieth century complicated how consumers purchased, cooked and understood their food. The first section of this chapter introduces the forces that shaped these bread standards, as our case study for the industrialization of America's food. The second section outlines the proliferation of food additives in food standards following the adoption of emulsifiers in the bread standards. By placing ingredients at the centre of research surrounding food identity standards, understanding can be gained of the forces that shaped food identity standards, and the American food landscape more broadly. Finally, the third section considers the long-term health effects of additives and consumer relationships to processed foods. The history of food identity standards is not simply the history of a little-known provision, but a lens through which to understand the huge technological, cultural and economic changes that are reflected in the food production and food preparation of the epoch. While chemical food additives and pure food legislation seem like oil and water, this research demonstrates how the Food and Drug Administration's (FDA's) adoption of chemical food additives in food identity standards created an emulsion, of sorts, that continues to affect America's food.

Standardizing America's bread

Emulsion: When two or more liquids may be virtually insoluble in each other and yet may be formed into a stable mixture by proper dispersion.

Atlas Chemical Company, 1949

In following the trail of emulsifiers, the breadcrumbs lead us to the intersection of advancements and changes in science, consumer habits, methods of bread production, gender roles and government food regulations. First, how did chemical emulsifiers end up in industrial bread recipes? It should be noted that emulsifiers generally are an ingredient that is nearly as old as bread itself. Historically, ingredients like eggs have been used to emulsify oil and water in preparations like mayonnaise, and the Greek physician Galen used beeswax as an emulsifier in the second century AD.[10] Chemically produced emulsifiers, on the other hand, were first created by the French chemist Barthelot in 1853. These chemical emulsifiers (the most recognizable types being mono and diglycerides) are made by modifying naturally occurring fats and oil molecules known as triglycerides. Chemical emulsifiers are made by combining vegetable oil, glycerine and an alkali into a hot slurry that is either cooled and used wet, or dried into flakes.[11] The earliest use for chemical emulsifiers in food was margarine, but food manufacturers soon saw widespread value in their ability to create small, uniform air bubbles and create smooth mixtures of fat and water.[12] When applied to bread specifically, emulsifiers change the size of gas bubbles in the fermenting dough. As the dough rises, the dough volume expands more than in natural fermentation, thus creating a softer crumb texture and a loaf that resists going stale longer.[13]

Just as chemical food additives were first being developed, America's food supply was rapidly industrializing. The emergence of rail lines led to the rise of new multistate corporations after 1875. While the greater connectedness of trade nationwide brought a larger variety of foods to consumers at lower prices, it also made it harder for small companies to compete. New national brands like Kellogg, Nabisco, Domino Sugar and Heinz used advertising and colourful packaging to build brand loyalty and preference.[14] By 1900, food manufacturing accounted for 20 per cent of America's overall manufacturing output.[15] The industrialization of food production was part of a larger shift that Chris Otter characterizes as the 'mineralization' of the economy. Sectors that had once been powered by wind and water changed to coal and oil. These new energy sources minimized the labour it took to produce food and power factories, led to the mechanization of farm equipment and formed the base of new chemical pesticides.[16]

One such example of this mineralization is the case of the Atlas Powder Company, an explosives company that would go on to produce and sell food additives. The Atlas Powder company was first incorporated in Delaware in 1912, as an offshoot of E.I. du Pont de Nemours and Company, after their explosives trust was broken up.[17] From 1912 to 1917, Atlas focused exclusively on explosives but later diversified into manufacturing other chemicals. Altas became the leading manufacturer of ammonium nitrate and during the First World War supplied 100,000 tons of it annually to the federal government.[18] In addition to serving as an explosive, nitrate of ammonium can also be used as a high-nitrogen fertilizer. Because Atlas had increased its production capabilities to meet wartime demands for this substance, once the war ended, Atlas sought to market the chemical in new ways. In 1919, Atlas published the book *Better Farming with Atlas Farm Powder*, which suggested that farmers use their explosive products to blast ditches, stumps, boulders and soil. The book also recommends Atlas products for soil treatment and fertilization, specifically nitrogen fertilizers (see Figure 12.1).[19]

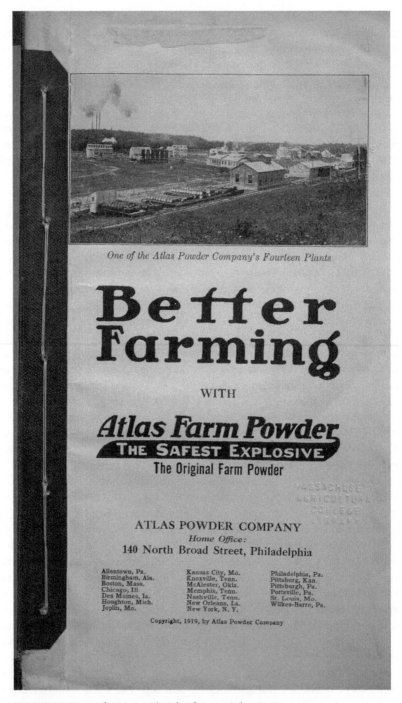

Figure 12.1 Better farming with Atlas farm powder, 1919.

Between the First and the Second World Wars, Atlas expanded their reach from farming chemicals to industrial food ingredients. Atlas discovered their forms of emulsifiers as a byproduct in the process of hydrogenating corn sugar to create the sugar alcohols mannitol and sorbitol.[20] Between 1938 and 1942, Atlas created four types of emulsifiers which they marketed with catchy names. Span and Arlacel were launched first, followed by Tween (and easy-mix formula with greater hydrophilic properties) and Myrj (meant to work without water). According to Atlas, these products were intended to disperse, wet and/or whip ingredients in food formulations. Atlas stated that Myrj was best suited for bread-making while Span and Tween were meant for use in ice cream and cake.[21] While bread, ice cream and cake were not new foods, Atlas' additives catered to the needs of new industrial preparations.

Atlas' branding of food additives for simple, staple foods signals the continued intensity with which the American food system was industrializing. Atlas was among a myriad of new food additive companies that offered food manufacturers new ways of producing foods whose recipes had remained fairly static for hundreds, if not thousands, of years. Within the history of the industrialization of America's food supply, bread specifically remained largely unchanged until the early twentieth century. Since the Neolithic period, bread had been made with the same basic ingredients: flour, water, salt and yeast. Sandwich-style sliced breads are often enriched with milk or fat for a richer, sweeter loaf. As late as 1890, 90 per cent of American bread was baked at home.[22] The 10 per cent of consumers who were buying store-bought bread were either the very wealthy who could afford high-quality loaves, or low-income immigrants who didn't have time to bake due to work obligations, and often settled for poor-quality adulterated bread.[23] Aaron Bobrow-Strain argues that the turn of the twentieth century brought new reverence for the idea of professionalism that contributed to the shift from homemade bread to store-bought.[24] While store-bought bread in the nineteenth century was viewed as adulterated and often unclean (partly for xenophobic reasons, as it was often produced by immigrants), bread manufacturers in the twentieth century touted the scientific cleanliness of their products and offered tours of their facilities.[25] As a result, consumers saw mass-produced bread as more scientifically advanced, purer and safer. Fears over germs led women's and consumer organizations to push bread manufacturers to sell their loaves wrapped. In 1912, bread producers responded with the first pre-wrapped bread, and by 1920 all store-bought bread was sold wrapped.[26] The wrapping of bread favoured larger, more automated bakeries, as they could afford to invest in wrapping materials and equipment. Additionally, large-scale bakeries that sold wrapped bread painted unwrapped bread made by smaller bakeries as unsanitary.

In 1928, the automatic bread slicing machine was invented in Missouri. This innovation further advantaged large bread manufacturers over local producers.[27] With the advent of wrapping and slicing, consumers shifted from choosing their bread using look and smell to seeking out 'squeezability'. At the same time, bakers were seeking ways to make production more cost-effective. In Harry Snyder's 1930 volume *Bread: A Collection of Popular Papers on Wheat, Flour and Bread*, he states,

The public is constantly demanding cheaper bread, and the baker is frequently called upon to explain why he does not make or sell cheaper bread, or some special kind of bread [. . .] The baker would like to make and sell and cheaper loaf if it were economically possible to do so.[28]

With consumer demands for more economical bread, and the importance of bread 'squeezability', food chemists were perfectly poised to address this need among bakers.

Industrialization coincided with shifts in how women related to their roles as wives, mothers and professionals. As Tracey Deutsch and Katherine J. Parkin note, women and food have long been linked, as the female responsibility for food preparation and the household's health has been a 'ubiquitous norm'.[29] At the turn of the twentieth century, the emergence of the ideas of scientific homemaking, home economics, household management and scientific motherhood led women (especially middle- and upper-class women) to believe that they were responsible for the health and morality of society.[30] They also embraced the advice of scientists and so-called experts thinking their counsel would allow them to best serve their families and communities. As a result, women with the means to purchase it believed that pre-made bread offered greater cleanliness but were wary of the use of new additives.

Historically speaking, women were right to be wary of food additives. During the nineteenth century, as food was being produced on a larger scale, American food producers and retailers increased their use of nefarious adulterants like lead colourings and cheapeners like chalk and sawdust. As more Americans moved to urban areas and subsistence farming lessened, these new city-dwellers relied on food purveyors to provide safe and pure foods. Many millers, butchers, milkmen, bakers and grocers seized this opportunity to increase their profits and began selling adulterated or contaminated goods.[31] By 1878, the market had become so corrupt that an industry guidebook for grocers states that it was nearly impossible to source unadulterated goods, even if the shop owner wanted to.[32] In response to the increasingly dishonest marketplace, the Pure Food and Drug Act (PFDA) was famously adopted in 1906 after Upton Sinclair's *The Jungle* generated feverish public outrage.[33]

Over the years, the PFDA became ineffectual, as manufacturers found loopholes in the law. In 1938, Congress and President Roosevelt repealed and replaced the PFDA with the new Federal Food, Drug, and Cosmetic Act (FDCA).[34] At its core, the stated objectives of the new law mirrored the goals of the PFDA; however, the new legislation broadened the scope of federal regulation in the existing categories of food and drugs, while also expanding oversight to cosmetics and medical devices.[35] In regulating food, the law brought several new approaches, the most innovative being the food identity standards provision. This provision allowed the FDA to create a recipe for common foods to protect consumers from additives and cheapeners. Food producers must adhere to the FDA's basic recipe in order to call their food by a name recognizable to consumers. This provision was meant to regulate products like 'bred-spred' a pectin and sugar mixture purporting to be jam but without any genuine fruit content. Under a standard of identity, bred-spred could not be called jam because it did not meet the minimum required level of fruit content.[36] Numerous scholars have argued that the food identity standards clause was the most significant regulatory breakthrough in the law, and journalists of the period wrote that the food identity standards provision was one of the strongest positive changes brought to the legislation.[37]

In the early years of the new standards of identity provision, the FDA implemented standards for staple foods like tomato products, canned fruits, jams and jellies, with little conflict over the formulation of the standards. In 1949, the FDA began drafting standards of identity for bread products and asked a congressional committee to explore public opinion about the use of emulsifiers in bread. The hearings occurred throughout the 1940s; they began in 1941, paused due to the Second World War, resumed in 1943 and paused once again, reopened for a third time in 1948 to consider 'new optional ingredients' and closed finally on 20 September 1949.[38] The committee found that consumers believed emulsifiers were used as an inexpensive substitute for wholesome ingredients and generally disliked any deviation from traditional baking techniques. Journalism of the period supports this sentiment by echoing the scepticism consumers felt over the use of additives in bread.[39] Holmes Alexander, a journalist writing in the *Los Angeles Times*, described the new recipes as 'one pound of this gook, plus five pounds of water, can be used to replace six pounds of natural fats and oils in bread'.[40] Despite a popular reverence for new technology, consumers distrusted the motives of industrial bread producers.

Consumer fears were echoed by government and industry voices. At a senate meeting of the Subcommittee on Agriculture and Forestry, a letter was read from C. B. Heinemann of the Independent Meat Packers Association. The letter stated,

> I would like to call your attention to the importance of food content of bread made with these emulsifiers. One pound of fat contains 4,080 calories. To replace this fat with 5 pounds of water would replace the caloric food value with water. This would short change the public in food value.[41]

While the Independent Meat Packers Association likely feared a decline in the use of animal fats in enriched bread, its concern over decreased nutritional density in foods was echoed by others. Congressman Frank Keefe, a Republican from Wisconsin, argued,

> It is apparent that such usage [of chemical emulsifiers] will grow as price competition invariably created through the nutritional debasement of the original food is developed. These conditions will force other manufacturers to adopt similar practices. It may be claimed by some that these chemical emulsifying agents improve the physical properties of certain foods. However the possibility of nutritional debasement and deception is so great that these factors should not be ignored when evaluating the true purposes behind the use of these materials.[42]

Outrage over the use of emulsifiers in bread continued to build, and in October of 1949 the General Federation of Women's Clubs petitioned Congress to adopt an amendment to the FDCA that would ban non-nutritive ingredients.[43] The petition was very specific and explained the exact ingredients, monoglycerides and diglycerides that their members believed were not suitable for use in bread. Though Congress did not adopt the proposed amendment, it is evident that this activism from consumers did not go unnoticed. In the process of setting the standard, members of Congress issued a statement advising the FDA to make their decision carefully: 'The introduction of chemicals into foods in order to make a cheaper product resemble a better one deserves a very thorough study.'[44]

In the end, the FDA elected to permit the use of emulsifiers in bread. When the identity standard for bread was adopted in 1955, the FDA permitted the use of lecithin, monoglycerides, diglycerides or adiacetyl tartaric acid esters of mono- and diglycerides, all different types of emulsifiers.[45] It believed that these ingredients were suitable for use in bread because they derived from natural fats and oils.[46] Despite the permission of numerous chemical additives, the FDA banned a new Atlas emulsifier called polyoxyethylene because it thought that it was unnatural and made with the intent to deceive consumers.[47] The FDA stated that the new bread standards would protect consumers from 'fad' ingredients, prevent fraud by setting requirements for the amount of flour used in bread and promote truthful labelling. Despite concerns about nutritional debasement levied during the congressional bread hearings, no specific health claims were made by the FDA about emulsifiers or the bread standards overall.

While the creation and application of emulsifiers in America's bread is the story of one additive in one food, the narrative demonstrates how food additives began to permeate America's food landscape despite widespread concerns about their implementation from consumer and government voices. As the next section will demonstrate, this pattern became more common as food additives experienced a renaissance in the post-war era, and the FDA looked for ways to manage the food industry's call for the increased use of these ingredients.

Food additives go mainstream

In 1953, *Fortune* magazine stated that the food industry 'was in relentless pursuit of convenience'.[48] As a part of this aim, between 1949 and 1959, chemists developed over 400 new food additives.[49] As new convenience, foods hit the post-war market with rapid speed, and the FDA regulated these products by giving them standards of identity. While the identity standards created before the Second World War were generally simple foods that adhered to the format of a recipe, the bread standards ushered in a change in how the FDA framed food identity standards. Many of these new foods were completely new inventions with no homemade analogue, which led the FDA to shift from writing identity standards like a recipe to writing longer standards that incorporated more legal and scientific terminology. Many food producers urged the FDA to allow new food additives into standardized foods in order to offer 'innovative' new products they felt consumers wanted.[50] The FDA's expansion of food standards as a means to regulate America's changing food marketplace meant that by the middle of the twentieth century half of all food purchased by Americans had a food identity associated with it.[51]

Between 1949 and 1954, chemical food additives were further incorporated into new food identities and amended into existing regulations. During this 5-year period, the greatest changes made were a cross-category use of emulsifiers and monosodium glutamate (MSG). Despite the efforts of women's groups to keep emulsifiers out of bread, the FDA wrote them into the new standards for bakery products along with processed cheese, mayonnaise and salad dressings.[52] The new standards for processed cheeses state that the use of emulsifiers was necessary because it allowed manufacturers to create a cheese that resembled a 'homogeneous plastic mass'.[53] The FDA also amended the canned vegetable standards to permit the use of MSG in over forty types of canned vegetables.[54]

As additives and industrial preparations expanded, the process for framing food standards changed dramatically. In 1954, the Hale Amendment to the Food, Drug, and Cosmetic Act was ratified. This amendment, which was sponsored by various members of the food industry, waived the requirement to hold a hearing for a proposed standard or amendment as long as no dissenting opinions were recorded.[55] Previously, the law had required that a public hearing be held in all cases, but the Hale Amendment only required that a hearing be conducted if the standard was challenged by someone who would be adversely affected.[56] Instead of requiring discussion in the framing process, individuals now had 30 days to file a dispute before the standard's planned implementation.[57] At the time, the *Food, Drug and Cosmetic Law Journal* wrote that interested parties would be advised to not take vacations because the dispute window was so short. While the window for comment was identical for both individuals and companies, the resources possessed by companies typically outmatched those possessed by individuals and grass-roots campaigns. This change reflects a desire to speed up the legislative process by creating fewer opportunities for discussion, a move that benefitted corporate interests.

The framing of food identity standards was further restructured in 1958 by the Food Additives Amendment to the FDCA, followed by the Colour Additives Amendment in 1960.[58] These new provisions regulated artificial ingredients by evaluating them separately from the foods they were used in and creating definitive restrictions for their use. Previously, the FDA had banned any ingredient thought to be injurious to health, even if a large dosage was required to induce maladies. Under the new additive amendments, food manufactures only had to prove the safety of ingredients in the amounts used in their products.[59] The Delaney Clause created an exception to this regulatory scheme by mandating that any substance shown to cause cancer in humans or animals be forbidden no matter the quantity (although this regulation did not extend to pesticides).[60] The food and chemical industries fought the Delaney Clause, calling it 'unscientific'.[61] In 1959, the *New York Times* estimated that these new regulations would cost the food industry $20 million over 5 years to test the additives already in the marketplace.[62] Though these amendments did not bring any direct changes to the food standards clause, they did influence how the FDA created subsequent food identities. By establishing separate oversight for artificial ingredients, the FDA no longer had to use food identities as a way to manage food additives, thus giving the agency an opportunity to refocus its approach to writing standards.[63]

The food standards that were passed after 1958 demonstrate the increasingly assertive role that food manufacturers had gained following passage of the Hale Amendment and the diminished focus on regulating additives brought by the Food Additive and Colour Additive amendments. The FDA created a standard for peanut butter which allowed manufacturers to extract the oil in the peanuts, hydrogenate it, add it back into the spread and still consider it part of the overall peanut content.[64] The FDA also adopted standards for frozen desserts after 19 years of disagreement regarding exactly how the regulations should be written.[65] Between 1942 and 1960, the hearings for these standards generated over 40,000 pages of testimony from government representatives, industry, academic experts and organized consumer groups.[66] In the end, identities were created for ice cream, frozen custard, ice milk, sherbet and water ices in which the FDA permitted the use of additives such as caseinates, gelling agents and emulsifiers across the board. Finally, during this time, the FDA revised their standards for canned fruits, jams, jellies and preserves, allowing the use of artificial sweeteners in many preparations.

In 1964, the FDA added standards for frozen raw breaded shrimp and frozen raw lightly breaded shrimp that Joseph M. Vallowe and H. Thomas Austern cite as a turning point in how identity standards were written.[67] Both scholars argue that these standards represent a new era in framing of food standards afforded by the separate oversight implemented by Food Additive and Colour Additive amendments. The identity for these foods offered a simpler format that stated how much shrimp was required (50 per cent shrimp for standard breading and 70 per cent shrimp for light breading) and stipulated that the breading substance must be 'safe and suitable'.[68] This standard exhibits a departure from the more technical standards of the previous decade and shows that by creating a separate means of regulating artificial ingredients, the FDA no longer needed to use food standards as a way to manage its jurisdiction over food additives.

From 1965 to 1967, the number of new standards and amendments declined. Because the FDA was not using identity standards to manage additives, the amendments made were typically small and for the most part affected the clarity of the label rather than the ingredients. In 1968, the FDA created an identity standard for soda water, and in keeping with the style of the breaded shrimp standard, offered a much looser regulatory scope. Although the name of the standard was for soda water, the standard essentially created an identity for carbonated soft drinks. The regulation states that the identity included proprietary beverages like cola, ginger ale and root beer, but did not oversee the individual recipes for these drinks. Because the new standard was so broad, it allowed manufacturers to use an array of ingredients including sweeteners, flavours made from fruit juice, natural flavours, artificial flavours, acidifying agents, buffering agents, viscosity-producing agents, stabilizing agents, foaming agents, quinine, chemical preservatives and defoaming agents.[69] It should be noted that not all new standards or revisions made at this time included chemical additives. In my review of the standards, the identity for canned peas is the lone example; this standard was changed to allow for dried green or red peppers, onions or garlic to be added to this food.[70]

While each of these standards in their own may seem like an inconsequential historical detail, together they reflect the industry and regulatory trends of the American food marketplace. In the span of two decades, the types of foods on American supermarket shelves had radically transformed. The FDA, in most cases, permitted the use of additives as the food industry argued they were necessary to produce the innovative foods the public wanted. These new foods transformed how

Americans ate and spent their time in the kitchen (especially for women who were still typically tasked with food preparation). While no immediate ill effects from these ingredients had been established during this time, there was widespread concern of the long-term risks. The contemporary discourse surrounding food additives in the 1950s and 1960s suggests that consumers and activists felt they were being used as guinea pigs by the food industry.[71] While cancer was seen as the main concern surrounding food additives, some doctors and consumers were most fearful of the new and untested nature of additives more broadly. The Delaney Clause promised to protect consumers from carcinogenic additives, yet by the end of the 1960s, these profound shifts in the American way of eating were having measurable effects in other areas of public health.

Processed foods and health

By 1969, the changes that had occurred to the American diet over the past two decades were beginning to have negative consequences. Because of the emergence of convenience and snack foods following the Second World War, many Americans were now suffering from malnutrition.[72] President Richard Nixon was alarmed by the high rates of hunger and malnourishment and organized the White House Conference of Food, Nutrition and Health in 1969 to assess the problem and generate solutions. Nixon's team of academic and industry advisors issued numerous recommendations to improve the health and diet of Americans, as well as help consumers make better choices. In the panel report 'The Provision of Food as It Affects the Consumer: Guidelines for Federal Action', Nixon's advisors argued that the current nutritional crisis could be alleviated by encouraging Americans to eat mostly 'nutritious and traditional food', improving nutrition education programs and ensuring that all foods provided a full ingredient list using plain language.[73] While food additives themselves did not cause malnutrition, the types of foods made possible by additives were thought to have diminished nutritional profiles.[74]

Popular culture discourse also began to reflect a growing concern over processed foods. By 1970, a plethora of books offering information about food additives were being published. Ruth Winter's 1970 text, *Beware of the Food You Eat* (with an introduction by Senator Walter Mondale) warned of the pesticides and additives that had permeated America's food:

> When Eve handed Adam the apple, it may have had a worm in it, but it didn't have any pesticides, wax coloring, or chemical fertilizer. We all know the consequences of taking a bite of the first apple, but what about the after effects of today's fruit?[75]

On top of concerns about agricultural chemicals described by Winter, the public was becoming more and more aware of the possible link between food additives and disease. Hundreds of articles appeared nationwide from the *New York Times* to the *Los Angeles Times* throughout the 1970s doubting the safety of food additives. Many of the articles questioned additives like saccharin, nitrates and nitrites, and suggested they could lead to increased cancer risks.[76] While the concern had moved from emulsifiers in bread to nitrates in baby food, and BHT/BHA in cooking oil, the belief that these compounds were meant to benefit food producers more than consumers remained.[77]

By the middle of the 1970s, the Health Research Group, a consumer advocacy organization funded by Ralph Nader's Public Citizen Inc., was calling for greater scrutiny of the health effects of food additives. Their publication 'Cancer Prevention and the Delaney Clause' argued that the FDA was not doing enough to prevent cancer or any other illnesses stemming from food additives. They claimed that Americans were consuming food additives at the rate of 5 pounds of food additives every year, with the latency period of many diseases lasting many years or decades.[78] With such increases in the consumption of food additives, and the limited scope of clinical trials, the Health Research Group stated that 'food additives are chemicals of small benefit' and argued that the Delaney clause should be strengthened and expanded.[79] They campaigned against specific additives like Red No. 2 and saccharin, which were both linked to increased cancer risk, arguing that the uncertainties and risks outweighed the benefits.[80]

Furthermore, Matthew Smith's work on the Feingold diet outlines how food additives were linked to hyperactivity in children by Dr Ben F. Feingold in his 1974 book, *Why Your Child Is Hyperactive*. Smith explains that hyperactive children were viewed as 'the proverbial canaries in the coal mine', suggesting that additives could be affecting the entire population in hidden or long-term ways.[81] Feingold advised parents to cut out foods with artificial colours and flavours, along with fruits that contained salicylates.[82] According to Smith, Feingold's argument gained widespread media attention and proved to be very divisive. Some families of hyperactive children saw results, while the food industry fought Feingold's assertions, and the medical community remained sceptical. Nevertheless, Feingold's theory further represents the increasing distrust of chemical additives that went mainstream during the 1970s.

Despite widespread wariness of food additives, it was difficult for consumers to cut convenience foods from their diet. Smith explains that implementing the Feingold diet was very time-consuming and difficult for working or single mothers to follow.[83] Outside of Feingold families, the changing gender dynamics ushered in by second-wave feminism impacted how women related to food procurement and preparation. While the homemakers who protested the use of emulsifiers in bread saw their roles as wives and mothers as a way to establish authority in the political realm, women during the mid-century period were receiving mixed messages about their role in society. The popular press encouraged women to pursue outside interests and paid work but also maintained expectations of women's domestic work.[84] Women's cookbooks and relationship manuals from the 1970s reminded readers that good food was the glue that held families together.

Because women were still viewed as responsible for feeding their families, processed foods offered women a way to fulfil their role while saving time and labour. In the years following the Second World War, marketers invested significant resources in selling women on the practicality and scientific superiority of frozen, canned and processed ingredients. A shopping manual from 1950 (that is dedicated by the homemaker authors, 'To the Men We Shop For') describes the benefits of convenience foods:

As long as so many women work at jobs away from home, we are going to see more and more ready-to-serve foods in frozen and canned form, especially main dishes. We shall also see new packaged mixes, those convenient foods that allow busy housekeepers to 'have their cake and eat it, too.'[85]

This sentiment was reiterated in a *New York Times* article from 1959, 'These [convenience foods] have given the housewife more time to spend with her family as well as the opportunity to work outside the home.'[86] While women were concerned about the ingredients in new convenience foods, the practicality of these dishes allowed them to fulfil their increasingly multifaceted roles of professionals, wives and mothers.

The proliferation of food additives in America's food identity standards during the mid-century period demonstrates the complicated (and sometimes contradictory) economic, cultural and legislative forces that underpinned the actions of food manufacturers, regulators and consumers. Food manufacturers created convenience products and used additives to preserve and produce these too-good-to-be-true foods. Consumers feared food additives but purchased processed foods because they offered a reprieve from taxing domestic responsibilities. By the time concerns about additives had reached the mainstream, processed food had already become bound up in the modern American lifestyle.[87]

Conclusion

Today, the Atlas Chemical Company no longer exists. Just as it emerged from the dismantling of DuPont's explosives monopoly, in the 1990s portions of Atlas were absorbed by AstraZeneca, while others became part of the Dutch company Azko Nobel. Though Atlas in name no longer exists as a standalone company, its influence in food production lives on. Today, industrial emulsifiers remain a common ingredient in processed food. Popular sliced bread manufacturers like Oroweat and Wonder continue to use chemical emulsifiers in their products. Additionally, mono and diglycerides are commonly found in many commercially produced baked goods, butter substitutes, icings, peanut butter, chocolate candies, coffee creamers and ice cream.[88] Despite their widespread use, a 2015 study linked emulsifiers to ulcerative colitis and Crohn's disease.[89]

Beyond emulsifiers, popular distrust of processed foods has only grown since the 1970s. Stores like Whole Foods Market now offer convenience foods like frozen dinners, natural American cheese slices and boxed macaroni and cheese with the promise of being free from most food additives. While 'natural' processed foods are on the rise, these foods require some processing in order to last in the unnatural world of long supply chains, supermarkets and modern consumer expectations. Shoppers that are able to afford the move towards natural convenience foods have more options than ever, while lower-income Americans remain tethered to the cost and time practicalities that conventional processed foods offer. A 2010 paper from *Nutrition Today* suggests that 'time poverty' is a barrier to preparing healthy meals, as low-cost, nutritious meals take longer to prepare than convenience foods.[90] A 2014 survey of Americans using food assistance programs by the non-profit organization Feeding America found that nearly 80 per cent of respondents purchased processed convenience foods because they were cheap and filling. This same study linked this practice to higher rates of dietary-related health conditions like diabetes and heart disease among low-income Americans.[91]

As Americans are more distrustful of food additives than ever, it is clear that processed convenience foods are not going anywhere. Consumers now expect food manufacturers to cleanse their product of additives, rather than eschewing processed foods altogether. Despite the visibility of fad diets like the #eatclean movement, actions by large food corporations like Kraft's 2015 decision to secretly remove artificial colours, flavours and preservatives from their boxed macaroni and cheese show that processed foods still remain staples of the American diet.[92] These expectations reflect the complicated relationship consumers developed over the twentieth century with processed foods. Though processed foods often bear no resemblance to the foods that one could prepare in a home kitchen, consumers still expect them to be just as wholesome. While consumers feared the additives that industrial food manufacturers favoured, the convenience of these foods was undeniable, especially for women juggling numerous professional and personal responsibilities.

In the end, consumer fears over emulsifiers in bread were ignored, ushering in the golden age of food additives. While food standards and additives seem like oil and water, the FDA emulsified them, writing them into nearly every food standard of the mid-century. Today, more than 300 food identity standards remain in effect, though they are most commonly invoked by one food giant against another to gain greater market share.[93] Just as the FDA practiced contradictory regulatory practices, consumers outwardly disliked additives while continuing to purchase foods containing them. Consumer reliance on the convenience of processed foods has remained, while dietary advice about the health risks of processed foods is often just as contradictory as consumer practices. Consumers receive messages linking food additives to increased risk of cancer and gastrointestinal diseases, while also being told to trust scientists on the safety of food chemicals.[94]

Using the bread standards as a case study, this chapter reveals the forces that went into the framing and function of food identity standards in the post-war period, the emergence of processed convenience foods and how consumers related to them. Analysing the power and influence that food companies exerted over the regulatory process helps account for the widespread use of additives, but it does not explain the continued popularity of these foods. Applying gender analysis helps explain why processed foods remained so popular despite popular distrust. Further intersectional analysis is needed to better understand the dilemma that women and lower-income consumers faced between cost, time and health in their food procurement practices during the middle of the twentieth century and beyond.

Notes

Introduction

1 David Bishai and Ritu Nalubola, 'The History of Food Fortification in the United States: Its Relevance for Current Fortification Efforts in Developing Countries', *Economic Development and Cultural Change* 51, no. 1 (2002), 45.

2 Mee Ryoung Song and Meeja Im, 'Moderating Effects of Food Type and Consumers' Attitude on the Evaluation of Food Items Labeled "Additive-Free"', *Journal of Consumer Behaviour* 17 (2018), e1–e12, https://doi.org/10.1002/cb.1671.

3 On current (2015) sales, see 'Rising Levels of Lactose Intolerance Predicted to Propel the Global Lactose Free Food Market Until 2020', *Business Wire*, 4 May 2016, https://www.businesswire.com/news/home/20160504005106/en/Rising-Levels-Lactose-Intolerance-Predicted-Propel-Global.

4 Imran Aziz, Federica Branchi and David Sanders, 'The Rise and Fall of Gluten!', *Proceedings of the Nutrition Society* 74 (2015), 221–26.

5 *Gluten-Free Products Market Size & Share, Industry Report, 2014–2025*, Grandview Research, May 2017, https://www.grandviewresearch.com/industry-analysis/gluten-free-products-market.

6 Nicoletta Pellegrini and Carlo Agostoni, 'Nutritional Aspects of Gluten-Free Products', *Journal of the Science of Food and Agriculture* 95 (2015), 2380–85.

7 Alexandra Livarda and Marijke van der Veen, 'Social Access and Dispersal of Condiments in North-West Europe from the Roman to the Medieval Period', *Vegetation History and Archaeobotany* 17, Suppl. 1 (2008), 201–9.

8 Steven Shapin, '"You Are What You Eat": Historical Changes in Ideas about Food and Identity', *Historical Research* 87 (2014), 380.

9 The key reference remains Alfred W. Crosby, *The Columbian Exchange: Biological and Cultural Consequences of 1492* (Westport, CT: Praeger, [1973] 2003). For a survey of Italian reactions, see David Gentilcore, 'The Impact of New World Plants, 1500–1800: The Americans in Italy', in *The New World in Early Modern Italy, 1492–1750*, ed. E. Horodowich and Lia Markey (Cambridge: Cambridge University Press, 2017), 190–205. For the problematic Italian reception of two foods in particular, see David Gentilcore, *Pomodoro! A History of the Tomato in Italy* (New York: Columbia University Press, 2010) and David Gentilcore, *Italy and the Potato: A History* (London: Continuum, 2012).

10 On changing medical and scientific ideas towards food and foods from the Middle Ages, see Ken Albala, *Eating Right in the Renaissance* (Berkeley: University of California Press, 2002); Marilyn Nicoud, *Les régimes de santé au moyen âge* (Rome: École Française de Rome, 2007); Heikki Mikkeli, *Hygiene in the Early Modern Medical Tradition* (Helsinki: Academia Scientiarum Fennica, 1999); Emma C. Spary, *Eating the Enlightenment: Food and the Sciences in Paris, 1670–1760* (Chicago,

   IL: University of Chicago Press, 2012); David Gentilcore, *Food and Health in Early Modern Europe: Diet, Medicine and Society, 1450–1800* (London: Bloomsbury, 2016).
11 Shapin, 'You Are What You Eat', 378.
12 Gyorgy Scrinis, *Nutritionism: The Science and Politics of Dietary Advice* (New York: Columbia University Press, 2013).
13 Harvey Levenstein, *Paradox of Plenty* (Oxford: Oxford University Press, 1993); Harvey Levenstein, *Fear of Food: A History of Why We Worry about What We Eat* (Chicago, IL: Chicago University Press, 2012)
14 Alberto De Bernardi, *Il mal della rosa. Denutrizione e pellagra nelle campagne italiane fra '800 e '900* (Milan: Franco Angeli, 1984); Arturo Warman, *Corn and Capitalism: How a Botanical Bastard Grew to Global Dominance*, trans. N. Westrate (Chapel Hill: University of North Carolina Press, 2003); Mary Katherine Crabb, 'An Epidemic of Pride: Pellagra and the Culture of the American South', *Anthropologica* 34 (1992), 89–103.
15 Laura Beil, 'Sweet Confusion: Does High Fructose Corn Syrup Deserve Such a Bad Rap?' *Science News* 183, no. 11 (2013), 22–25.
16 Alexander Bay, *Beriberi in Modern Japan: The Making of a National Disease* (Rochester, NY: University of Rochester Press, 2012); K. Codell Carter, 'The Germ Theory, Beriberi, and the Deficiency Theory of Disease', *Medical History* 21 (1977), 119–36; Anne Hardy, 'Beri-beri, Vitamin B1 and World Food Policy, 1925–1970', *Medical History* 39 (1995), 61–77.
17 Although most critiques of the global food economy emphasize the environmental costs of importing food thousands of miles (for instance, in order to have seasonal produce, such as asparagus, out of season), some compelling arguments about the health benefits of a local diet have been made. Richard A. Cone and Emily Martin, 'Corporeal Flows: The Immune System, Global Economies of Food, and Implications for Health', *Ecologist* 27 (1997), 107–11; Michael Mikulak, *The Politics of the Pantry: Stories, Food, and Social Change* (Montreal: McGill-Queen's University Press, 2013).
18 Colin Spencer, 'The British Isles', in *The Cambridge World History of Food*, ed. K. Kiple and K. Ornelas (Cambridge: Cambridge University Press, 2000), 1217–26; Andrea Broomfield, *Food and Cooking in Victorian England: A History* (Westport, CT: Praeger, 2007).
19 Paul Clayton and Judith Rowbotham, 'An Unsuitable and Degraded Diet?', *Journal of the Royal Society of Medicine* part 1, 101, no. 6 (2008), 282–89; part 2, 101, no. 7 (2008), 350–57; and part 3, 101, no. 9 (2008), 454–62.
20 Robert Millward and Frances Bell, 'Economic Factors in the Decline of Mortality in Late Nineteenth Century Britain', *European Review of Economic History* 2, no. 3 (1998), 263–88; Robert Woods, *The Demography of Victorian England and Wales* (Cambridge: Cambridge University Press, 2000).
21 David Bishai and Ritu Nalubola, 'The History of Food Fortification in the United States: Its Relevance for Current Fortification Efforts in Developing Countries', *Economic Development and Cultural Change* 51, no. 1 (2002), 37–53; Y. Park, C. Sempos, C. Barton, J. Vanderveen and E. Yetley, 'Effectiveness of Food Fortification in the United States: The Case of Pellagra', *American Journal of Public Health* 90, no. 5 (2000), 727–38.
22 Klaus Grunert, 'European Consumers' Acceptance of Functional Foods', *Annals of the New York Academy of Sciences*, no. 1190 (2010), 166–73. See also, Navdeep Kaur

and Devinder Pal Singh, 'Deciphering the Consumer Behaviour Facets of Functional Foods: A Literature Review', *Appetite*, no. 112 (2017), 167–87.

23 For the article that started it all, see S. Boyd Eaton and Melvin Konner, 'Paleolithic Nutrition: A Consideration of Its Nature and Current Implications', *New England Journal of Medicine* 312, no. 5 (1985), 283–89.

24 Charlotte Biltekoff, 'Consumer Response: The Paradoxes of Food and Health', *Annals of the New York Academy of Sciences* 1190 (2010), 174–78.

25 Surinder Phull, 'The Mediterranean Diet: Socio-Cultural Relevance for Contemporary Health Promotion', *Open Public Health Journal* 8 (2015), 35–40.

26 Lauren Renée Moore, ' "But We're Not Hypochondriacs": The Changing Shape of Gluten-Free Dieting and the Contested Illness Experience', *Social Science and Medicine* 105 (2014), 76–83.

27 As one industry spokesperson put it, 'There are few markets where you can win "a customer for life", and who is willing to pay a big premium for the right product. But this is one of them'. 'Lactose-Free Gains Ground Globally', *Dairy Industries International* 77, no. 6 (2012), 8.

28 Susan Raatz, LuAnn Johnson and Matthew Picklo, 'Consumption of Honey, Sucrose, and High-Fructose Corn Syrup Produces Similar Metabolic Effects in Glucose-Tolerant and Intolerant Individuals', *Journal of Nutrition* 145, no. 10 (2015), 2265–72; 'Sickly Sweetener: High Fructose Corn Syrup', *Economist*, Saturday, 29 May 2010, issue 8684, 69; Ashby Jones, ' "Corn Sugar" Goes on Trial as Suit Debates High-Fructose Corn Syrup', *Wall Street Journal*, 20 September 2011; Julie Jargon, 'McDonald's to Remove High-Fructose Corn Syrup from Sandwich Buns', *Wall Street Journal*, 2 August 2016.

29 Sharon Friel et al., 'Shaping the Discourse: What Has the Food Industry Been Lobbying for in the Trans Pacific Partnership Trade Agreement and What Are the Implications for Dietary Health?', *Critical Public Health* 26, no. 5 (2016), 518–29.

30 Deborah Lupton, *Food, the Body and the Self* (London: Sage, 1996), 72–73.

31 James Harvey Young, 'The Pig That Fell into the Privy: Upton Sinclair's The Jungle and the Meat Inspection Amendments of 1906', *Bulletin of the History of Medicine* 59 (1985), 467–80; James Harvey Young, *Pure Food, Securing the Federal Pure Food and Drug Act of 1906* (Princeton, NJ: Princeton University Press, 1989); Jeffrey Haydu, 'Frame Brokerage in the Pure Food Movement, 1879–1906', *Social Movement Studies* 11 (2012), 97–112.

32 Haydu, 'Frame Brokerage', 101.

33 Ibid., 104–5; Upton Sinclair, *The Jungle* (New York: Doubleday, 1906). Sinclair famously declared that 'I aimed at the public's heart and by accident hit its stomach'. For more on how the relationship between meat and human health has been understood, see David Cantor, Christian Bonah and Matthias Dörries, eds, *Meat, Medicine and Human Health in the Twentieth Century* (London: Pickering and Chatto, 2010).

34 Philip Conford, *The Origins of the Organic Movement* (Edinburgh: Floris Books, 2001); Richard Moore-Colyer, 'Towards "Mother Earth": Jorian Jenks, Organicism, the Right and the British Union of Fascists', *Journal of Contemporary History* 39 (2004), 353–71.

35 Moore-Colyer, 'Towards "Mother Earth" ', 365–66.

36 Warren Belasco, *Appetite for Change: How the Counterculture Took on the Food Industry* (Ithaca, NY: Cornell, [1989] 2007).

37 Ian Mosby, '"That Won-Ton Soup Headache": The Chinese Restaurant Syndrome, MSG and the Making of American Food, 1968–1980', *Social History of Medicine* 22 (2009), 133–51.
38 Mikulak, *Politics of the Pantry*.
39 Rima Apple, *Mothers and Medicine: A Social History of Infant Feeding* (Madison: University of Wisconsin Press, 1987); Jacqueline H. Wolf, *Don't Kill Your Baby: Public Health and the Decline of Breastfeeding in the Nineteenth and Twentieth Centuries* (Columbus: Ohio State University Press, 2001); Rima Apple, *Perfect Motherhood: Science and Childrearing in America* (New Brunswick, NJ: Rutgers University Press, 2006).
40 Maia Boswell-Penc has put arguments about the purity of breastmilk versus the artificiality of formula in context by highlighting the issue of 'breastmilk toxicity', caused by environmental contamination. Maia Boswel-Penc, *Tainted Milk: Breastmilk, Feminisms, and the Politics of Environmental Degradation* (New York: University of New York Press, 2006).
41 C. West, 'Introduction of Complementary Foods to Infants', *Annals of Nutrition and Metabolism* 70 (2017), 47–54
42 Karin Garrety, 'Social Worlds, Actor-Networks and Controversy: The Case of Cholesterol, Dietary Fat and Heart Disease', *Social Studies of Science* 27 (1995), 727–73; Mark W. Bufton and Virginia Berridge, 'Post-War Nutrition Science and Policy Making in Britain c. 1945–1994: The Case of Diet and Heart Disease', in *Food, Science, Policy and Regulation in the Twentieth Century*, edited by David F. Smith and Jim Phillips (London: Routledge, 2000), 207–21; Frances Steel, 'A Source of Our Wealth, Yet Adverse to Our Health? Butter and the Heart Link in New Zealand to c. 1990', *Social History of Medicine* 18 (2005), 475–93; David Cantor, 'Confused Messages: Meat, Civilization and Cancer Education in the Early Twentieth Century', in *Meat, Medicine and Human Health in the Twentieth Century*, ed. David Cantor, Christian Bonah and Matthias Dorries (London: Pickering and Chatto, 2010), 111–26; Élodie Giroux, 'The Framingham Study and the Constitution of a Restrictive Concept of Risk Factor', *Social History of Medicine* 26 (2013), 94–113.
43 Matthew Smith, *Hyperactive: The Controversial History of ADHD* (London: Reaktion, 2012).
44 Matthew Smith, *An Alternative History of Hyperactivity: Food Additives and the Feingold Diet* (New Brunswick, NJ: Rutgers University Press, 2011).
45 National Advisory Committee on Hyperkinesis and Food Additives, *Final Report to the Nutrition Foundation* (New York: Nutrition Foundation, 1980).
46 Rima Apple, *Vitamania: Vitamins in American Culture* (New Brunswick, NJ: Rutgers University Press, 1996); Harmke Kamminga, '"Axes to Grind": Popularising the Science of Vitamins, 1920s and 1930s', in *Food, Science, Policy and Regulation in the Twentieth Century*, ed. David F. Smith and Jim Phillips (London: Routledge, 2000), 83–100.
47 Ann F. La Berge, 'How the Ideology of Low Fat Conquered America', *Journal of the History of Medicine and the Allied Sciences* 62 (2008), 139–77.
48 David F. Smith and Jim Phillips, 'Food Policy and Regulation: A Multiplicity of Actors and Experts' in *Food, Science, Policy and Regulation in the Twentieth Century*, ed. David F. Smith and Jim Phillips (London: Routledge, 2000), 1.
49 Michael Pollan, *In Defence of Food: The Myth of Nutrition and the Pleasures of Eating* (London: Allen Lane, 2008).
50 Warren Belasco, 'Future Notes: The Meal-in-a-Pill', *Food and Foodways* 8, no. 4 (2000), 253–71.

1 The Pre-History of the Paleo Diet:
Cancer in Nineteenth-Century Britain

1 'Dr. Loren Cordain', http://thepaleodiet.com/dr-loren-cordain/, accessed 29
   September 2017.
2 'Breast Cancers and Other Cancers: Disease of Western Civilization?', http://
   thepaleodiet.com/breast-cancer-and-other-cancers-diseases-of-western-civilization/,
   accessed 29 September 2017.
3 Ibid.
4 Ibid.
5 Charles E. Rosenberg, 'Pathologies of Progress: The Idea of Civilization as Risk',
   Bulletin of the History of Medicine 72, no. 4 (1998), 714.
6 Ibid., 273.
7 Roy Porter, *The Greatest Benefit to Mankind. A Medical History of Humanity
   from Antiquity to the Present* (London: Fontana Press, 1999), 574; Siddhartha
   Mukherjee, *The Emperor of All Maladies: A Biography of Cancer* (New York: Scribner,
   2011), 241.
8 There are, of course, exceptions. Frances Burney's 1811 mastectomy has received
   detailed scrutiny from feminist scholars such as J. Epstein and S. Mediratta: J. E.
   Epstein, 'Writing the Unspeakable: Fanny Burney's Mastectomy and the Fictive Body',
   Representations 16, no. 1 (1986), 131–66; S. Mediratta, 'Beauty and the Breast: The
   Poetics of Physical Absence and Narrative Presence in Frances Burney's Mastectomy
   Letter (1811)', *Women: A Cultural Review* 19, no. 2 (2008), 188–207. Cancer and
   gender in the nineteenth century has also been studied: I. Löwy, ' "Because of Their
   Praiseworthy Modesty, They Consult Too Late": Regimes of Hope and Cancer of
   the Womb, 1800–1910', *Bulletin of the History of Medicine* 85 (2001), 356–83; O.
   Moscucci, 'Gender and Cancer in Britain, 1860–1910: The Emergence of Cancer as a
   Public Health Concern', *American Journal of Public Health* 95, no. 8 (2005), 1312–21;
   Gender and Cancer in England, 1860–1948 (Basingstoke: Palgrave Macmillan, 2016).
   Finally, cancer in nineteenth-century America has received more attention than in the
   United Kingdom: R. A. Aronowitz, *Unnatural History: Breast Cancer and American
   Society* (Cambridge: Cambridge University Press, 2007).
9 George Weisz and Jesse Olszynko-Gryn, 'The Theory of Epidemiologic
   Transition: The Origins of a Citation Classic', *Journal of the History of Medicine and
   Allied Sciences* 65 (2010), 287–326.
10 Abdel Omran, 'The Epidemiological Transition: A Theory of the Epidemiology of
   Population Change', *The Milbank Quarterly* 83 (1971), 731–57.
11 Anon., 'Cancer Increasing at an Alarming Rate', *Vogue*, 15 April 1909, 726.
12 For example, contemporary concerns that contaminated milk communicated typhoid.
   See, Jacob Steere-Williams, 'The Perfect Food and the Filth Disease: Milk-Borne
   Typhoid and Epidemiological Practice in late Victorian Britain', *Journal of the History
   of Medicine and Allied Sciences* 65, no. 4 (2010), 514–45; and Keir Waddington, 'The
   Dangerous Sausage: Diet, Meat and Disease in Victorian and Edwardian Britain',
   Cultural and Social History 8, no. 1 (2011), 51–71.
13 David Cantor, 'Confused Messages: Meat, Civilization, and Cancer Education in the
   Early Twentieth Century', in *Meat, Medicine and Human Health in the Twentieth
   Century*, ed. David Cantor, Christian Bonah and Matthias Dörries (London: Pickering
   & Chatto, 2010), 111.

14 Leukaemia and other malignancies that do not manifest tumours or growths were not defined as cancers in the nineteenth century. It was only in the early twentieth century that they were designated cancers. See, Emm Barnes Johnstone and Joanna Baines, *The Changing Faces of Childhood Cancer: Clinical and Cultural Visions Since 1940* (Basingstoke: Palgrave Macmillan, 2015).

15 Scholars have argued that in the eighteenth century, the 'externally unbounded' body became offensive and modernity became increasingly implicated in the practice of disciplining the corporeal. The messy, disorganized cancerous body posed, therefore, a fundamental challenge to the creation of the new 'bourgeois body' in the long nineteenth century. See, Barbara Duden, *The Woman beneath the Skin: A Doctor's Patients in Eighteenth-Century German*, trans. Thomas Dunlap (Cambridge, MA: Harvard University Press, 1991), 13.

16 These were the Cancer Ward at the Middlesex Hospital in 1792, and 'The Society and Institution for Investigating the Nature and Cure of Cancer' in 1802. Both were established in London. See, John Howard, *The Plan Adopted by the Governors of the Middlesex-Hospital for the Relief of Persons Afflicted with Cancer: With Notes and Observations* (London: H. L. Galabin, 1792); Bruce Schoenberg, 'A Program for the Conquest of Cancer: 1802', *Journal of the History of Medicine and Allied Sciences* XXX (1975), 3–22.

17 Thomas Denman, *Observations on the Cure of Cancer, with Some Remarks upon Mr. Young's Treatment of That Disease* (London: E. Cox, 1816), 3.

18 Alanna Skuse, *Constructions of Cancer in Early Modern England: Ravenous Natures* (London: Palgrave Macmillan, 2015), 25.

19 John Abernethy, *Surgical Observations on Tumours* (London: Longman, Hurst, Rees, Orme, and Brown, 1811), 74.

20 Thomas Pope, 'On Cancer', *Association Medical Journal* 3 (1855), 859.

21 Alanna Skuse, 'Wombs, Worms and Wolves: Constructing Cancer in Early Modern England', *Social History of Medicine* 27 (2014), 632.

22 HC Deb 08 February 1841 vol 56 cc375–451.

23 See, Laura Otis, 'The Metaphoric Circuit: Organic and Technological Communication in the Nineteenth Century', *Journal of the History of Ideas* 63, no. 1 (2002), 127.

24 Henry T. Butlin, 'Carcinoma Is a Parasitic Disease. Being the Bradshaw Lecture Delivered before the Royal College of Surgeons of England', *British Medical Journal* 2 (1905), 1566.

25 Charles Walker, 'Theories and Problems of Cancer: Part III', *Science Progress in the Twentieth Century* 7, no. 26 (1912), 223–238, 228.

26 Ibid.

27 Woods Hutchinson, 'The Cancer Problem: Or, Treason in the Republic of the Body', *The Contemporary Review*, July 1899, 113.

28 James Braithwaite, 'Excess of Salt as a Cause of Cancer', *British Medical Journal* 2 (1902), 1376.

29 P. W. Hislop and P. Clennell Fenwick, 'Cancer in New Zealand', *British Medical Journal*, 2 (1909), 1225.

30 See, John M. Eyler, 'The Conceptual Origins of William Farr's Epidemiology: Numerical Methods and Social Thought in the 1830s', in *Times, Places, and Persons: Aspects of the History of Epidemiology*, ed. Abraham M. Lilienfeld (Baltimore, MD: Henry E. Sigerist Supplements to the Bulletin of the History of Medicine 4, 1980), Ian Hacking, *The Taming of Chance* (Cambridge: Cambridge University Press, 1990); Eileen Magnello and Anne Hardy, eds, *The Road to Medical Statistics* (Amsterdam: Brill, 2002).

31 Edward Higgs, 'Registrar General's Reports for England and Wales, 1838–1858', *Online Historical Population Reports*, http://histpop.org/, accessed 13 October 2016.

32 Edward Higgs, 'The Annual Report of the Registrar-General, 1839–1920: A Textual History', in *The Road to Medical Statistics*, ed. Eileen Magnello and Anne Hardy (Amsterdam: Brill, 2002), 55.

33 George Graham, 'Statistical Nosology', *Fourth Annual Report of the Registrar-General* (England, 1840–1841), 93–105.

34 Brydges P. Henniker, 'Introduction', *Forty-Second Annual Report of the Registrar-General* (England, 1879), xxx.

35 William MacGregor, 'An Address on Some Problems of Tropical Medicine', *The Lancet* 156 (1900), 1055–61; W. Renner, 'The Spread of Cancer among the Descendants of the Liberated Africans or Creoles of Sierra Leone', *British Medical Journal* 2, no. 2075 (1910), 977–84.

36 Hugh P. Dunn, 'The Increase of Cancer', *Pall Mall Gazette*, 12 May 1884.

37 Ibid.

38 H. Herasey, 'The Rarity of Cancer among the Aborigines of British Central Africa. Squamous Carcinoma: Acinous Carcinoma: Physiological Reasons for Immunity from Cancer of the Breast: Columnar Carcinoma', *British Medical Journal* 2, no. 2396 (1906), 1562–63, 1562.

39 Anon., 'Cancer in the Colonies', *British Medical Journal* 1 (1906), 812.

40 Renner, 'The Spread of Cancer among the Descendants of the Liberated Africans or Creoles of Sierra Leone', 588.

41 Anon., 'Cancer in the Colonies', 812.

42 Ibid., 812.

43 Ibid.

44 In his 1883 'Address in Pathology', the parasitologist Charles Creighton wrote that smallpox was 'peculiarly an African disease'. This particularity was a biological one – 'the loathsomeness, the peculiar odour, and the no less peculiar scars of small-pox, might of themselves suggest another skin than ours.'

45 Leo Loeb, 'The Cancer Problem', *Interstate Medical Journal* XVII (1910), 1.

46 E. F. Bashford, 'An Address Entitled Are the Problems of Cancer Insoluble?', *British Medical Journal* 2 (1905), 1510.

47 William Hill-Climo, 'Cancer in Ireland: An Economic Question', *The Empire Review* VI (1903), 410.

48 W. Roger Williams, 'Cancer in Egypt and the Causation of Cancer', *British Medical Journal* 2 (1902), 917.

49 Hill-Climo, 'Cancer in Ireland', 411.

50 https://diseasesofmodernlife.org/, accessed 25 August 2017.

51 Rosenberg, 'Pathologies of Progress', 718.

52 Macgregor, 'An Address on Some Problems of Tropical Medicine', 979.

53 Anon., 'Is Race Extinction Staring Us in the Face?', *New York Times*, 15 October 1911, 11.

54 'An anti-toxic diet, that is a diet which discourages the development of putrefactive poisons in the intestine, is specially to be commended as a means of combating cancer . . . During the last 45 years the writer has had unusual opportunities for observation in relation to the influence of a non-flesh dietary upon the occurrence of cancer. Of many thousands of flesh-abstainers with whom he has been acquainted, he has known during this period of only four cases of cancer in persons who had been for a long time flesh abstainers . . . There can be no doubt that among the thousands of

persons under observation who escape the disease, as the writer believes through flesh abstaining, there must have been a considerable number who were especially susceptible to cancer because of heredity and who were able to overcome this special susceptibility by a non-flesh dietary'. John Harvey Kellogg, *The New Dietetics, What to Eat and How: A Guide to Scientific Feeding in Health and Disease* (Battle Creek: Modern Medicine Publishing Co., 1921), 793.

55   Anon., 'Overeating and Cancer', *British Medical Journal* 1, no. 2045 (1900), 596.
56   Ibid.
57   Macgregor, 'An Address on Some Problems of Tropical Medicine', 982.
58   Anon., 'Is Race Extinction Staring Us in the Face?', 11.
59   Ian Miller, *Reforming Food in Post-Famine Ireland: Medicine, Science and Improvement, 1845–1922* (Manchester: Manchester University Press, 2014).
60   Hill-Climo, 'Cancer in Ireland: An Economic Question', 413. Commenters from Linnaeus to Lapouge suggested European populations could be separated along biological lines. Mediterranean peoples were understood as physically inferior – 'Homo Alpinus' rather than 'Homo Europaeus' – and seen as closer in quality to the less-civilized races of warmer climes. Northern Italians sometimes said that Calabria evoked Africa; the South was cast as a form of 'other' world. Daniel Pick, *Faces of Degeneration. A European Disorder, c. 1848–1918* (Cambridge: Cambridge University Press, 1989), 114. The Irish were similarly racialized, caricatured in the British press with simian noses, long upper lips, huge projecting mouths and sloping foreheads. L. P. Curtis, *Apes and Angels: The Irishman in Victorian Caricature* (Washington, DC: Smithsonian Books, 1971), 29.
61   Hill-Climo, 'Cancer in Ireland: An Economic Question', 413.
62   Anon., 'Cancer in Ireland: An Economical Question', *British Medical Journal* 2 (1903), 1544.
63   Ibid.
64   HC Deb 07 April 1897 vol. 48 cc677–711.
65   In their review of Hill-Climo's argument, the *British Medical Journal* was deeply unimpressed that 'such an important medical proposition' had been first printed 'in a lay journal, in which it cannot be conveniently subjected to skilled criticism'. They recognized the impact such a claim could make on the imaginations of the *Empire Review*'s middle-class readership. While they were damming about the veracity of Hill-Climo's claims, the damage had been done. Anon., 'Cancer in Ireland: An Economical Question', 1544.
66   Hill-Climo, 'Cancer in Ireland: An Economic Question', 414.
67   Ibid., 413.
68   'Chronic Diseases Are Killing More in Poorer Countries', https://www.nytimes.com/2014/12/04/world/asia/chronic-diseases-are-killing-more-in-poorer-countries.html?_r=0, accessed 30 September 2017.

2 Nutrition, Starvation and Diabetic Diets:
A Century of Change in the United States

1   Thursday, 25 January, 10:00 am, discussion at University of Texas San Antonio, Retama Auditorium, San Antonio, Texas.

2 Frederick M. Allen, *Total Dietary Regulation in the Treatment of Diabetes* (New York: The Rockefeller Institute for Medical Research, 1919).

3 Elliott P. Joslin, *A Diabetic Manual for the Mutual Use of Doctor and Patient* (Philadelphia, PA: Lea & Febiger, 1941), 10, https//catalog.hathitrust.org/Record/001578358.

4 Elijah Muhammad, *How to Eat to Live, Book 1* (Phoenix: Secretarius MEMPS, 1967, 1997), 30.

5 Richard K. Bernstein, *The Diabetes Diet: Dr. Bernstein's Low-Carbohydrate Solution*, 1st edn (New York: Little, Brown, 2005), vii.

6 David F. Burg, *Chicago's White City of 1893* (Lexington: University Press of Kentucky, 2015). During the 1893 Chicago's World Fair, Chicago was dubbed the 'White City' due to the white stucco buildings, neoclassical architecture, bright streetlights and more.

7 'Full Text of "World's Columbian Exposition, Chicago, IL, 1893"', accessed 2 February 2018, https://archive.org/stream/worldscolumbian00awargoog/worldscolumbian00awargoog_djvu.txt.

8 Wilbur Olin Atwater, *Foods: Nutritive Value and Cost* (Washington, DC: US Dept. of Agriculture, 1894).

9 W. O. Atwater, *The Chemical Composition of American Food Materials* (Washington, DC: 1896), http://hdl.handle.net/2027/uva.x030348906.

10 Michael Bliss, *The Discovery of Insulin* (Chicago, IL: University of Chicago Press, 1982). Insulin is discovered in Toronto in 1921 and widely available for public use by 1922.

11 *Dietetic and Hygienic Gazette* (New York: Gazette, 1896), 417.

12 Atwater, *Chemical Composition of American Food Materials*. As this text explained, Atwater produced 'a tabular summary of analysis made in the United States of materials used for the food of man', 3.

13 John Christopher Feudtner, *Bittersweet : Diabetes, Insulin, and the Transformation of Illness* (Chapel Hill: University of North Carolina Press, 2003), 23–24; Bliss, *Discovery of Insulin*, 23–24.

14 Allen, *Total Dietary Regulation in the Treatment of Diabetes*. See especially Chapter 1.

15 Ibid., 19.

16 Ibid., 23–24, 31, 37, 62.

17 Bliss, *Discovery of Insulin*, 23–24.

18 'Display Ad 1 – Eating to Live Longer', *New York Times*, 15 March 1915.

19 Bernard Zinman et al., 'Diabetes Research and Care Through the Ages', *Diabetes Care* 40, no. 10 (October 2017), 1302–13, https://doi.org/10.2337/dci17-0042.

20 *Dietetic and Hygienic Gazette*, 416.

21 Atwater, *Chemical Composition of American Food Materials*, 3.

22 Orlando H. Petty and William Hoy Stoner, *Diabetes, Its Treatment by Insulin and Diet: A Handbook for the Patient*, 3rd rev. edn (Philadelphia, PA: F.A. Davis Company, 1926), 34.

23 Bliss, *Discovery of Insulin*, 23–24; Mexican Cookbook Collection, UTSA Special Collection, *El Cocinero Mexicano, ó, Coleccion de Las Mejores Recetas Para Guisar Al Estilo Americano: Y de Las Mas Selectas Segun El Metodo de Las Cocinas Española, Italiana, Francesa e Inglesa* (Mexico: Imprenta de Galvan, a cargo de Mariano Arevalo, Calle de Cadena num. 2, 1831).

24 Arthur Scott Donkin, *On the Relation between Diabetes and Food and Its Application to the Treatment of the Disease* (New York: G. P. Putnam's Sons, 1875), 151.

25 Bliss, *The Discovery of Insulin*, 23.
26 Charles Gatchell, *'Doctor, What Shall I Eat?': A Handbook of Diet in Disease, for the Profession and the People* (Milwaukee, WI: Cramer, Aikens & Cramer, 1880), http://archive.org/details/63831160R.nlm.nih.gov.
27 First Presbyterian Church, ed., *The Texas Cook Book: A Thorough Treatise on the Art of Cookery* (St. Louis, MO: The Association, R.P. Studley, 1883).
28 Elliott P. Joslin, 'The Treatment of Diabetes Mellitus', *Canadian Medical Association Journal* 6, no. 8 (August 1916), 673–84. See p. 677.
29 'Full Text of "World's Columbian Exposition, Chicago, IL., 1893"', 9.
30 Atwater, *Chemical Composition of American Food Materials*, 1896, 5.
31 Joslin, *Diabetic Manual for the Mutual Use of Doctor and Patient*, 76, http://archive.org/details/adiabeticmanual00unkngoog; Joslin, 'The Treatment of Diabetes Mellitus', 196.
32 To be sure, Stoner and Petty recognized that insulin was required for the most severe patients, and diabetic cures without insulin were impossible for severe diabetics. Petty and Stoner, *Diabetes, Its Treatment by Insulin and Diet*, 60.
33 Allen, *Total Dietary Regulation In the Treatment of Diabetes*.
34 Ibid., vi.
35 Allan Mazur, 'Why Were "Starvation Diets" Promoted for Diabetes in the Pre-Insulin Period?', *Nutrition Journal* 10 (11 March 2011), 2, https://doi.org/10.1186/1475-2891-10-23.
36 'Fasting Treatment for Diabetes', *The British Medical Journal* 1, no. 2882 (25 March 1916), 458.
37 Allen, *Total Dietary Regulation In the Treatment of Diabetes*.
38 'Fasting Treatment for Diabetes'.
39 This list is a summary of library and archival holdings (available in 2016) according to WorldCat. The issue of provenance is unclear; however, because of the popularity of the text between 1915 and 1922, I suspect the libraries acquired them then.
40 As quoted in Mazur, 'Why Were "Starvation Diets" Promoted for Diabetes in the Pre-Insulin Period?', 4, and found in Elliott P. Joslin, 'Present-Day Treatment', *American Journal of the Medical Sciences* 150, no. 4 (1915), 485–96, see p. 486.
41 Bliss, *Discovery of Insulin*; Feudtner, *Bittersweet*; Jeremy A. Greene, *Prescribing by Numbers: Drugs and the Definition of Disease*, 1st edn (Baltimore, MD: Johns Hopkins University Press, 2008).
42 Bliss, *Discovery of Insulin*, 13.
43 Henry John respected Allen's work and dedicated this manual to him. As John's dedication read, 'To Dr. Frederick M. Allen, The most indefatigable worker I have ever met; a man who has devoted his life to the attainment of an ideal and has given us a deeper insight into the problem of diabetes through his extensive researches, in humbleness and admiration I dedicate this volume', (p. 7).
44 Henry Jerry John, *Diabetic Manual for Patients* (St. Louis, MO: The C.V. Mosby Company, 1928), 55; Joslin, *Diabetic Manual for the Mutual Use of Doctor and Patient*, //catalog.hathitrust.org/Record/001565827; Petty and Stoner, *Diabetes, Its Treatment by Insulin and Diet*.
45 H. Gray and Jean M. Stewart, 'Quantitative Diets versus Guesswork in the Treatment of Obesity and Diabetes', *The Scientific Monthly* 32, no. 1 (1931), 46–53.
46 Gray and Stewart recommend Atwater and Bryant's *The Chemical Composition of American Food Products*, 1906, for its comprehensiveness, as well as Elliot Joslin's *Diabetic Manual* (1929) for its simplicity. See page 47 and image 52.

47 Gray and Stewart, 'Quantitative Diets versus Guesswork in the Treatment of Obesity and Diabetes'.

48 Ibid., 46.

49 'The Founders: Story of the Novo Nordisk founders, August and Marie Krogh, Hans Christian Hagedorn, August Kongsted', accessed 5 March 2018, http://www. novonordisk.com/about-novo-nordisk/novo-nordisk-history/the-founders.html. See also H. R. Wiedemann, 'The Pioneers of Pediatric Medicine. Karl Stolte (1881–1951)', *European Journal of Pediatrics* 152, no. 2 (1993), 81.

50 L. Sawyer and E. A. M. Gale, 'Diet, Delusion and Diabetes', *Diabetologia* 52, no. 1 (January 2009), 3, https://doi.org/10.1007/s00125-008-1203-9.

51 Feudtner, *Bittersweet*, 95.

52 Edward Tolstoi, *Living with Diabetes* (New York: Gramercy, 1952), 3. See also, 'Diet, Delusion and Diabetes | SpringerLink', accessed 3 March 2018, https://link.springer. com/article/10.1007/s00125-008-1203-9.

53 Chris Feudtner, 'The Want of Control: Ideas, Innovations, and Ideals in the Modern Management of Diabetes Mellitus', *Bulletin of the History of Medicine* 69, no. 1 (Spring 1995), 88.

54 Abraham Rudy, *Practical Handbook for Diabetic Patients, with 180 International Recipes (American, Jewish, French, German, Italian, Armenian, etc.)* (Boston: M. Barrows, 1929), 91, http://hdl.handle.net/2027/coo.31924003513623.

55 Joslin, *Diabetic Manual for the Mutual Use of Doctor and Patient*, 1941, 41.

56 Lev Grossman, 'Persons of the Year 2002 – TIME', *Time*, accessed 5 March 2018, http://content.time.com/time/specials/packages/article/ 0,28804,2022164_2021937_2 021901,00.html.

57 'decolonize YOUR DIET', accessed 1 March 2018, http://decolonizeyourdiet.org/ about.

58 Luz Calvo and Catriona Rueda Esquibel, *Decolonize Your Diet: Plant-Based Mexican-American Recipes for Health and Healing* (Vancouver: Arsenal Pulp Press, 2015).

59 Elliott P. Joslin, *The Treatment of Diabetes Mellitus* (Philadelphia, PA: Lea & Febiger, 1946); Edward Tolstoi, *The Practical Management of Diabetes*, American Lecture Series, No. 199. American Lectures in Metabolism; Variation: American Lecture Series, No. 199. American Lectures in Metabolism (Springfield, IL: Thomas, 1953); Allen, *Total Dietary Regulation in the Treatment of Diabetes*. Although Joslin and Tolstoi differed in their theories of care, both presented data on patients to support their theory. Likewise, Allen's work in the pre-insulin era included case studies, but also illustrates the limitations of case study analysis versus data collection.

60 'Radical New Method of Treating Diabetes: The Allen Plan, Which Upsets Old Traditions, Is Being Given a Thorough Test at the Rockefeller Institute – Five Salient Points of the System', *New York Times*, 1916, sec. MAGAZINE SECTION.

61 'Radical New Method of Treating Diabetes'.

62 E. K. Caso, 'Calculation of diabetic diets', *Journal of the American Dietetic Association* 26 (1950), 575–83.

63 Greene, *Prescribing by Numbers*, 98–105.

64 O. B. Crofford, S. Genuth and L. Baker, 'Diabetes Control and Complications Trial (DCCT): Results of Feasibility Study', *Diabetes Care* 10, no. 1 (1987), 1–19.

65 M. Porta, *Embedding Education into Diabetes Practice* (Basel: Karger Medical and Scientific Publishers, 2005), VII.

66 Sawyer and Gale, 'Diet, Delusion and Diabetes', 1.

3 Allergic to Innovation? Dietary Change
and Debate about Food Allergy in the United States

1 Heneage Ogilvie, 'Foreword' to Richard Mackarness, *Eat Fat and Grow Slim* (London: Harvil Press, 1958), 1–2.

2 See Kenneth F. Kiple, 'The Question of Paleolithic Nutrition and Modern Health: From the End to the Beginning', in *The Cambridge World History of Food*, Volume II, ed. Kenneth F. Kiple (Cambridge: Cambridge University Press, 2001), 1704–10.

3 Richard Mackarness, 'Stone Age Diet for Functional Disorders', *Medical World* 91 (1959), 14–19. The famed Franco-American microbiologist René Dubos Dubos (1901–1982) also warned that dietary change could cause health problems, though of a different type. Two of Dubos's concerns were the toxicity of new foodstuffs and the inappropriateness of high-calorie diets for people living sedentary lifestyles. René Dubos, 'Medical Utopias', *Daedalus* 88 (1959), 410–24. See also Alan C. Logan, Martin A. Katzman and Vincent Balanzá-Martínez, 'Natural Environments, Ancestral Diets, and Microbial Ecology: Is There a Modern "Paleo-Deficit Disorder"? Part I and II', *Journal of Physiological Anthropology* 34 (2015), https://jphysiolanthropol. biomedcentral.com/articles/10.1186/s40101-015-0041-y and https://jphysiolanthropol. biomedcentral.com/articles/10.1186/s40101-014-0040-4, accessed 20 October 2017.

4 Richard Mackarness, *Not All in the Mind: How Unsuspected Food Allergy Can Affect Your Body AND Your Mind* (London: Pan Books, 1976).

5 Clemens von Pirquet, 'Allergie', *Münchener Medizinische Wochenschrift* 30 (1906), 1457–58; Mark Jackson, *Allergy: The History of a Modern Malady* (London: Reaktion, 2006).

6 Much of food allergy's controversial nature rested on the fact that the skin tests used to diagnose most allergies were not effective for food allergies. As such, elimination diets (where patients were prescribed a very simple diet consisting of hypoallergenic foods and introduced challenge foods individually) were preferred. Since the evidence provided by elimination diets relied on patient testimony, it was thought to be less reliable. Matthew Smith, *Another Person's Poison: A History of Food Allergy* (New York: Columbia University Press, 2015).

7 Mark Jackson, '"Allergy con Amore": Psychosomatic Medicine and the "Asthmogenic Home" in the Mid-Twentieth Century', in *Health and the Modern Home*, ed. M. Jackson (London: Routledge, 2007), 153–74.

8 Ibid.

9 Mackarness began *Not All in the Mind* with the story of a patient who would have been given a lobotomy had he not successfully intervened with his Stone Age diet. Mackarness, *Not All in the Mind*, 11–24.

10 Jackson, *Allergy*; Paul Blanc, *How Everyday Products Make People Sick: Toxins at Home and in the Workplace* (Berkeley: University of California Press, 2007); Gregg Mitman, *Breathing Space: How Allergies Change Our Lives and Landscapes* (New Haven, CT: Yale University Press, 2007); Michelle Murphy, *Sick Building Syndrome and the Problem of Uncertainty: Environmental Politics, Technoscience, and Women Workers* (Durham, NC: Duke University Press, 2005).

11 Harvey Levenstein, *Fear of Food: A History of Why We Worry about What We Eat* (Chicago, IL: University of Chicago Press, 2012); Geoff Andrews, *The Slow Food Story: Politics and Pleasure* (Montreal: McGill-Queen's University Press, 2008);

Warren Belasco, *Appetite for Change: How the Counterculture Took on the Food Industry* (Ithaca, NY: Cornell University Press, 2006); Harvey Levenstein, *Paradox of Plenty: A Social History of Eating in Modern America* (New York: Oxford University Press, 1993).

12 Steve Kroll-Smith and H. Hugh Floyd, *Bodies in Protest: Environmental Illness and the Struggle over Medical Knowledge* (New York: NYU Press, 2000); Peter Radetsky, *Allergic to the Twentieth Century: The Explosion in Environmental Allergies – From Sick Buildings to Multiple Chemical Sensitivity* (Boston, MA: Little, Brown, 1997); Richard A. Cone and Emily Martin, 'Corporeal Flows: The Immune System, Global Economies of Food, and Implications for Health', *Ecologist* 27 (1997), 107–11.

13 The Stone Age diet has recently been transformed into the paleo diet. Although most adherents adopt it to lose weight, proponents also claim that it can reduce allergies and improve digestion. Most nutrition experts, however, remain sceptical of it and related diets, ranging from the similarly high-protein Atkins diet to the raw food diet.

14 Charles Rosenberg, 'Pathologies of Progress: The Idea of Civilization at Risk', *Bulletin of the History of Medicine* 72 (1998), 714–30; Roy Porter, 'Civilisation and Disease: Medical Ideology in the Enlightenment', in *Culture, Politics and Society in Britain, 1660–1800*, ed. Jeremy Black and Jeremy Gregory (Manchester: Manchester University Press, 1991).

15 Levenstein, *Fear of Food*, viii.

16 Ibid., 2

17 For instance, Rima Apple, *Vitamania: Vitamins in American Culture* (New Brunswick, NJ: Rutgers University Press, 1996); Michael Pollan, *The Omnivore's Dilemma* (New York: Penguin, 2006); Marion Nestle, *Food Politics* (Berkeley: University of California Press, 2002); Michael Mikulak, *The Politics of the Pantry: Stories, Food, and Social Change* (Montreal: McGill-Queen's University Press, 2013); Gyorgy Scrinis, *Nutritionism: The Science and Politics of Dietary Advice* (New York: Columbia University Press, 2013).

18 US Food and Drug Administration, 'Food Allergen Labeling and Consumer Protection Act of 2004 (FALCPA), Public Law 108–282, Title II', https://www.fda.gov/Food/GuidanceRegulation/GuidanceDocumentsRegulatoryInformation/Allergens/ucm106187.htm, accessed 9 October 2017.

19 Mackarness, *Not All in the Mind*, 59. Keen to replicate his self-experimentation, Rinkel tried eggs again 5 days later and suffered yet another acute attack. Presumably he avoided them after that.

20 See volume 6 of *Annals of Allergy* (1948) for examples of allergenic products.

21 Helen Morgan, *You Can't Eat That! A Manual and Recipe Book for Those Who Suffer Either Acutely or Mildly (and Perhaps Unconsciously) from Food Allergy* (New York: Harcourt, Brace and Company, 1939), 7.

22 Ibid., 5.

23 Ibid., 247. Although Cone and Martin have asked questions about the health implications of consuming food from far-flung regions of the globe, Alvarez suggested that exotic alternatives, such as rice, chickpea, dates, sesame seed and rapeseed oils, might provide needed nutrients to those allergic to local foods. Ibid., xvi; Cone and Martin, 'Corporeal Flows'.

24 Ibid., 248, 282–87.

25 Ibid., 300.

26 Ibid., 301.

27   For more on how American food became 'industrialized', see Gabriella W. Petrick, 'Industrial Food', in *The Oxford Handbook of Food History*, ed. Jeffrey M. Pilcher (Oxford: Oxford University Press, 2012).

28   Belasco, *Appetite for Change*, 37–41.

29   Jackson, *'Allergy con Amore'*, 160–61.

30   For more on trust in the food supply, see Karin Zachman and Per Østby, 'Food, Technology and Trust: An Introduction', *History and Technology* 27 (2011), 1–10.

31   Randolph's concerns about corn predated when high-fructose corn syrup, recently linked to increases in American obesity rates, became widely used in the 1970s.

32   Paul Roberts, *The End of Food* (New York: Houghton Mifflin, 2008), 20.

33   See chart in Brad Plumer, 'A Brief History of U.S. Corn in One Chart', *Washington Post* (16 August 2012), https://www.washingtonpost.com/news/wonk/wp/2012/08/16/a-brief-history-of-u-s-corn-in-one-chart/?utm_term=.edbdd9da25a1, accessed 17 October 2017. Productivity lagged until 1930, when hybrid strains describes were developed. Increased corn yields also led to more volatility in production during times of drought. After peaking in 2010 at 160 bushels per acre, production slipped to just over 120 bushels per acre in 2012, due to a severe drought in the American Midwest.

34   By 2005, demand for ethanol, derived from corn, drove production even more. Today, 30 per cent of American corn is also used for biofuel. Roberts, *End of Food*, 206.

35   Jeffrey A. Gwirtz and Maria Nieves Garcia-Casal, 'Processing Maize Flour and Corn Meal Food Products', *Annals of the New York Academy of Sciences* 1312 (2014), 66–75.

36   Beatrice Trum Hunter, *The Sugar Trap and How to Avoid It* (Boston, MA: Houghton Mifflin, 1982), 23.

37   Theron G. Randolph, *Environmental Medicine: Beginnings and Bibliographies of Clinical Ecology* (Fort Collins, CO: Clinical Ecology, 1987), 27. Rinkel was also allergic to corn.

38   Ibid., 26.

39   Ironically, given his subsequent troubles with the food industry, the research on which this initial article was based was funded by food manufacturer Swift and Company. Theron G. Randolph, 'Cornstarch as Allergen, Sources of Contact in Food Containers', *Journal of the American Dietetic Association* 24 (1948), 841–46; Theron G. Randolph and L. B. Yeager, 'Corn Sugar as an Allergen', *Annals of Allergy* 7 (1949), 651–61; Theron G. Randolph, J. P. Rollins and C. K. Walter, 'Allergic Reactions from Ingestion or Intravenous Injection of Corn Sugar', *Journal of Laboratory and Clinical Medicine* 24 (1949), 1741; Suzanne White Junod, 'The Rise and Fall of Federal Food Standards in the United States: The Case of the Peanut Butter and Jelly Sandwich', in *The Food and Drug Administration*, ed. Meredith A. Hickman (New York: Nova, 2003), 35–48.

40   Harry S. Bernton, 'Food Allergy with Special Reference to Corn and Refined Corn Derivatives', *Annals of Internal Medicine* 36 (1951), 177–85.

41   Theron G. Randolph and Ralph W. Moss, *Allergies: Your Hidden Enemies* (New York: Harper Collins, 1981), 5.

42   Herbert Rinkel, Theron G. Randolph and Michael Zeller, *Food Allergy* (Springfield, IL: Charles C. Thomas, 1951).

43   Will C. Spain, 'Review of *Food Allergy*', *Quarterly Review of Biology* 28 (1953), 97–98.

44   Theron G. Randolph to Harry G. Clark, 3 July 1951, Box 7, Folder 8, Theron G. Randolph Papers, 1935–1991, H MS c183, Harvard Medical Library in the Francis A. Countway Library of Medicine, Centre for the History of Medicine, Boston.

45 Arthur Coca to Theron G. Randolph, 9 June 1953, Box 7, Folder 11, Theron
    G. Randolph Papers, 1935–1991, H MS c183, Harvard Medical Library in the Francis
    A. Countway Library of Medicine, Centre for the History of Medicine, Boston.
46 Theron G. Randolph to Arthur Coca, 16 July 1953, Box 7, Folder 11, Theron
    G. Randolph Papers, 1935–1991, H MS c183, Harvard Medical Library in the Francis
    A. Countway Library of Medicine, Centre for the History of Medicine, Boston.
47 Ibid.; Mitman, *Breathing Space*, 189.
48 Randolph, *Environmental Medicine*, 58.
49 Letter (30 October 1974) from Elizabeth B. Magner (Geln Ellyn, IL) to James O. Kelly,
    Exec. Secretary of AAA, American Academy of Allergy, Asthma and Immunology
    Records, 1923–2011. University of Wisconsin-Milwaukee Libraries, Archives
    Department. Emphasis in original.
50 Rachel Carson, *Silent Spring* (New York: Houghton Mifflin, 1962). There were
    earlier concerns about food chemicals, but these tended to concentrate on chemicals
    used illicitly, rather than those included on purpose. Randolph warnings about
    environmental chemicals also preceded those of Carson but were not as eloquently
    expressed. Theron G. Randolph, 'Human Ecology and Susceptibility to the Chemical
    Environment', *Annals of Allergy* 19 (1961), 518–40, 657–77, 779–99, 908–29.
51 Levenstein, *Paradox of Plenty*.
52 Alison Downham and Paul Collins, 'Colouring Our Foods in the Last and Next
    Millennium', *International Journal of Food Science and Technology* 35 (2000), 5–22.
53 Stephen D. Lockey, 'Allergic Reactions Due to Dyes in Foods', Speech presented to the
    Pennsylvania Allergy Society, 1948.
54 William R. Hoobler, 'Some Early Symptoms Suggesting Protein Sensitization in
    Infancy', *American Journal of Diseases of Children* 12 (2016), 129–35; T. Wood Clarke,
    'The Relation of Allergy to Character Problems in Children', *Annals of Allergy* 8
    (1950), 21–38; Frederic Speer, 'Allergic Tension-Fatigue in Children', *Annals of Allergy*
    12 (1954), 168–71.
55 Matthew Smith, *Hyperactive: The Controversial History of ADHD* (London:
    Reaktion, 2012).
56 Feingold opted for a popular publication after being rebuffed by his medical
    colleagues. Benjamin F. Feingold, *Why Your Child Is Hyperactive* (New York: Random
    House, 1974).
57 Matthew Smith, *An Alternative History of Hyperactivity: Food Additives and the
    Feingold Diet* (New Brunswick, NJ: Rutgers University Press, 2011).
58 Feingold, *Hyperactive*, 135.
59 Ibid., 162.
60 E. K. Silbergeld and A. M. Goldberg, 'Hyperactivity: A Lead-Induced Behavior
    Disorder', *Environmental Health Perspectives* 7 (1974), 227–32.
61 H. W. Mielke and S. Zahran, 'The Urban Rise and Fall of Air Lead (pb) and the Latent
    Surge and Retreat of Societal Violence', *Environment International* 43 (2012), 48–55.
62 Andrew F. Smith, *Peanuts: The Illustrious History of the Goober Pea*
    (Urbana: University of Illinois Press, 2002), 30–44; Pedro A. Alvarez and Joyce
    I. Boye, 'Food Production and Processing Considerations of Allergenic Food
    Ingredients: A Review', *Journal of Allergy* (2012), https://www.hindawi.com/journals/
    ja/2012/746125/; Jon Krampner, *Creamy and Crunchy: An Informal History of Peanut
    Butter, the All-American Food* (New York: Columbia University Press, 2012); Beatriz
    Cabanillas and Natalija Novak, 'Effects of Daily Food Processing on Allergenicity',
    Critical Reviews in Food Science and Nutrition 11 (2017), 1–12.

63 S. K. Sathe and G. M. Sharma, 'Effects of Processing on Food Allergens', *Molecular Nutrition and Food Research* 53 (2009), 970–78.
64 Norelle R. Reilly, 'The Gluten-Free Diet: Recognizing Fact, Fiction, and Fad', *Journal of Pediatrics* 175 (2016), 206–10.
65 Elizabeth M. Whalen and Frederick J. Stare, *Panic in the Pantry* (New York: Antheum, 1975).

4 Dietary Change and Epidemic Disease: Fame, Fashion and Expediency in the Italian Pellagra Disputes, 1852–1902

1 Law no. 427, 'Sulla prevenzione e cura della pellagra, 21 luglio 1902'. Luigi Perisutti, 'La legge contro la pellagra', in *Atti del secondo congresso pellagrologico italiano: Bologna, 26–28 Maggio 1902*, ed. Gio. Battista Cantarutti (Udine: Fratelli Tosolini e G. Jacob, 1902), 303–19; J. W. Babcock and W. B. Cutting, *Pellagra* (Washington, DC: Government Printing Office, 1911), 46–49.
2 Luigi Perisutti and Giovanni Battista Cantarutti, 'Inchiesta sulla pellagra nel regno e sui provvedimenti diversi per la cura preventiva della stessa', *Bollettino di notizie agrarie* 31 (1900), 1385–86.
3 Discussed in Alberto De Bernardi, *Il mal della rosa. Denutrizione e pellagra nelle campagne italiane fra '800 e '900* (Milan: Franco Angeli, 1984), 252–53; De Bernardi, 'Pellagra, Stato e scienza medica: la curabilità impossibile', in *Storia d'Italia. Annali 7. Malattia e medicina*, ed. Franco Della Peruta (Turin: Einaudi, 1984), 703–4.
4 Giovanni Levi, 'L'energia disponibile', in *Storia dell'economia italiana*, vol. 2. *L'età moderna: verso la crisi*, ed. R. Romano (Turin: Einaudi, 1991), 141–68. By contrast, the reception of other New World food plants in Italy, like the tomato and potato, had been slow and problematic. See David Gentilcore, 'The Impact of New World Plants, 1500–1800: The Americans in Italy', in *The New World in Early Modern Italy, 1492–1750*, ed. E. Horodowich and Lia Markey (Cambridge: Cambridge University Press, 2017), 190–205.
5 Aldino Monti, *I braccianti* (Bologna: il Mulino, 1998); Vera Zamagni, *The Economic History of Italy, 1860–1990: Recovery after Decline* (Oxford: Clarendon Press, 1993), 47–74.
6 Piero Bevilacqua, 'Società rurale e emigrazione', in *Storia dell'emigrazione italiana*, ed. P. Bevilacqua, A. De Clementi and E. Franzina (Rome: Donzelli, 2001), vol. 1, 95–112.
7 Harmke Kamminga and Andrew Cunningham, eds, *The Science and Culture of Nutrition, 1840–1940* (Amsterdam: Rodopi, 1995), editors' introduction, 2.
8 David Wootton, *Bad Medicine: Doctors Doing Harm Since Hippocrates* (Oxford: Oxford University Press, 2007), 14.
9 Ibid., 26.
10 Two early works remain fundamental: Elizabeth Etheridge, *The Butterfly Caste: A Social History of Pellagra in the South* (Westport, CT: Greenwood, 1972); Daphne Roe, *A Plague of Corn: The Social History of Pellagra* (Ithaca, NY: Cornell University Press, 1973). See also, Alfred Jay Bollet, 'Politics and Pellagra: The Epidemic of Pellagra in the U.S. in the Early Twentieth Century', *Yale Journal of Biology and Medicine* 65 (1992), 211–21.
11 The US medical response to pellagra and ensuing debates about it have been well studied. See Charles Bryan, *James Woods Babcock and the Red Plague of Pellagra*

(Columbia: University of South Carolina Press, 2014); Alan Kraut, *Goldberger's War: The Life and Work of a Public Health Crusader* (New York: Hill and Wang, 2003); Chris Leslie, '"Fighting an Unseen Enemy": The Infectious Paradigm in the Conquest of Pellagra', *Journal of Medical Humanities* 23 (2002), 187–202; Harry Marks, 'Epidemiologists Explain Pellagra: Gender, Race, and Political Economy in the Work of Edgar Sydenstricker', *Journal of the History of Medicine and Allied Sciences* 58 (2003), 34–55.

12　The key work remains De Bernardi's *Il mal della rosa*. Also illustrative of this approach are Giorgio Porisini, 'Agricoltura, alimentazione e condizioni sanitarie. Prime ricerche sulla pellagra in Italia dal 1880 al 1940', *Cahiers internationaux d'histoire économique et sociale* 3 (1984), 1–50; Roberto Finzi, 'Quando e perché fu sconfitta la pellagra in Italia', in *Salute e classi lavoratrici in Italia dall'Unità al fascismo*, ed. M. L. Betri and A. Gigli Marchetti (Milan: Franco Angeli, 1982), 391–430. More recently, from a demographical perspective, Monica Ginnaio, *L'impact démographique des crises sanitaires et nutritionelles des societés anciennes: le cas de la pellagre en Italie* (Villeneuve d'Ascq: Atelier national de reproduction des theses, 2010).

13　A notable exception is De Bernardi's 'Pellagra, Stato e scienza medica', 681–704. Most attention here has been devoted to pellagrous insanity and its treatment in the asylum context. For instance, Roberto Finzi, 'La psicosi pellagrosa in Italia fra la fine dell'800 e gli inizi del '900', in *Follia, psichiatria e società. Istituzioni manicomiali, scienza psichiatrica e classi sociali nell'Italia moderna e contemporanea*, ed. A. De Bernardi (Milan: Franco Angeli, 1982), 284–97; Massimo Ferrari, 'Pellagra e pazzia nelle campagne reggiane', *Sanità, scienza e storia* 1, no. 1 (1985), 169–212; David Gentilcore and Egidio Priani, '"San Servolo Lunatic!": Segregation and Integration in the Life Cycle of Pellagra Patients at Venice's Provincial Asylums (1842–1912)', in *Segregration and Integration in the History of the Hospital*, ed. K. Stevens Crawshaw and K. Vongsathorn (Rotterdam: Clio Medica, in press).

14　David Gentilcore, '"Italic Scurvy", "Pellarina", "Pellagra": Medical Reactions to a New Disease in Italy, 1770–1830', in *A Medical History of Skin: Scratching the Surface*, ed. J. Reinarz and K. Siena (London: Pickering and Chatto, 2013), 57–69.

15　To rephrase K. Codell Carter's formulation, in *The Rise of Causal Concepts of Disease: Case Histories* (Aldershot: Ashgate, 2003), 22.

16　Gentilcore, 'Medical Reactions', 65; Andrea Bisaglia, *Sulla pellagra: osservazioni* (Padua: Minerva, 1830), 24.

17　K. Codell Carter, 'Ignaz Semmelweis, Carl Mayrhofer, and the Rise of Germ Theory', *Medical History* 29 (1985), 33–53.

18　Carter, *Causal Concepts*, 50.

19　Cesare Fenili, 'Filippo Lussana e la lotta alla pellagra', in *Filippo Lussana (1820–1897): da Cenate alle neuroscienze*, ed. Giosuè Berbenin and Lorenzo Lorusso (Bergamo: Fondazione per la storia economica e sociale di Bergamo, 2008), 97–127.

20　Filippo Lussana, 'Dottrine di G. Liebig su l'alimentazione; ed annotazioni su l'eziologia della pellagra e su la metamorfica produzione epatica dell'adipe', *Gazzetta Medica Italiana: Lombardia* III, no. 2 (November 1852), 408.

21　Filippo Lussana and Carlo Frua, *Su la pellagra: memoria* (Milan: Giuseppe Bernardoni, 1856), 26–128.

22　Lussana and Frua, *Su la pellagra*, 124. All translations are my own, unless indicated otherwise.

23　On his publications, Pier Luigi Baima Bollone, *Cesare Lombroso ovvero il principio dell'irresponsabilità* (Turin: Società Editrice Internazionale, 1992), n. 4, 60–66.

The most sophisticated intellectual biography is Delia Frigessi's *Cesare Lombroso* (Turin: Giulio Einaudi, 2003).

24 Cesare Lombroso, *Studi clinici ed esperimentali sulla natura, causa e terapia della pellagra* (Bologna: Fava and Garagnani, 1869).

25 Ibid., 12.

26 Ibid., 386.

27 Ibid., 349.

28 On Moleschott, see Harmke Kamminga, 'Nutrition for the People, or the Fate of Jacob Moleschott's Context for a Humanist Science', in *The Science and Culture of Nutrition, 1840-1940*, ed. H. Kamminga and A. Cunningham (Amsterdam: Rodopi, 1995), 15-47; on Lombroso and Moleschott's materialist science, see Frigessi, *Lombroso*, 54-66.

29 Lussana and Frua, *Su la pellagra*, in their discussion of ergotism in maize, 87-121. First suggested by Ludovico Balardini, Lombroso's insight was to shift the focus away from Balardini's and Lussana's *sponsorium maidis* to *penicillium glaucum*, different kinds of fungi that attack maize. Lombroso would later pinpoint the toxic exact agent responsible as something he labelled 'pellagrozeine'.

30 Cit. in Delia Frigessi, 'Cesare Lombroso tra medicina e società', in *Cesare Lombroso cento anni dopo*, ed. S. Montalto and P. Tappero (Turin: UTET, 2009), 9.

31 Raf de Bont, ' "Writing in Letters of Blood": Manners in Scientific Dispute in Nineteenth-Century Britain and the German Lands', *History of Science* 51 (2013), 309-35.

32 Filippo Lussana, *Sulle cause della pellagra* (Padua: Prosperini, 1872), 8.

33 Ibid., 18.

34 Ibid., 20.

35 Cesare Lombroso, 'Sulle cause della pellagra: lettera polemica al Prof. Lussana', *Giornale di dermatologia* [vol. number unknown] (1872), 1-32.

36 Ibid., 7.

37 Ibid., 1.

38 Ibid., 25.

39 Ministero di Agricoltura, Industria e Commercio, *La pellagra in Italia*, in the *Annali di agricoltura* 18 (Rome, 1879), 324-25.

40 Clodomiro Bonfigli, 'La pellagra nella provincia di Ferrara', *Bollettino del manicomio provinciale di Ferrara* 10, no. 5 (1878).

41 Adello Vanni and Luigi Missiroli, 'Bonfigli contro Lombroso: della polemica sulla etiopatogenesi della pellagra', *Rivista sperimentale di freniatria* 111, no. 6 (1987): 1383-96.

42 Cesare Lombroso, *La pellagra in Italia in rapporto alla pretesa insufficienza alimentare: lettera polemica . . . al dott. Bonfigli* (Turin: Celanza, 1880). With Lombroso now ensconced in Turin with his own laboratory, most of the book was written by two of his assistants, Agostino Caudana and Giovanni Battista Laura. Paolo Novaria, 'Cesare Lombroso professore a Torino. Un percorso tra i documenti dell'Archivio storico dell'università', in *Gli archivi della scienza. L'Università di Torino e altri casi italiani*, ed. S. Montaldo and P. Novaria (Milan: Franco Angeli, 2011), 40-55.

43 Clodomiro Bonfigli, 'Sulla pellagra: lettere polemiche . . . al dott. C. Lombroso', *Raccoglitore Medico* series 4, 11 (1879), 51, 154, 252-55.

44 Ibid., 316.

45 Clodomiro Bonfigli, 'Le questioni sulla pellagra . . . Appendice alle lettere polemiche', *Raccoglitore Medico*, series 4, vol. 16 (1881); Cesare Lombroso, 'Degli ultimi studi

sulla pellagra', *Archivio di Psichiatria, Scienza Penali e Antropologia Criminale*, 2 (1881), 115.

46 Lombroso, *Pellagra* (1880).

47 Filippo Lussana, 'Una allucinazione del professor Lombroso', *Gazzetta Medica Italiana: Lombardia* (offprint, Milan: Rechiedei, 1883).

48 Ibid., 3.

49 Ibid., 6.

50 In their otherwise excellent study of Bonfigli and the treatment of pellagrous insanity at the insane asylum in Ferrara, Magda Beltrami and Mara Guerra pit Lombroso's 'exclusively technical' approach against Bonfigli's 'acute' socially aware perspective, with the latter as victim. *'Legati mani e piedi con rozze funi'. Le carte raccontano la pellagra a Ferrara, 1859–1933* (Ferrara: Tresogni, 2015), 24–28.

51 On history of science and science studies approaches, see Lorraine Daston, 'Science studies and the history of science', *Critical Inquiry* 35 (2009), 798–813.

52 Thomas Brante and Aant Elzinga, 'Towards a Theory of Scientific Controversies', *Social Studies* 2 (1990), 33–46.

53 Silvano Montaldo, 'Cento anni dopo: il punto della situazione', in *Cesare Lombroso cento anni dopo*, ed. S. Montaldo and P. Tappero (Turin: UTET, 2009), xi.

54 Helen Zimmern, 'Criminal Anthropology in Italy', *Appletons' Popular Science Monthly* 52 (April 1898), 750.

55 Mauro Forno, 'Scienziati e mass media: Lombroso e gli studiosi positivisti nella stampa tra Otto e Novecento', in *Cesare Lombroso. Gli scienziati e la nuova Italia*, ed. S. Montaldo (Bologna: il Mulino, 2010), 213.

56 Silvano Montaldo, 'La partecipazione degli scienziati alla vita politica', in *Cesare Lombroso. Gli scienziati e la nuova Italia*, ed. S. Montaldo (Bologna: il Mulino, 2010), 173.

57 Gaetano Strambio, 'Da Legnano a Mogliano Veneto: un secolo di lotta contro la pellagra', *Memorie del Real Istituto Lombardo di Scienze e Lettere* 17 (1890), 320.

58 Tirsi Mario Caffaratto, 'Lo stato della cultura e della pratica medica in Piemonte nell'ultimo periodo dell'Ottocento', in *La scienza accademica nell'Italia post-unitaria: discipline scientifiche e ricerca universitaria*, ed. Vittorio Ancarani (Milan: Franco Angeli, 1989), 271.

59 Carter, *Causal Concepts*, 104.

60 S. E. D. Shortt, 'Physicians, Science, and Status: Issues in the Professionalization of Anglo-American Medicine in the Nineteenth Century', *Medical History* 27 (1983): 53.

61 Michael Warboys, *Spreading Germs: Disease Theories and Medical Practice in Britain, 1865–1900* (Cambridge: Cambridge University Press, 2000), 2–3.

62 Vanni and Missiroli, 'Bonfigli contro Lombroso'.

63 According to the German clinician Bernard Naunyn (1839–1925), in his *Erinnerungen, Gedanken und Meinungen* (Munich: J. F. Bergmann, 1925), 225, cit. in J. Büttner, 'The Origin of Clinical Laboratories', *European Journal of Clinical Chemistry and Clinical Biochemistry* 30 (1992), 590.

64 Cesare Lombroso, *Trattato profilattico e clinico della pellagra* (Turin: Bocca, 1892).

65 De Bernardi, 'Pellagra, stato e scienza medica', 690–92.

66 Lombroso, *Trattato profilattico e clinico*, vii, viii, xviii. Lombroso made the same points in his short preface to a French abridgement of this work, published in 1908, and continued to uphold the veracity of his thesis until his death the following year. The preface to Auguste Marie's *La pellagre* (Paris: V. Giard, 1908) was retained in the

English translation, made by the two US doctors who first encountered the disease in the southern United States, C. H. Lavinder and J. W. Babcock, which also include an additional 'prefatory note' Lombroso made shortly before his death: *Pellagra* (Columbia, SC: State Co., 1910), 7–9, 11–12.

67 Cesare Lombroso, 'Sulla pellagra maniaca e sua cura', *Giornale italiano delle malattie veneree e della pelle* 3 (1868), 137.

68 Letter from Gris to Lombroso, c. 1885, cit. in Livio Vanzetto, *I ricchi e i pellagrosi: un secolo di storia dell'Istituto 'Costante Gris' di Mogliano Veneto* (Abano Terme: Francisci, 1992), 122–27, 136.

69 Tristam Engelhardt and Arthur Caplan, eds, *Scientific Controversies: Case Studies in the Resolution and Closure of Disputes in Science and Technology* (Cambridge: Cambridge University Press, 1987), editors' introduction, 12.

70 Cesare Vigna, 'Sulla pellagra nella provincia di Venezia', *La pellagra: Annali di agricoltura* 18 (Rome: Ministero di Agricoltura, Industria e Commercio, 1879), 448.

71 David Gentilcore and Egidio Priani, *Venetian Mental Asylums Database (VMAD), 1842–1912.* UK Data Service, 2016. SN: 8058, http://doi.org/10.5255/UKDA-SN-8058-1.

72 Archivio della Fondazione di San Servolo, Venice (AFSSV), *San Servolo: Maniaci*, b. 91 (1882), patient Antonio P.

73 Egidio Priani, ' "Shrouded in a Dark Fog": The Diagnosis of Pellagra and General Paralysis of the Insane between Italy and United Kingdom, 1840–1900', *History of Psychiatry* 28, no. 2 (2017), 166–81.

74 AFSSV, *San Servolo: Maniaci*, b. 91 (1882), patient Taddeo A.; AFSSV, San Clemente, *Posizioni alienate: uscite*, b. 192 (1882), patient Teresa S.

75 Vincenzo Camurri, 'L'etiologia della pellagra nel giudizio dei medici condotti in Italia', in *Atti del quinto congresso pellagrologico italiano*, ed. G. B. Cantarutti (Udine: Tosolini, 1912), 220–35.

76 Giuseppina Bock Berti, 'Flippo Lussana', *Dizionario biografico degli italiani* 66 (2006), sub voce: http://www.treccani.it/enciclopedia/filippo-lussana_(Dizionario-Biografico)/; Lorenzo Lorusso et al. 'Filippo Lussana (1820–1897): From Medical Practitioner to Neuroscience', *Neurological Science* 33 (2012), 703–8.

77 Egisto Taccari, 'Clodomiro Bonfigli', *Dizionario biografico degli italiani*, 12 (1971), sub voce: http://www.treccani.it/enciclopedia/clodomiro-bonfigli_(Dizionario-Biografico)/; Anna Lia Bonella, *L'ospedale dei pazzi a Roma dai papi al '900* (Rome: Dedalo, 1994), vol. 2, 162.

78 David Gentilcore, 'Louis Sambon and the Clash of Pellagra Etiologies in Italy and the United States, 1904–15', *Journal of the History of Medicine and Allied Sciences* 71, no. 1 (2015), 23–24.

79 Aristide Stefani, *Relazione sull'opera della Commissione pellagrologica provinciale di Padova nell'anno 1910* (Padua: Penada, 1911), 10–11.

80 Casimir Funk, 'The Etiology of the Deficiency Diseases: Beri-Beri, Polyneuritis in Birds, Epidemic Dropsy, Scurvy, Experimental Scurvy in Animals, Infantile Scurvy, Ship Beri-Beri, pellagra', *Journal of State Medicine* 20 (1912), 341–68.

81 Ibid., 342, 363.

82 Francesco Coletti, 'Una vittoria nel silenzio', *Corriere della Sera*, 11 July 1922, 1, cit. in Luigi Messedaglia, 'Mais e pellagra: un dramma di vita rurale' (1927), in idem, *La gloria del mais e altri scritti sull'alimentazione Veneta*, ed. Corrado Barberis and Ulderico Bernardi (Castabissara, Vicenza: Angelo Colla, 2008), 251.

5 Conceptualizing the Vitamin and Pellagra as an Avitaminosis: A Case-Study Analysis of the Sedimentation Process of Medical Knowledge

1 Casimir Funk, 'The Etiology of the Deficiency Diseases', *Journal of State Medicine* 20 (1912), 341–68.
2 Gerald F. Combs, Jr., *The Vitamins. Fundamental Aspects in Nutrition and Health*, 3rd edn. (Amsterdam: Elsevier Academic Press, 2008), 13.
3 F. Gowland Hopkins, *Newer Aspects of the Problem of Nutrition* (New York: Columbia University Press, 1922), 15–16.
4 F. Gowland Hopkins, 'Feeding Experiments Illustrating the Importance of Accessory Factors in Normal Dietaries', *Journal of Physiology* 44 (1912), 425–60.
5 Elmer V. McCollum and Marguerite Davis, 'The Necessity of Certain Lipins in the Diet during Growth', *Journal of Biological Chemistry* 15 (1913), 167–75.
6 George Wolf and Kenneth J. Carpenter, 'Early Research into the Vitamins: The Work of Wilhelm Stepp', *Journal of Nutrition* 127 (1997), 1255–59.
7 See Casimir Funk, *The Vitamines* (Baltimore, MD: Williams & Wilkins, 1922), 19–25 and 128–29 for a summary of this research.
8 Henry Fraser and A. T. Stanton, 'An Inquiry Concerning the Etiology of Beriberi', *The Lancet* 173 (1909), 451–55.
9 Henry Fraser and A. T. Stanton, 'The Etiology of Beri-beri', *Transactions of the Royal Society of Tropical Medicine and Hygiene* 5 (1910), 257–67.
10 Casimir Funk, 'On the Chemical Nature of the Substance Which Cures Polyneuritis in Birds Induced by a Diet of Polished Rice', *Journal of Physiology* 43 (1911), 395–400.
11 Funk, *The Vitamines*, 26; Hopkins, 'Feeding Experiments', 425; McCollum and Davis, 'The Necessity of Certain Lipins', 174–75.
12 Elmer V. McCollum, 'The "Vitamin" Hypothesis and the Diseases Referable to a Faulty Diet', *Journal of the American Medical Association* 71 (1918), 937.
13 Funk, *The Vitamines*, 35–36.
14 McCollum, 'The "Vitamin" Hypothesis', 937, 939.
15 Elmer V. McCollum, Nina Simmonds and J. Ernestine Becker, 'Studies on Experimental Rickets. XXI', *Journal of Biological Chemistry* 53 (1922), 293–312.
16 Conrad A. Elvehjem, 'Pellagra: A Deficiency Disease', *Proceedings of the American Philosophical Society* 93 (1949), 335–39.
17 Victor Babeş, *Cercetări Nouă asupra Pelagrei* (Bucharest: Librăria Socec & Comp şi C. Sfetea, 1914), 1.
18 A. Marie, *Pellagra*, trans. C. H. Lavinder and J. W. Babcock (Columbia, SC: State Co., 1910), 59.
19 Daphne Roe, 'Pellagra', in *The Cambridge World History of Food*, ed. Kenneth F. Kiple and Kriemhild Conee Ornelas (Cambridge: Cambridge University Press, 2000), 962; H. H. Draper, 'Human Nutritional Adaptation: Biological and Cultural Aspects', in *The Cambridge World History of Food*, ed. Kenneth F. Kiple and Kriemhild Conee Ornelas (Cambridge: Cambridge University Press, 2000), 1473.
20 Filippo Lussana and Carlo Frua, 'Su la Pellagra', in *Pellagra*, ed. Kenneth J. Carpenter (Stroudsburg: Hutchinson Ross, 1981), 13.
21 Ibid., 13.

22 Ismael Salas, 'Etiology and Prophylaxis of Pellagra', in *Pellagra*, ed. Kenneth J. Carpenter (Stroudsburg: Hutchinson Ross, 1981), 19–20.

23 Aldo Perroncito, *Eziologia della Pellagra* (Florence: Societa Tipografica Fiorentina, 1913), 3, 11.

24 Cesare Lombroso, *Studi Clinici ed Esperimentali sulla Natura, Causa e Terapia della Pellagra* (Bologna: Tipi Fava e Garagnani, 1869), 75–78.

25 Victor Babeş, *Cauzele Cancerului – Tratamentul Pelagrei* (Bucharest: Institutul de Arte Grafice Carol Göbl, 1900), 7.

26 C. H. Lavinder, *Pellagra* (Washington, DC: Government Printing Office, 1908), 8.

27 Ioan Neagoe, *Raportul Doctorului Ioan Neagoe asupra Misiunei Sale în Străinătate pentru a Studia Midloacele de Combatere a Pelagrei din Numitele Ţeri* (Bucharest: Imprimeria Statului, 1889), 14–15.

28 Ioan Neagoe, *Studiu asupra Pelagrei* (Bucharest: Institutul de Arte Grafice Carol Göbl, 1900), 331–32.

29 Ioan Neagoe, *Pelagra şi Administraţia Noastră* (Bucharest: Tip. Munca, 1906), 10.

30 Neagoe, *Studiu asupra Pelagrei*, 332.

31 Neagoe, *Pelagra şi Administraţia Noastră*, 10.

32 Neagoe, *Studiu asupra Pelagrei*, 333.

33 Babeş, *Tratamentul Pelagrei*, 7.

34 Ibid.

35 Adolf Urbeanu, *Despre Caracteristica Alimentaţiei Ţeranului Român* (Bucharest: Imprimeria Statului, 1903), 6.

36 Ibid., 7.

37 Ibid., 9.

38 Edith Willcock and F. Gowland Hopkins, 'The Importance of Individual Amino-Acids in Metabolism', *Journal of Physiology* 35 (1906), 88–102.

39 Thomas Osborne and Lafayette Mendel, 'Nutritive Properties of Proteins of the Maize Kernel', *Journal of Biological Chemistry* 18 (1914), 1–16.

40 Pietro Albertoni and Pietro Tullio, *L'alimentation Maidique chez L'individu sain et chez le Pellagreux* (Turin: Impr. V. Bona, 1914).

41 Lavinder, *Pellagra*, 8; Stewart R. Roberts, *Pellagra* (St. Louis, MO: C. V. Mosby Company, 1913), 234–41; George M. Niles, *Pellagra: An American problem* (Philadelphia, PA: W. B. Saunders, 1912), 37.

42 Extensive quote from Aristide Stefani in 'Sull'eziologia della pellagra', *Rivista Pellagrologica Italiana* 16 (1916), 21–23.

43 Ibid., 21.

44 Ibid.

45 C. H. Lavinder, 'The Salient Epidemiological Features of Pellagra', *Public Health Reports* 26 (1911), 1468.

46 Funk, 'The Etiology of the Deficiency Diseases', 341, 362, 366.

47 Rupert Blue, 'The Problem of Pellagra in the United States', *Transactions of the National Association for the Study of Pellagra. Second Triennial Meeting at Columbia, South Carolina, October 3 and 4, 1912* (Columbia, SC: R. L. Bryan, 1914), 1–7.

48 F. M. Sandwith, 'Can Pellagra Be a Disease Due to a Deficiency in Nutrition?', *Transactions of the National Association for the Study of Pellagra. Second Triennial Meeting at Columbia, South Carolina, October 3 and 4, 1912* (Columbia, SC: R. L. Bryan, 1914), 96–100.

49 Robert Wilson, Jr. 'A Case of Beri-beri Presenting an Initial Erythema Resembling Pellagra', *Transactions of the National Association for the Study of Pellagra. Second Triennial Meeting at Columbia, South Carolina, October 3 and 4, 1912* (Columbia, SC: R. L. Bryan, 1914), 321–22.

50 Eleanora B. Saunders, 'The Coexistence of Pellagra and Beri-beri', *Transactions of the National Association for the Study of Pellagra. Second Triennial Meeting at Columbia, South Carolina, October 3 and 4, 1912* (Columbia, SC: R. L. Bryan, 1914), 325–31.

51 Edward B. Wedder, 'Dietary Deficiency as the Etiological Factor in Pellagra', *Archives of Internal Medicine* 18 (1916), 137–73.

52 Funk, 'The Etiology of the Deficiency Diseases', 341, 362, 366.

53 Ibid., 341.

54 Ibid., 167.

55 Casimir Funk, 'Studies on Pellagra. I', *Journal of Physiology* 47 (1913), 389–92.

56 Casimir Funk, *Die Vitamine* (Wiesbaden: J. F. Bergmann, 1914).

57 Ibid., 119.

58 Joseph Goldberger, 'The Treatment and Prevention of Pellagra', *Public Health Reports* 29 (1914), 2822.

59 Ibid., 2821.

60 Joseph Goldberger, C. H. Waring and David G. Willets, 'The Prevention of Pellagra: A Test Diet among Institutional Inmates', *Public Health Reports* 30 (22 October 1915), 3117–31.

61 Joseph Goldberger and G. A. Wheeler, 'Experimental Pellagra in the Human Subject Brought about by a Restricted Diet', *Public Health Reports* 30 (12 November 1915), 3336–39.

62 Joseph Goldberger, G. A. Wheeler and Edgar Sydenstricker, 'A Study of the Relation of Diet to Pellagra Incidence in Seven Textile-Mill Communities of South Carolina in 1916', *Public Health Reports* 35 (19 March 1920), 648–713.

63 Babeș, *Cercetări Nouă asupra Pelagrei*, 4–5.

64 Ottorino Rossi, 'Avitaminosi e Pellagra. Dubbi e Proposte', *Quaderni di Psichiatria* 2 (April 1915), 146–63.

65 Eugenio Bravetta, *Vitamine e Pellagra* (Udine: Tipografia Domenico del Bianco, 1915).

66 Paolo Ramoino, 'Contributo allo Studio delle Alimentazioni Incomplete. Nota III', *Pathologica* 7 (April 1915), 158–61.

67 Antonino Clementi, *Osservazioni sugli effetti delle alimentazioni esclusive maidica e orizanica, con Speciale riguardo al problema delle vitamine* (Siena: Tip. Ditta C. Nava, 1916).

68 Pietro Rondoni, *Alimentazione Maidica e Vitamine (Con Dimonstrazioni)* (Florence: Soc. Tip. Fiorentona, 1915).

69 Ibid., 6–7; Pietro Rondoni, *Ricerche sulla Alimentazione Maidica, con Speciale Riguardo alla Pellagra* (Florence: Soc. Tip. Fiorentona, 1915), 791.

70 See the concluding remarks from Rossi, 'Avitaminosi e Pellagra', 162.

71 Mircea Scrob, *From Mămăligă to Bread as the 'Core' Food of Romanian Villagers: A Consumer-Centered Interpretation of a Dietary Change (1900–1980)* (Budapest: Central European University, unpublished PhD dissertation).

72 Rondoni, *Ricerche sulla Alimentazione Maidica*, 792.

73 P. van den Brandt et al., 'The Contribution of Epidemiology', *Food and Chemical Toxicology* 40 (2002), 394.

6 Food and Diet as Risk: The Role
of the Framingham Heart Study

This research was conducted with funding from CAPES – Higher Education Improvement Coordination, Ministry of Education, Brazil. Process number: 8752-12-5.

1 Robert A. Aronowitz, *Making Sense of Illness: Science, Society, and Disease* (Cambridge: Cambridge University Press, 1998); Charles E. Rosenberg, 'Banishing Risk: Continuity and Change in the Moral Management of Disease', in *Health and Morality: Interdisciplinary Perspectives*, ed. Allan M. Brandt and Paul Rozin (New York: Routledge, 1997).
2 Kirstie Blair, '"Proved on the Pulses": Heart Disease in Victorian Culture, 1830–1860', in *Framing and Imagining Disease in Cultural History*, ed. George Sebastian Rousseau, Miranda Gill, David Haycock and Malte Herwig (New York: Palgrave Macmillian, 2003).
3 Thomas R. Dawber and William B. Kannel, 'The Framingham Study: An Epidemiological Approach to Coronary Heart Disease', *Circulation* 34, no. 4 (1966), 553–55.
4 Mervyn Susser, 'Epidemiology in the United States after World War II: The Evolution of Technique', *Epidemiological Reviews* 7 (1985), 147–77.
5 Allan M. Brandt and Paul Rozin, eds, *Health and Morality: Interdisciplinary Perspectives* (New York: Routledge, 1997).
6 Howard M. Leichter, '"Evil Habits" and "Personal Choices": Assigning Responsibility for Health in the 20th Century', *Milbank Quarterly* 81, no. 4 (2003), 603–26.
7 Michel Foucault, 'Technologies of the Self', in *Technologies of the Self: A Seminar with Michel Foucault*, ed. Luther H. Martin, Huck Gutman and Patrick H. Hutton (Amherst: University of Massachusetts Press, 1988).
8 Alain Desrosières, *The Politics of Large Numbers: A History of Statistical Reasoning* (Cambridge, MA: Harvard University Press, 1998).
9 Ian Hacking, *The Emergence of Probability: A Philosophical Study of the Early Ideas about Probability* (New York: Cambridge University Press, 1975); Ian Hacking, *The Taming of Chance* (New York: Cambridge University Press, 1990).
10 Gyorgy Scrinis, *Nutritionism: The Science and Politics of Dietary Advice* (New York: Columbia University Press, 2013), 5.
11 US Department of Agriculture, *Food for Fitness – A Daily Food Guide*, leaflet no. 424 (Washington, DC: US Department of Agriculture, Agricultural Research Service, 1958).
12 Gary Taubes, 'The Soft Science of Dietary Fat', *Science* 291, no. 5513 (2001), 2536–45.
13 Gary Taubes, *Good Calories, Bad Calories: Fats, Carbs, and the Controversial Science of Diet and Health* (New York: Anchor Books, 2008).
14 Walter C. Willet, 'Editorial: The Dietary Pyramid: Does the Foundation Need Repair?', *American Journal of Clinical Nutrition* 68 (1998), 218–19.
15 Maiko R. Spiess, 'Doenças Cardíacas e Risco: o Framingham Heart Study' (Doctoral Dissertation, Política Científica e Tecnológica, Universidade Estadual de Campinas, 2014).
16 Daniel Levy and Susan Brink, *A Change of Heart: How the People of Framingham, Massachusetts, Helped Unravel the Mysteries of Cardiovascular Disease* (New York: Vintage Books, 2005).

17   Thomas R. Dawber, *The Framingham Heart Study* (Cambridge, MA: Harvard University Press, 1980); Gerald M. Oppenheimer, 'Framingham Heart Study: The First 20 Years', *Progress in Cardiovascular Disease* 53, no. 1 (2010), 55–61.

18   Gerald M. Oppenheimer, 'Becoming the Framingham Study 1947–1950', *American Journal of Public Health* 95, no. 4 (2005), 602–10.

19   Shanti Mendis, 'The Contribution of the Framingham Heart Study to the Prevention of Cardiovascular Disease: A Global Perspective', *Progress in Cardiovascular Disease* 53, no. 1 (2010), 10–14.

20   Aronowitz, *Making Sense of Illness*; William G. Rothstein, *Public Health and the Risk Factor: A History of an Uneven Medical Revolution* (Rochester, NY: University of Rochester Press, 2003); Gerald M. Oppenheimer, 'Profiling Risk: The Emergence of Coronary Heart Disease Epidemiology in the United States (1947–70)', *International Journal of Epidemiology* 35, no. 3 (2006), 720–30.

21   Élodie Giroux, 'The Framingham Study and the Constitution of a Restrictive Concept of Risk Factor', *Social History of Medicine* 26, no. 1 (2013), 94–112; Karin Garrety, 'Social Worlds, Actor-Networks and Controversy: The Case of Cholesterol, Dietary Fat and Heart Disease', *Social Studies of Science* 27, no. 5 (1997), 727–73.

22   William B. Kannel, Thomas R. Dawber, Abraham Kagan, Nicholas Revotskie and Joseph Stokes, 'Factors of Risk in the Development of Coronary Heart Disease – Six Year Follow-Up Experience. The Framingham Study', *Annals of Internal Medicine* 55, no. 1 (1961), 33–48.

23   Dawber, *Framingham Heart Study*.

24   Oppenheimer, *Becoming the Framingham Study*.

25   Joseph W. Mountin, 'Changing Concepts of Basic Local Public Health Services', *American Journal of Public Health* 39, no. 11 (1949), 1417–28.

26   William P. Castelli, interview with Maiko R. Spiess. Personal interview. Framingham, MA, 2013.

27   Ann F. La Berge, 'How the Ideology of Low Fat Conquered America', *Journal of the History of Medicine and Allied Sciences* 63, no. 2 (2008), 139–77.

28   Taubes, *Good Calories, Bad Calories*.

29   Levy and Brink, *Change of Heart*.

30   Dawber, *Framingham Heart Study*.

31   Ibid.

32   Thomas R. Dawber, Felix E. Moore and George V. Mann, 'Coronary Heart Disease in the Framingham Study', *American Journal of Public Health* 47, no. 4 (1957), 4–24.

33   Thomas R. Dawber, Georgiana Pearson, Patricia Anderson, George V. Mann, William B. Kannel, Dewey Shurtleff and Patricia McNamara, 'Dietary Assessment in the Epidemiologic Study of Coronary Heart Disease: The Framingham Study', *American Journal of Clinical Nutrition* 11, no. 3 (1962), 226–34.

34   Dawber et al., *Coronary Heart Disease in the Framingham Study*.

35   George V. Mann, Georgiana Pearson, Tavia Gordon and Thomas Dawber, 'Diet and Cardiovascular Disease in the Framingham Study I. Measurement of Dietary Intake', *American Journal of Nutrition* 11, no. 3 (1962), 200–25.

36   Ancel Keys and Margaret Keys, *Eat Well and Stay Well* (New York: Doubleday, 1959).

37   Daniel Levy, interview with Maiko R. Spiess. Personal interview. Framingham, MA, 2013.

38   Castelli, *Interview*.

39   Levy and Brink, *Change of Heart*.

40 Sejal S. Patel, 'Methods and Management: NIH Administrators, Federal Oversight, and the Framingham Heart Study', *Bulletin of the History of Medicine* 86, no. 1 (2012), 94–121.
41 Levy and Brink, *Change of Hearts*.
42 Castelli, *Interview*.
43 Levy and Brink, *Change of Heart*.
44 Spiess, *Doenças Cardíacas e Risco*.
45 David S. Jones, Scott H. Podolsky and Jeremy A. Greene, 'The Burden of Disease and the Changing Task of Medicine', *New England Journal of Medicine* 366, no. 25 (2012), 2333–38.
46 Michel Callon, 'Some Elements of a Sociology of Translation: Domestication of Scallops and the Fishermen of St. Brieuc Bay' in *The Sociological Review Monograph 38 – Sociology of Monsters: Essays on Power, Technology, and Domination*, ed. John Law (London: Routledge, 1986).
47 Taubes, *Good Calories, Bad Calories*.
48 Scrinis, *Nutritionism*.

7 From John Yudkin to Jamie Oliver: A Short but Sweet History on the War against Sugar

 1 Sarah Boseley, 'Jamie Oliver's Sugar Rush: A Crusade to Save Britain's Health', *Guardian*, 27 August 2015; Lucy Siegle, 'Just What the Doctor Ordered: Jamie Oliver Declares War on Sugar', *Guardian*, 30 August 2015.
 2 'Eat Fat, Cut the Carbs and Avoid Snacking to Reverse Obesity and Type 2 Diabetes', *National Obesity Forum and Public Heath Collaboration*, 23 May 2016.
 3 Henry Bodkin, 'Eat Fat to Get Thin: Official Diet Advice Is "Disastrous" for Obesity Fight, New Report Warns', *Telegraph*, 23 May 2016.
 4 Gary Taubes, 'What If It's All Been a Big Fat Lie?' *New York Times*, 7 July 2002; P. K. Nguyen, 'A Systematic Comparison of Sugar Content in Low-Fat vs Regular Versions of Foods', *Nutrition and Diabetes* 6, no. 1 (2016), 193; Anahad O'Conner, 'How the Sugar Industry Shifted Blame to Fat', *New York Times*, 12 September 2016.
 5 Barbara Griggs, *The Food Factor in Disease: Why We Are What We Eat* (Harmondsworth: Penguin, 1986), 277.
 6 Julia Llewellyn Smith, 'John Yudkin: The Man Who Tried to Warn Us about Sugar', *Telegraph*, 17 February 2017.
 7 Sidney W. Mintz, *Sweetness and Power: The Place of Sugar in Modern History* (New York: Penguin, 2008), xxix.
 8 Ibid., 190.
 9 Denis P. Burkitt, *Refined Carbohydrate Foods and Disease* (London: Academic Press, 1975), 37.
10 Ibid., 37.
11 Haven Emerson and Louise D. Larimore, 'Diabetes Mellitus: A Contribution to Its Epidemiology Based Chiefly on Mortality Statistics', *Archives of Internal Medicine* 35, no. 5 (1924), 585–630.
12 Ann F. La Berge, 'How the Ideology of Low Fat Conquered America', *Journal of the History of Medicine and Allied Sciences* 63, no. 2 (2008), 139–77; Harry

Marks, *The Progress of Experiment: Science and Therapeutic Reform, 1900–1990* (Cambridge: Cambridge University Press, 1997).

13 Howard Rusk, 'Overweight Persons Termed Top Health Problem in U.S.', *New York Times*, 17 April 1952, 44.

14 Ancel Keys, 'Diet and the Epidemiology of Coronary Heart Disease', *Journal of the American Medical Association* 164, no. 17 (1957), 1912–19.

15 Yudkin, *Diet and Coronary Thrombosis*, 162.

16 Ibid., 155.

17 John Yudkin, *Pure, White and Deadly: How Sugar Is Killing Us and What We Can Do to Stop It* (London: Penguin, 1998), foreword.

18 Gyorgy Scrinis, *Nutritionism: The Science and Politics of Dietary Advice* (New York: Columbia University Press, 2013), 2.

19 Ibid., 3.

20 Ann F. La Berge, 'How the Ideology of Low-Fat Conquered America', *Journal of the History of Medicine and Allied Sciences* 63, no. 2 (2008), 150.

21 Scrinis, *Nutritionism*, 83.

22 The deriding of Yudkin's career has attracted substantial attention in recent years with the renewed sugar debate; see, for example, Ian Leslie 'The Sugar Conspiracy', *Guardian*, 7 April 2016; Gary Taubes 'What if it's all been a big fat lie?'

23 'Special article: Food and Food Values. From the Scientist to the Administrator, Nutrition as an Aid to Health', *Times*, 28 August 1942, 5.

24 Professor John Yudkin Collection, Kings College: London, GB0100 KCLCA K/PP36. Yudkin's research interests are apparent in both his publications and also in this collection of personal reference cards kept by Yudkin. The cards demonstrate his remarks on every article he read and the progression of his research interests from 1954 to 1971.

25 'Products to Aid Slimming: B. M. A. Inspection Urged', *Times*, 18 July 1958, 6.

26 Ibid.

27 John Yudkin, *This Slimming Business* (London: MacGibbon & Kee, 1958).

28 Victoria Brittain, 'Not So Sweet on Sugar', *Times*, 26 June 1972, 9.

29 John Yudkin, A. M. Brown and J. C. Mackenzie, 'Knowledge of Nutrition amongst Housewives of a London Suburb', *Nutrition* 17, no. 1 (1963), 1.

30 Ibid., 4.

31 Ibid., 5.

32 Yudkin, *This Slimming Business*, 12.

33 John Yudkin, *Lose Weight, Feel Great* (London: MacGibbon and Kee, 1964), 8.

34 Ibid., 9.

35 Ibid., 9.

36 Ibid., 10.

37 John Yudkin, 'Dietary Fat and Dietary Sugar', *Lancet* 284, no. 7349 (1964), 4.

38 John H. Speedby, 'Letters to the Editor', *Lancet* 284, no. 7356 (22 August 1964), 412.

39 Ibid., 412.

40 Harvey Levenstein, *Fear of Food: A History of Why We Worry about What We Eat* (Chicago, IL: University of Chicago Press, 2012), 146.

41 Yudkin, *Pure, White and Deadly*, 162.

42 Joan Brumberg, *Fasting Girls: The History of Anorexia Nervosa* (New York: Vintage, 2000), 25.

43 La Berge, *How the Ideology of Low-Fat Conquered America*, 141.

44 Hillel Schwartz, *Never Satisfied: A Cultural History of Diets, Fantasies and Fads* (New York: Anchor, 1990); Harvey Levenstein, *Fear of Food: A History of Why We Worry about What We Eat* (Chicago, IL: University of Chicago Press, 2013).

45 Mintz, *Sweetness and* Power, 12; see also, Caroline De la Pena, *Empty Pleasures: The Story of Artificial Sweeteners from Saccharin to Splenda* (Chapel Hill: University of North Carolina Press, 2010).

46 Warren Belasco, *Appetite for Change: How the Counterculture Took on the Food Industry* (New York: Cornell Paperbacks, 2007), 48.

47 Matthew Smith, *An Alternative History of Hyperactivity: Food Additives and the Feingold Diet* (New Brunswick: Rutgers University Press, 2011).

48 US Senate Select Committee on Nutrition and Human Needs, *Dietary Goals for the United States*, 2nd edn (Washington, DC: US Government Printing Office, December 1977), 4.

49 Ibid.

50 'Dietary Recommendations for Diabetic's for the 1980s' (1979), Report by the Nutrition Sub-Division of the Medical Advisory Committee, *British Diabetic Association* (Joan Walker Collection, University of Leicester).

51 'Instruction for Diabetic Patients' (1943), Royal Free Hospital: London, 3; see also, R. D. Lawrence (1955), 'The Diabetic Life: It's Control by Diet and Insulin', in *A Precise Practical Manual for Practitioners and Patients* (London: J & A Churchill).

52 La Berge, *How the Ideology of Low-Fat Conquered America*, 149.

53 J. M. Price et al. 'Bladder Tumours in Rats Fed Cyclohexylamine or High Doses of a Mixture of Cyclamate and Saccharin', *Science* 167, no. 3921 (1960), 1131–32.

54 Lawrence K. Altman, 'Listing Saccharin as Drug Considered', *New York Times*, 11 March 1977, 18.

55 Ibid.

56 Richard D. Lyons, 'Plan to Restrict Saccharin Debated', *New York Times*, 19 May 1977, 8.

8 The Popularization of a New Nutritional Concept: The Calorie in Belgium, 1914–1918

1 Deborah Levine underlines the prompt usage of 'calorie' by various institutions in the 1890s, opposed to the general public's attitude ('The Curious History of the Calorie in U.S. policy', *American Journal of Preventive Medicine* 52, no. 1 [2017], 125–29).

2 For example, Yves Segers, 'Food Recommendations and Change in a Flemish Cookbook, Ons Kookboek, 1920–2000', *Appetite* 45 (2005), 4–14.

3 For example, Katarzyna Cwiertka, 'Propagation of Nutritional Knowledge in Poland, 1863–1939', in *Order and Disorder: The Health Implications of Eating and Drinking in 19th and 20th Centuries*, ed. Alexander Fenton (East Linton: Tuckwell Press, 2000), 96–111.

4 For example, Jane Philippot, 'How Healthy Are Government Dietary Guidelines? Part 1. Origin and Evolution of Dietary Guidelines', *The Nutrition Practitioner* (Summer 2009), 1–15.

5 Anna Landau – Czajka and A. Kreczmar, 'Diet Patterns in 19th and 20th Century School Manuals', *Acta Poloniae Historica* 85 (2010), 265–84.

6 For example, Anneke Van Otterloo, 'Dutch Food Culture and Its Cookery
   Teachers: The Rise, Diffusion and Decline of a Tradition (1880-1980)', in *The
   Diffusion of Food Culture in Europe from the Late 18th Century to the Present Day*, ed.
   Derek Oddy and Lydia Petranova (Prague: Academia, 2005), 96-106.

7 For example, Adel den Hartog, 'The role of Nutrition in Food Advertisements: The
   Case of the Netherlands', in *Food Technology, Science and Marketing*, ed. Adel den
   Hartog (East Linton: Tuckwell Press, 1995), 268-80.

8 Josep Bernabeu-Mestre et al., 'La divulgación radiofónica de la alimentación y le
   higiene infantil en la España de la Segunda Republica (1933-1935)', *Salud Colectiva* 7,
   suppl. 1 (2011), 49-60.

9 'Calorie' (with capital c) refers to kilocalorie, which never appeared in my sources.
   Throughout this text, I will use 'calorie'.

10 To this testified a report on food in one of the Brussels general hospitals, L. Stiénon,
   Rapport sur l'alimentation (Brussels: Hôpitaux de Bruxelles, 1902), 2.

11 Gyorgy Scrinis, 'On the Ideology of Nutritionism', *Gastronomica* 8, no. 1 (2008), 43.

12 David Frankenfield, 'On Heat, Respiration, and Calorimetry', *Nutrition* 26 (2010),
   939-50 (here: 945).

13 Nick Cullather, 'The Foreign Policy of the Calorie', *American Historical Review* 112,
   no. 2 (2007), 339. The mentioning of 'caloric value of food' via Google Book's Ngram
   Viewer, 1890-1930, English language, confirms the decisive role of the war (https://
   books.google.com/ngrams/graph?content=caloric+value+of+food, 25 June 2017).

14 Peter Scholliers, 'Food Recommendations in Domestic Education, Belgium 1890-
   1940', *Paedagogica Historica* 49, no. 5 (2013), 645-63.

15 Sophie De Schaepdrijver, 'A Civilian War Effort: The *Comité National de Secours et
   d'Alimentation* in Occupied Belgium, 1914-1918', in *Remembering Herbert Hoover and
   the Commission for Relief in Belgium* (Brussels: Fondation Universitaire, 2007), 24-37.

16 The relation between science and *the* public is lively debated, see, for example,
   Bernadette Bensaude-Vincent, *L'opinion publique et la science* (Paris: La
   Découverte, 2013).

17 A solid argument for using newspapers: Adrian Bingham, 'Reading
   Newspapers: Cultural Histories of the Popular Press in Modern Britain', *History
   Compass* 10, no. 2 (2012), 144.

18 On censured and clandestine press during the war, see the *Belgian War Press*, https://
   warpress.cegesoma.be/en/node/11 (accessed in June 2017); on the Brussels press, see
   Pierre Van den Dungen, 'Milieux de presse bruxellois pendant la Grande Guerre', *Les
   Cahiers de la Fonderie* 32 (2005), 15-20.

19 *Het Archief* (www.hetarchief.be), accessed between April and July 2016 and in
   March 2017. The databank includes 360,000 pages of censored and clandestine press
   (newspapers, weekly and monthly magazines and pamphlets in French, Dutch and
   German).

20 *Belgicapress, Royal Library of Belgium* (www.kbr.be/belgicapress), accessed in March
   2016 and April 2017. The databank contains seventy-seven widely read newspapers.

21 *Delpher*, Royal Library of the Netherlands (www.delpher.nl/), accessed in August
   2016; *Gallica*, Bibliothèque Nationale de France (www.gallica.bnf.fr), accessed in
   June 2017. In both cases, I first selected 'calorie(s)', then 'voeding' or 'alimentation'.
   Delpher supplies a searchable databank, but Gallica does not, forcing me to select ten
   newspapers.

22 James Hargrove, 'History of the Calorie in Nutrition', *The Journal of Nutrition* 136
   (2006), 2957-61.

23 Doctor of science Albert J. J. Van de Velde (1871–1956) was the director of the Ghent municipal laboratory.

24 Prior to the war, Dr Louis Delattre (1870–1938) published accessible and humourous books on healthy and tasty nourishment meant for a large audience.

25 Louis Baudry de Saunier (1865–1938) was a scientific journalist with special interest in technology (e.g. automobiles, radio broadcasting).

26 'Food units' refer to carbohydrates, proteins, fats and the like.

27 Aarnout J. C. Snijders, *Onze voedingsmiddelen* (Zutphen: Thieme, 1889) with editions in 1896 and 1911.

28 Parisian-based Dr Francis Heckel (1872–1944 ?) specialized in obesity.

29 For example, Baudry de Saunier wrote, 'Les vitamines, de découverte récente, les savants ignorent encore ce qu'elles sont' (*L'Illustration*, 1 June 1918, 23).

30 For example, in *Le Peuple*, 28 September 1895; *Gazette de Charleroi*, 15 January 1907; and *Journal de Bruxelles*, 1 October 1908.

31 Abbé Berger, *L'alimentation populaire en temps de guerre* (Enghien: Office d'Editions, 1915).

32 All 142 articles include 'calorie', but 'calorie' was not always used in dietary recommendations.

33 Cullather, 'Foreign Policy'.

34 The *Commission Scientifique Interalliée du Ravitaillement* (Inter-Allied Food Council) met in Paris on 25 March 1917 and in Rome on 20 April 1917, and it continued its actions until after the war.

9 Nutritional Reform and Public Feeding in Britain, 1917–1919

1 See, for example, *The Daily Telegraph*, 26 June 1916.

2 For scholarly discussion of public feeding schemes in wartime in international contexts, see Peter Scholliers, 'Restaurants Économiques a Bruxelles Pendant La Grande Guerre', in *Manger et Boire entre 1914 et 1918*, ed. Caroline Poulain (Dijon and Gand: Bibliothèque de Dijon & Editions Snoeck, 2014), 111–18; Hans-Jurgen Teuteberg, 'Food Provisioning on the German Home Front 1914–1918', in *Food and War in Twentieth Century Europe*, ed. Ina Zweiniger-Bargielowska, Rachel Duffett and Alain Drouard (Farnham: Ashgate, 2011), 59–72; Alice Weinreb, *Modern Hungers: Food and Power in Twentieth-Century Germany* (New York: Oxford University Press, 2017), 79–80; Bertram Gordon, 'Fascism, the Neo-Right and Gastronomy: A Case in the Theory of the Social Engineering of Taste', in *Taste: Proceedings of the Oxford Symposium on Food and Cookery*, ed. Tom Jaine (London: Prospect Books, 1988), 82–97.

3 Thomas Jones, *The Unbroken Front, Ministry of Food 1916–1944* (London: Everybody's Books, 1944), 40.

4 Karen Hunt's 'The Politics of Food and Women's Neighborhood Activism in First World War Britain', *International Labor and Working-Class History* 77, no. 1 (2010), briefly discusses communal kitchens through the prism of gender-based activism. National kitchens are mentioned fleetingly in P. B. Johnson's *Land Fit for Heroes* (Chicago: University of Chicago Press, 1968). See also L. Margaret Barnett, *British Food Policy during the First World War* (London: Allen & Unwin, 1985), 151, and

Derek Oddy, *From Plain Fare to Fusion Food: British Diet from the 1890s to the 1990s* (Woodbridge: Boydell Press, 2003), 76.

5   Ian Gazeley and Andrew Newell, 'The First World War and Working-Class Food Consumption in Britain', *European Review of Economic History* 17, no. 1 (2013), 72.

6   Adrian Gregory, *The Last Great War: British Society and the First World War* (Cambridge: Cambridge University Press, 2008), 192–98.

7   Minutes of the Committee on Cookery, 22 March 1917, Glasgow and West of Scotland College of Domestic Science records, Glasgow Caledonian University Archives.

8   See William Chance, *Industrial Unrest: Reports of the Commissioners (July 1917)* (London: P. S. King & Son, 1917), 12–14; 32–33.

9   Dilwyn Porter, 'Jones, (William) Kennedy (1865–1921)', *Oxford Dictionary of National Biography* (Oxford: Oxford University Press, 2004).

10 Brigid Allen, 'Miles, Eustace Hamilton (1868–1948)', *Oxford Dictionary of National Biography* (Oxford: Oxford University Press, 2004).

11 Elsa Richardson, 'Sun-Fired Foods and Nutritional Science: Eustace Miles and Vegetarian Reform', *Food Anxieties in Twentieth-Century Britain and Ireland*, University of Ulster, Belfast, 7 April 2017.

12 Richardson, 'Sun-Fired Foods'.

13 R. Hippisley Cox, H. J. Bradley and Eustace Miles, *Public Kitchens, their Organisation and Importance* (London: Simpkin, Marshall, Hamilton, Kent, 1917), 4.

14 Ibid., 3.

15 Ibid., 13.

16 Ministry of Food, *National Kitchens Handbook* (London: Stationery Office, 1917), 17.

17 Spencer to Rhondda, 16 January 1918. TNA, MAF 60/310.

18 Spencer memo on the future of national kitchens, October 1918. TNA, MAF 60/310.

19 Frank Trentmann, 'Coping with Shortage: The Problem of Food Security and Global Visions of its Coordination', c. 1890s–1950', in *Food and Conflict in the Age of the Two World Wars*, ed. Trentmann and Fleming Just (Houndmills: Palgrave Macmillan, 2006), 17–18.

20 Cox, Bradley and Miles, *Public Kitchens*, 15.

21 Marianne Colloms and Dick Weindling, 'West Hampstead's Tennis World Champion (and Food Fanatic)', *West Hampstead Life*, 25 June 2014.

22 Richardson, 'Sun-Fired Foods'.

23 G. K. Chesterton, *Irish Impressions* (London: Collins, 1919), 5.

24 Colloms and Weindling, 'West Hampstead's Tennis World Champion'.

25 Cox, Bradley and Miles, *Public Kitchens*, 15.

26 Ibid., 16.

27 Ministry of Food, *National Kitchens Handbook*, 27.

28 Colin Spencer, *The Heretic's Feast: A History of Vegetarianism* (Hanover: University Press of New England, 1995), 359.

29 Adam Shprintzen, *The Vegetarian Crusade: The Rise of an American Reform Movement, 1817–1921* (Chapel Hill: University of North Carolina Press, 2003), 3–27.

30 Gazeley and Newell, 'First World War and Working-Class Food Consumption in Britain', 73. For a comparison between British and German experiences of feeding, see Avner Offer, *The First World War: An Agrarian Interpretation* (Oxford: Clarendon Press, 1989).

31 Cox, Bradley and Miles, *Public Kitchens*, 18.

32 These concerns were summarized in the Report of the Interdepartmental Committee on Physical Deterioration (London, 1904), accessible in its original format at https://archive.org/details/b21358916.

33 Cox, Bradley and Miles, *Public Kitchens*, 4.

34 Ibid., 15.

35 Ibid., 19.

36 Ministry of Food, *National Kitchens Handbook*, 14.

37 Alexandra Harris, *Romantic Moderns: English Writers, Artists and the Imagination from Virginia Woolf to John Piper* (London: Thames & Hudson, 2015), 3.

38 John Carey, *The Intellectuals and the Masses: Pride and Prejudice among the Literary Intelligentsia, 1880–1939* (London: Faber, 1992), 152.

39 Arnold Bennett, 'Thoughts on National Kitchens', *Daily News*, 1918, 2.

40 Ibid., 4.

41 Maud Pember Reeves, *Round about a Pound a Week* (London: G. Bell, 1913).

42 James Vernon, *Hunger: A Modern History* (Cambridge, MA: Harvard University Press, 2007), 181.

43 C. S. Peel, *Life's Enchanted Cup: An Autobiography, 1872–1933* (London: John Lane, 1933), 59.

44 Conference of Teachers of Domestic Science pamphlet (undated), Glasgow and West of Scotland College of Domestic Science records, Glasgow Caledonian Archives.

45 Elizabeth Waldie, *Mrs Waldie's Collection of Economical Recipes Suitable for War Cookery and Notes on Meaning of Economy as Regards Food and Fuel* (Glasgow: s.n., 1917), 9–28.

46 *Glasgow Herald*, 16 October 1915. See also J. Struthers to J. A. McCallum, 9 June 1917, Minutes of the Committee on Cookery, 17 May 1917, Glasgow and West of Scotland College of Domestic Science records, Glasgow Caledonian University Archives.

47 Liverpool training school of cookery minutes, April–November 1917. John Moores University Archives, F. L. Calder collection.

48 Chalmers Wilson, memorandum on food economy campaign (Scotland), 6 April 1917, Glasgow and West of Scotland College of Domestic Science records, Glasgow Caledonian University Archives.

49 Liverpool training school of cookery minutes, May 1918. John Moores University Archives, F. L. Calder collection.

50 Ibid.

51 Minutes of departmental committee meeting, 11 April 1918. TNA, MAF 60/310.

52 Minutes of the Committee on Cookery, 14 June 1918, Glasgow and West of Scotland College of Domestic Science records, Glasgow Caledonian University Archives.

53 *Glasgow Evening News*, 15 April 1919.

54 Liverpool training school of cookery minutes, November 1917. John Moores University Archives, F.L. Calder collection.

55 Glasgow Corporation Minutes, Minutes of Special Committee on National Kitchens Order 1918, 23 August 1918.

56 John Pearce, 'Be British – Play the Game', undated correspondence, TNA, MAF 60/310.

57 Trentmann, 'Coping with Shortage', 18–19.

58 Minutes of the Joint Meeting of the Finance and Educational Methods Committees, 14 June 1918, Glasgow and West of Scotland College of Domestic Science records, Glasgow Caledonian University Archives.

59 *Glasgow Evening News*, 25 April 1919.

60 Ministry of Food National Kitchens Branch, Kitchens Advisory Committee minutes, 26 February 1919. TNA, MAF 60/329.

61 Ministry of Food National Kitchens Branch, Kitchens Advisory Committee minutes, 3 March 1919. TNA, MAF 60/329.

62 Ministry of Food National Kitchens Branch, Kitchens Advisory Committee minutes, 12 March 1919. TNA, MAF 60/329.

63 Ministry of Food National Kitchens Branch, Kitchens Advisory Committee minutes, 30 April 1919. TNA, MAF 60/329.

64 Ministry of Food National Kitchens Branch, Kitchens Advisory Committee minutes, 30 April 1919. TNA, MAF 60/329.

65 Kennedy Jones memo on national kitchens, 30 September 1919. TNA, MAF 60/310.

66 Ministry of Food National Kitchens Branch, Kitchens Advisory Committee minutes, 26 May 1919. TNA, MAF 60/329.

67 Kennedy Jones memo on national kitchens, 30 September 1919. TNA, MAF 60/310.

68 Ibid.

10 The Sin of Eating Meat: Fascism, Nazism and the Construction of Sacred Vegetarianism

1 Heather Arndt Anderson, *Breakfast* (Lanham, MD: Rowman and Littlefield, 2013), 22–27.

2 Detlef Briesen, 'What Is a Healthy Diet? Some Ideas about the Construction of Healthy Food in Germany Since the Nineteenth Century', in *Eating Traditional Food: Politics, Identity and Practices*, ed. Brigitte Sébastia (London: Routledge, 2017).

3 Francesco Buscemi, 'From Physical Illness to Social Virtue: The Italian Way to Vegetarianism in the Newspaper *La Stampa* from 1867 to the Present', in *Vegetarians' Dilemma: Rethinking Food Choice Throughout Time* (Fayetteville: University of Arkansas Press, in press).

4 Alberto Capatti, *Vegetit: Le Avanguardie Vegetariane in Italia* (Lucca: Cinquesensi, 2016).

5 Richard H. Schwartz, *Judaism and Vegetarianism* (Herndon, VA: Lantern, 2001); Rosalba Mattei and Irene Basili, 'L'Alimentazione Vegetariana', in *Manuale di Nutrizione Clinica*, ed. Rosalba Mattei (Milan: Franco Angeli, 2003); Francesco Buscemi, 'Edible Lies: How Nazi Propaganda Represented Meat to Demonise the Jews', *Media, War and Conflict* 9, no. 2 (2016), 180–97.

6 Zbynek Zeman, *Nazi Propaganda* (Oxford: Oxford University Press, 1964); David Welch, *The Third Reich: Politics and Propaganda* (Abingdon: Psychology Press, 2002); David Welch, 'Nazi Propaganda and the Volksgemeinschaft: Constructing a People's Community', *Journal of Contemporary History* 39, no. 2 (2004), 213–38; Jeffrey Herf, *The Jewish Enemy: Nazi Propaganda during World War II and the Holocaust* (Harvard, MA: Harvard University Press, 2006); Giuseppe Finaldi, *Mussolini and Italian Fascism* (London: Routledge, 2013).

7 Aaron Gillette, *Racial Theories in Fascist Italy* (London: Routledge, 2002); Richard Gray, *About Face: German Physiognomic Thought from Lavater to Auschwitz* (Detroit, MI: Wayne State University Press, 2004).

8 Gerald Kirwin, 'Allied Bombing and Nazi Domestic Propaganda', *European History Quarterly* 15, no. 3 (1985), 341–62; Victoria de Grazia, *How Fascism Ruled Women*

(Berkeley: University of California Press, 1992); Barbara Spackman, *Fascist Virility: Rhetoric, Ideology and Social Fantasy in Italy* (Minneapolis: University of Minnesota Press, 1996).

9 Randall Bytwerk, *Julius Streicher: Nazi Editor of the Notorious Anti-Semitic Newspaper Der Stürmer* (Lanham, MD: Cooper Square Press/Rowman & Littlefield, 2001); Randall Bytwerk, 'The Argument for Genocide in Nazi Propaganda', *Quarterly Journal of Speech* 91, no. 1 (2005), 37–62; Rolf Giesen, *Nazi Propaganda Films: A History and Filmography* (Jefferson, NC: McFarland, 2003); Steven Ricci, *Cinema and Fascism: Italian Film and Society, 1922–1943* (Berkeley: University of California Press, 2008).

10 Boria Sax, *Animals in the Third Reich: Pets, Scapegoat, and the Holocaust* (London: Continuum, 2000).

11 Alexander Nützenadel, 'Dictating Food: Autarchy, Food Provision, and Consumer Politics in Fascist Italy 1922–1943', in *Food and Conflict in Europe in the Age of the Two World Wars*, ed. Frank Trentmann and Flemming Just (Basingstoke: Palgrave Macmillan, 2006).

12 Buscemi, 'Edible Lies'.

13 Bernhard Forchtner and Ana Tominc, 'Kalashnikov and Cooking-Spoon: Neo-Nazism, Veganism and a Lifestyle Cooking Show on YouTube', *Food, Culture and Society* 20, no. 3 (2017), 415–41.

14 Ignazio Silone, *Il Fascismo: Origini e Sviluppo* (Milano: SugarCo, 1992); Simonetta Falasca Zamponi, *Lo Spettacolo del Fascismo* (Soveria Mannelli: Rubbettino, 2003); Sergio Romano, 'La Marcia su Roma Cominciò a Fiume', *Il Corriere della Sera*, 3 July 2004. http://www.corriere.it/cultura/speciali/2014/prima-guerra-mondiale//notizie/marcia-roma-comincio-fiume-bf4dfe04-02a3-11e4-af6d-a9a93b39a7aa.shtml.

15 Giordano Bruno Guerri, *D'Annunzio: L'Amante Guerriero* (Milan: Mondadori, 2009).

16 Renzo De Felice, *La Carta del Carnaro nei Testi di Alceste de Ambris e Gabriele D'Annunzio* (Bologna: Il Mulino, 1973).

17 De Felice, *La Carta del Carnaro.*

18 Claudia Salaris, *Alla Festa della Rivoluzione: Artisti e Libertari con D'Annunzio a Fiume* (Bologna: Il Mulino, 2002).

19 Salaris, *Alla Festa*, 70.

20 Michael Arthur Leeden, *D'Annunzio a Fiume* (Bari: Laterza, 1975).

21 Nicholas Fellows, *Democracy and Dictatorships in Germany: 1919–1963* (London: Hachette UK, 2017); Lavinia Stan and Lucian Turcescu, *Church, State, and Democracy in Expanding Europe* (Oxford: Oxford University Press, 2011); Derek McGhee, *Homosexuality, Law and Resistance* (Abingdon: Routledge, 2001).

22 Raffaello Uboldi, *La Presa del Potere di Benito Mussolini* (Milan: Mondadori, 2010).

23 Denis Mack Smith, *Mussolini* (Milan: Rizzoli, 1981).

24 Buscemi, 'Edible Lies'.

25 Sandro Pozzi, *Guido Keller: Nel Pensiero nelle Gesta* (Milan: Mediolanum, 1933).

26 Ibid.

27 Ibid., 209.

28 Salaris, *Alla Festa.*

29 Leeden, *D'Annunzio*, 196.

30 Guido Keller, 'Amore La Nuova Scuola', *La Testa di Ferro*, 13 (June 1920), 1–20.

31 Salaris, *Alla Festa*, 51.

32 Linea Verde, 'Interview with Giordano Bruno Guerri', *Rai 1*, Italian TV programme, 3 May 2015.

33 Salaris, *Alla Festa*, 201.

34 Ibid., 202.

35 Gabriele D'Annunzio, 'O Italia o Morte. Comando di Fiume d'Italia', *Bollettino Ufficiale*, 12 September, year 1, n. 1, 1919.

36 Pozzi, *Guido Keller*, 49.

37 Ibid., 63.

38 Nick Fiddes, *Meat: A Natural Symbol* (London: Routledge, 1991); Carol J. Adams, *The Sexual Politics of Meat (20th Anniversary Edition): A Feminist-Vegetarian Critical Theory* (New York: Continuum, 2010).

39 Carolyn Marvin and David W. Ingle, *Blood Sacrifice and the Nation: Totem Rituals and the American Flag* (Cambridge: Cambridge University Press, 1999).

40 Fiddes, *Meat*.

41 Buscemi, 'Edible Lies'.

42 Adams, *The Sexual*.

43 Yoga, *Primo Quaderno dello Yoga* (Fiume: Ed. Mino Somenzi – Città di Vita, 1920).

44 Giovanni Comisso, *Le Mie Stagioni* (Treviso: Edizioni di Treviso, 1951).

45 Comisso, *Le Mie*, 74–75; Salaris, *Alla Festa*, 200.

46 Salaris, *Alla Festa*, 200–1.

47 Giovanni Comisso, *Il Porto dell'Amore* (Treviso: Stamperia di Antonio Vianello, 1924), 161.

48 Eugenio Coselschi, *La Marcia di Ronchi* (Florence: Vallecchi, 1929), 203–4.

49 Yoga, *Primo Quaderno*.

50 Luigi Urettini, *Il Giovane Comisso e le sue Lettere a Casa (1914–1920)* (Abano Terme: Francisci, 1985), 215–16; Salaris, *Alla Festa*, 29–30.

51 Fiddes, *Meat*.

52 Pozzi, *Guido Keller*, 22.

53 Ufficio Stampa e Propaganda, 'Ai Veneti!!' (Fiume: Ufficio Stampa e Propaganda del Comando città di Fiume, Sezione per il Veneto – Palazzo Baccich, February 1920).

54 John Cornwell, *Hitler's Scientists* (London: Penguin, 2013).

55 James Cross Giblin, *The Life and Death of Adolf Hitler* (New York: Clarion, 2002), 105

56 Robert N. Proctor, *The Nazi War on Cancer* (Princeton, NJ: Princeton University Press, 1999), 134.

57 Sax, *Animals*.

58 Adams, *The Sexual*.

59 Buscemi, 'Edible Lies'.

60 Zygmunt Bauman, *Postmodernity and Its Discontents* (Cambridge: Polity Press, 1997).

61 'Insolenza dei Macellai Croati', *La Vedetta d'Italia*, 24 September 1919, 2.

62 Buscemi, 'Edible Lies'.

63 Nicholas Goodrick-Clarke, *The Occult Roots of Nazism: Secret Aryan Cults and Their Influence on Nazi Ideology* (New York: New York University Press, 2004).

64 Peter Staudenmaier, *Between Occultism and Nazism: Anthroposophy and the Politics of Race in the Fascist Era* (Leiden: Brill, 2004), 4.

65 Karl Toepfer, *Empire of Ecstasy: Nudity and Movement in German Body Culture, 1910–1935* (Berkeley: University of California Press, 1997), 37–38.

66 Carroll P. Kakel, *The American West and the Nazi East: A Comparative and Interpretive Perspective* (Basingstoke: Palgrave Macmillan, 2011), 42; Jean-Denis Lepage, *Hitler Youth 1922–1945: An Illustrated History* (London: McFarland & Company, 2009), 17.

67   Ben Kiernan, *Blood and Soil: A World History of Genocide and Extermination from Sparta to Darfour* (New Haven, CT: Yale University Press), 418.

68   Peter B. Clarke, *Encyclopedia of New Religious Movements* (London: Routledge, 2006), 394.

69   Coselschi, *La Marcia*.

70   Yoga, *Primo*; Ferdinando Gerra, *L'Impresa di Fiume, vol. 2* (Milan: Longanes, 1974); Salaris, *Alla Festa*.

71   Comisso, *Le Mie*, 83–84.

72   'Contro la Pesca con la Dinamite', *La Vedetta d'Italia*, 2 September 1919, 6.

73   Yoga, *Primo*, 6.

74   Guido Armellini, *Le immagini del Fascismo nelle Arti Figurative* (Milan: Fabbri editore, 1980).

75   Capatti, *Vegetit*.

76   Sandro Consolato, 'Gicomo Boni: L'Archeologo Vate della Terza Roma', in *Esoterismo e Fascismo*, ed. Gianfranco De Turris (Rome: Edizioni Mediterranee, 2006), 185.

77   Ibid., 186.

78   Ibid., 185–86.

79   Enrica Garzilli, *L'Esploratore del Duce: Le Avventure di Giuseppe Tucci e la Politica Italiana in Oriente da Mussolini ad Andreotti*, Vol. 1 and 2 (Milan: Asiatica Association, 2012); 'Tucci, L'Indiana Jones all'Italiana', *Il Tempo*, 14 October 2013. http://www.iltempo.it/cultura-spettacoli/2013/10/14/gallery/tucci-lindiana-jones-allitaliana-910670/.

80   Buscemi, 'From Physical Illness'.

81   Renato Paresce, 'L'Arte fra gli Artigli di Albione', *La Stampa*, 9 August 1933, 3.

82   La Stampa, 'Donne, Birra ed Autografi', *La Stampa*, 26 June 1931, 6.

83   Italo Zingarelli, 'Dovete essere Belle ma Esser Anche Sane', *La Stampa*, 11 October 1937, 3.

84   Luciano Magrini, 'India Primeva e Rinnovata: Dove Insegnano Gandhi e Tagore, e Dove I Missionari Italiani Catechizzano gli Idolatri', *La Stampa*, 23 August 1926, 3.

85   Marco Impiglia, 'Mussolini Sportivo', in *Sport e Fascismo*, ed. Maria Canella and Sergio Giuntini (Milan: Franco Angeli, 2009), 27.

86   Capatti, *Vegetit*.

87   Hasia R. Diner, *Hungering for America. Italian, Irish and Jewish Foodways in the Age of Migration* (Cambridge, MA: Harvard University Press, 2001).

88   Miriam Mafai, *Pane Nero* (Milan: Mondadori, 1987).

89   Eric Voegelin, *Die Politische Religionen* (Wien: Wilhelm Fink Verlag, 1996).

90   Michael Burleigh, *The Third Reich: A New History* (New York: Hill and Wang, 2000).

91   Richard Steigmann-Gall, *The Holy Reich: Nazi Conceptions of Christianity, 1919–1945* (Cambridge: Cambridge University Press, 2003); Roger Griffin, 'Religious Politics: A Concept Comes of Age', *Leidschrift Historisch Tijdschrift* 26, no. 2 (2011), 7–18.

92   Emilio Gentile, *Le Religioni della Politica: Tra Democrazie e Totalitarismi* (Bari: Laterza, 2014).

93   Herbert W. Schneider, *Making the Fascist State* (Oxford: Oxford University Press, 1928).

94   Steigmann-Gall, *The Holy*.

95   Buscemi, 'Edible Lies'.

96   Valentina Napolitano, *Migrant Hearts and the Atlantic Return: Transnationalism and the Roman Catholic Church* (New York: Fordham University Press, 2016), 25.

97   Mattei and Basili, 'L'Alimentazione'; Buscemi, 'Edible Lies'.

11 'Milk Is Life': Nutritional Interventions and Child Welfare: The Italian Case and Post-War International Aid

1 See, among others, Erna Melanie Dupuis, *Nature's Perfect Food. How Milk Became America's Drink* (New York; London: New York University Press, 2002); Richie Nimmo, *Milk, Modernity and the Making of the Human. Purifying the Social* (Abingdon, Oxon: Routledge, 2010); Aleck Ostry, 'The Early Development of Nutrition Policy in Canada', in *Children's Health Issues in Historical Perspective*, ed. Cheryl Krasnick Warsh and Veronica Strong-Boag (Waterloo, ON: Wilfrid Laurier University Press, 2005).

2 Peter J. Atkins, 'The Milk in Schools Scheme, 1934–45: "Nationalization" and Resistance', *History of Education* 34, no. 1 (2005), 1–21; Ido de Haan, 'Vigorous, Pure and Vulnerable: Child Health and Citizenship in the Netherlands Since the End of the Nineteenth Century', in *Cultures of Child Health in Britain and the Netherlands in the Twentieth Century*, ed. Marijke Gijswijt-Hofstra and Hilary Marland (Amsterdam; New York: Rodopi, 2003), 45.

3 James A. Gillespie, 'International Organizations and the Problem of Child Health 1945–1960', *Dynamis*, no. 23 (2003), 115–142, 135.

4 Atkins, 'The Milk in Schools Scheme'; Peter J. Atkins, 'Fattening Children or Fattening Farmers? School Milk in Britain, 1921–1941', *Economic History Review* LVIII, no. 1 (2005), 57–78; Virginia Thorley, 'Australian School Milk Schemes to 1974: For the Benefit of Whom?', *Health and History* 16, no. 2 (2014), 63–86; Susan Levine, *School Lunch Politics. The Surprising History of America's Favorite Welfare Program* (Princeton, NJ: Princeton University Press, 2008), 49, 93.

5 Atkins, 'The Milk in Schools Scheme', 20; Didier Nourrisson, 'Le lait à l'école. Pédagogie de la voie lactée', in *À votre santé! Éducation et santé sous la IVe République*, ed. Didier Nourrisson (Saint-Étienne: Publications de l'Université de Saint-Étienne, 2002), 96.

6 Alice Autumn Weinreb, *Matters of Taste: The Politics of Food and Hunger in Divided Germany 1945–1971* (PhD. diss., University of Michigan, 2009), 268–70.

7 On UNRRA Italian Mission, see Luigi Rossi, 'L'UNRRA strumento di politica estera agli albori del bipolarismo', in *L'Amministrazione per gli Aiuti Internazionali. La ricostruzione dell'Italia tra dinamiche internazionali e attività assistenziali*, ed. Andrea Ciampani (Milan: Franco Angeli, 2002); Silvia Salvatici, '"Not Enough Food to Feed the People". L'UNRRA in Italia (1944–1945)', *Contemporanea*, no. 1 (2011), 83–100; Michele Affinito, *La storia della missione esplorativa dell'UNRRA in Italia (1944–1945). Con, in appendice, il volume di Spurgeon Milton Keeny 'A Mission is born. Italy July 1944–May 1945'* (Naples: Università degli studi Suor Orsola Benincasa, 2012).

8 On Montini, see in particular Luca Barbaini, *Cattolicesimo, modernità, europeismo in Lodovico Montini* (Rome: Edizioni di storia e letteratura, 2013).

9 Lodovico Montini, 'Nutrizione e assistenza in Italia', extract of *Quaderni della Nutrizione* no. 1 (1950), 1–13, 5. See also *L'Amministrazione per gli Aiuti Internazionali. Origini, ordinamento, funzioni, attività* (Rome: A.b.e.t.e., 1952), 4–12; Domenica La Banca, *Welfare in Transizione. L'esperienza dell'ONMI (1943–1950)* (Naples; Rome: Ed. Scientifiche italiane, 2013), 183–97.

10 Archivio Centrale dello Stato (hereafter, ACS), Ministero dell'Interno (hereafter, MI), Amministrazione per le Attività Italiane e Internazionali (hereafter, AAI), Presidenza,

b. 71, Lettera di S. M. Keeny a Maurice Pate, 29 luglio 1947. This evaluation was probably based on the entire population aged up to 18 years.

11 Amministrazione per gli Aiuti Internazionali, *L'attività assistenziale dell'Amministrazione aiuti internazionali nel quadriennio 1945–48. Tavole statistiche estratte dall'Annuario Statistico Italiano 1944–48* (Rome: Istituto Poligrafico dello Stato, 1949), 9.

12 In 1953, the AAI was renamed *Amministrazione per le Attività Assistenziali Italiane e Internazionali* (AAI-Administration for Italian and International Welfare Activities), thus conforming to its internal changes through the affirmation of its role within the development and promotion of Italian welfare, and the cooperation with international bodies.

13 Andrea Ciampani, 'La costituzione dell'AAI: relazioni internazionali, ricostruzione sociale e attività assistenziali', in *L'Amministrazione per gli Aiuti Internazionali*, ed. Andrea Ciampani (Milan: Franco Angeli, 2002), 105–6.

14 Comitato Italiano Unicef, ed., *Fondo delle nazioni unite per l'infanzia (U)* (Padua: Cedam, 1957), 93. More generally on UNICEF's activities in Italy, see A. Villani, *Dalla parte dei bambini. Italia e Unicef tra ricostruzione e sviluppo* (Padua: Cedam, 2016).

15 Ciampani, 'La costituzione dell'AAI', 141.

16 For discussion on these questions, see Gillespie, 'International Organizations and the Problem of Child Health', 133–40; Corinne A. Pernet, 'L'Unicef et la lutte contre la malnutrition en Amérique centrale dans les années 1950: entre coopération et compétition', *Relations internationales* no. 161 (2015), 27–42.

17 Carol Helstosky, *Garlic and Oil: Food and Politics in Italy* (Oxford, NY: Berg, 2004), 63–125.

18 ACS, MI, AAI, Presidenza, b. 60, Appunto per l'on. Montini sul latte in polvere ICEF. Situazione attuale, prospettive ed impegni per il futuro, 10 luglio 1948.

19 For an overview of the dairy industry in Italy after the Second World War, see Emanuele Felice, 'Il settore lattiero-caseario in Italia dal dopoguerra al Duemila', in *Una storia di qualità: Il Gruppo Granarolo fra valori etici e logiche di mercato*, ed. Giuliana Bertagnoni (Bologna: il Mulino, 2004).

20 On the development of the MCP, see Maggie Black, *The Children and the Nations: The Story of Unicef* (New York: UNICEF, 1986), 46–48.

21 'Centrali del latte e sanità pubblica', *Il Latte* no. 8 (1946), 5–6.

22 ACS, MI, AAI, Presidenza, b. 184, Relazioni sulle centrali del latte del programma MCP, settembre 1972.

23 Cassa per Opere Straordinarie di Pubblico Interesse nell'Italia Meridionale, 'Strutture e mercati dell'agricoltura meridionale', in *Latte e derivati. Caratteri, prospettive e fabbisogni della produzione lattiero-casearia*, vol. 3, ed. Carlo Aiello (Rome: Cassa per il Mezzogiorno, 1960), 52–53.

24 ACS, MI, AAI, Presidenza, b. 184, Relazioni sulle centrali del latte del programma MCP, cit.

25 Comitato Italiano Unicef, ed., *Fondo delle nazioni unite per l'infanzia*, 98.

26 Filippo Usuelli, *Gli assillanti problemi demografici ed alimentari in Italia e nel mondo* (S.l.: S.n., 1953), 6–7.

27 Maria Cao-Pinna, 'Le classi povere', in *Atti della Commissione parlamentare di inchiesta sulla miseria in Italia e sui mezzi per combatterla*, vol. 2, ed. Camera dei Deputati, *Indagini tecniche. Condizioni di vita delle classi misere* (Milan: Unione tipografica, 1953), 46, 93, 97–102.

28 Poor families accounted for 35 per cent of the global population of southern Italy, compared to 8.7 per cent of central Italy and 2.3 per cent of northern Italy. See Paolo Braghin, *Le diseguaglianze sociali. Analisi empirica della situazione di diseguaglianza in Italia*, vol. 1 (Milan: Sapere, 1973), 207, 210.

29 Ibid., 223.

30 Virgilio Bacchetta, *Alimentazione e stato di nutrizione dei bambini italiani dopo la guerra* (Spoleto: Tip. Panetto e Petrelli, 1951), 20–48.

31 See, for example, Carlo Arnaudi, 'Aspetti del problema del latte alimentare', *Il Latte* no. 10 (1951), 417–21; Giovanni Della Torre, *Il latte alimentare e le sue proprietà* (Milan: Hoepli, 1956), 210.

32 'Il Convegno nazionale per la valorizzazione del latte e dei suoi derivati', *Il Latte* no. 5 (1955), 293–302, 301.

33 Alto Commissariato dell'Alimentazione, 'L'approvvigionamento del latte alimentare nelle singole provincie della Repubblica', *Il Mondo del Latte* no. 6 (1950), 273–80; Saladino Cramarossa, 'Criteri informatori della legislazione sanitaria nei paesi a più alto consumo di latte', in *Il latte alimento per tutti nel pensiero di fisiologi, igienisti e clinici italiani*, ed. Istituto Nazionale della Nutrizione del Consiglio Nazionale delle Ricerche, Amministrazione per le Attività Assistenziali Italiane e Internazionali (Rome: AAI, 1957).

34 Sabato Visco, 'Problemi alimentari delle comunità', *Assistenza d'Oggi* no. 3 (1955), 16–31, 21–22; Amministrazione per le attività assistenziali italiane e internazionali, *Gli alimenti e il bambino* (Brescia: La Scuola, 1961), 75; A. M. Calvi, *L'alimentazione nelle collettività infantili* (Rome: Tip. F. Failli, 1966), 19, 27.

35 Lodovico Montini, 'Introduzione', in *Il latte alimento per tutti*, ed. Istituto Nazionale della Nutrizione del Consiglio Nazionale delle Ricerche, Amministrazione per le Attività Assistenziali Italiane e Internazionali (Rome: AAI, 1957), 6.

36 UNRRA Italian Mission, Welfare Division, Nutrition Branch, *The School Lunch Manch* (s.l.: s.n., 1946).

37 Giorgio Cigliana, 'Lodovico Montini e gli aiuti internazionali', *Studium* no. 3 (1990), 357–369, 366.

38 Telesforo Bonadonna, Dino Desiderio Nai and Filippo Usuelli, 'Problemi del latte e prospettive economiche', *Il Latte* no. 9 (1950), 291–92, 291. The distribution of milk in schools was supported even by Pope Pius XII, who pointed out its advantages in terms of industrialization and public health, and hoped for its implementation on a larger scale. See 'XIV Congresso internazionale di latteria – Roma 24–28 settembre 1956', *Il Mondo del Latte* no. 10 (1956), 665–74, 665–66.

39 'Comitato Nazionale di Coordinamento studi per il Latte e i suoi Derivati', *Il Mondo del Latte* no. 9 (1950), 485–89.

40 'Relazione del presidente sull'attività svolta dall'Associazione Italiana Lattiero-Casearia durante l'anno 1951', *Il Mondo del Latte* no. 6 (1952), 323–36, 334; 'Il XIV Congresso Internazionale del latte in Italia nel 1946 [sic]. Il Prof. Sabato Visco membro della FIL', *Il Latte* no. 8 (1953), 428.

41 'Le Giornate di studio sul latte alimentare a Amalfi', *Il Latte* no. 11 (1954), 637; 'Il XIV Congresso Internazionale del latte e derivati', *Il Mondo del Latte* no. 9 (1956), 591–95.

42 A council on scientific and economic issues was created within the committee to monitor the relations among the committee itself, CNR, INN, ACA, ACIS and the Ministries of Agriculture, Education, Industry and Trade, Foreign Trade and Finance. See 'Sette anni di vita del Comitato Italiano del Latte nella relazione del suo illustre Presidente', *Il Latte* no. 8 (1957), 532–34, 533.

43 'Il Convegno nazionale per la valorizzazione del latte e dei suoi derivati', 301.

44 Law 27 November 1956, no. 1367, art. 3.

45 Renato Longardi, 'Una maglia di lana e una tazza di latte!', *L'Unità*, 13 December 1951, 6.

46 Comitato Italiano Unicef, ed., *Fondo delle nazioni unite per l'infanzia*, 94.

47 Ibid., 95.

48 ACS, MI, AAI, Presidenza, b. 60, Resoconto della riunione tenuta a Napoli con alcuni membri dell'Unicef il 14 luglio 1948.

49 ACS, MI, AAI, Presidenza, b. 60, Appunto per l'On. Montini sul latte in polvere ICEF, cit.

50 Montini, 'Nutrizione e assistenza in Italia', 7.

51 Letizia Pagliai, *Giorgio La Pira e il piano latte. La funzione sociale della Centrale* (Florence: Polistampa, 2010), 125–30.

52 More generally on the AAI food programme, see S. Inaudi, 'Assistenza ed educazione alimentare: l'Amministrazione per gli aiuti internazionali, 1947–1965', *Contemporanea* no. 3 (2015), 373–400.

53 Ibid., 388–93. See also Amministrazione per le Attività Assistenziali Italiane e Internazionali, *Programmi di assistenza alimentare e di educazione alimentare svolti con il contributo degli Stati Uniti e la cooperazione delle Nazioni Unite. Accordi e statistiche* (Rome: Tip. F. Failli, 1961). The vitamin intake, instead, should have been provided by the organizations involved, which, according to the agreement, were committed to supplementing the meals with fruit and vegetables produced locally.

54 Alimentazione italiana, 'Quod superest. . .', *L'Alimentazione Italiana* II, no. 2 (1956).

55 Levine, *School Lunch Politics*, 93.

56 Sabato Visco, 'Nuovi aspetti di assistenza alimentare nei programmi AAI', *L'Alimentazione Italiana* II, no. 10 (1956).

57 Sabato Visco, 'Mezzi per favorire un maggior consumo del latte e dei derivati', *Il Mondo del Latte* no. 4 (1955), 224–27, 227.

58 'La discussione e le conclusioni del convegno di Livorno', *Il Latte* no. 8 (1955), 525–29.

59 Visco, 'Mezzi per favorire un maggior consumo del latte e dei derivati', 226–27.

60 Bruno Angelillo, 'Il latte in alcuni suoi aspetti igienico-sanitari', in *2 Convegno nazionale sul latte nel quadro alimentare dell'Italia. Milano 14 Ottobre 1968* (Rome: FIAMCLAF, 1968), 43.

61 See, for example, ACS, MI, AAI, Presidenza, b. 66, Unicef, Comité du programme, Recommandations du directeur général relatives à des affectations de crédits supplémentaires à l'Italie pour la conservation du lait (E/ICEF/R.314), 28 mars 1952 and ACS, MI, AAI, Archivio generale, Raccolta Circolari, b. 4, Circolare no. 1129, 26 agosto 1957.

62 ACS, MI, AAI, Presidenza, b. 111, Promemoria. Il latte nei programmi assistenziali AAI, 19 maggio 1961. The distribution at territorial level was very variable between years for numerous reasons.

63 Francesco Mancini, 'Il latte nella refezione scolastica', in *Il latte alimento per tutti*, ed. Istituto Nazionale della Nutrizione del Consiglio Nazionale delle Ricerche, Amministrazione per le Attività Assistenziali Italiane e Internazionali (Rome: AAI, 1957), 106.

64 Ibid., 103.

65 'Assistenza alimentare AAI – Programmi speciali', *L'Alimentazione Italiana* III, no. 7 (1957); Mancini, 'Il latte nella refezione scolastica', 104.

66 Giorgio Mingoni, 'Iniziative assistenziali italiane ed internazionali', *L'Alimentazione Italiana* II, no. 8 (1956).

67 Giovanni Galizzi and Giorgio Cingolani, 'Lineamenti della produzione e del consumo di latte in Italia', *Annali della Facoltà di Agraria* no. 2 (1960), 126–59, 139–40.

68 Guido De Marzi, 'Istituito un Comitato di studio per i problemi della nutrizione', *Assistenza d'Oggi* no. 3 (1955), 60–63, 61–62; Manlio Pompei, 'Una politica per il latte', *Il Giornale d'Italia*, 30 June 1961.

69 Visco, 'Mezzi per favorire un maggior consumo del latte e dei derivati', 226.

70 Maria Cao-Pinna, 'Qualche linea di informazione sull'Accordo e di raffronto con l'Accordo UNRRA', *Assistenza d'Oggi* no. 5/6 (1955), 8–19, 18–19.

71 Carla Colombelli, 'Il cibo dell'infanzia', in *Storia d'Italia, Annali 13, L'alimentazione*, ed. Alberto Capatti, Alberto De Bernardi and Angelo Varni (Turin: Einaudi, 1998), 641–43.

72 Inaudi, 'Assistenza ed educazione alimentare', 392–94.

73 Montini, 'Introduzione', 11.

74 Ibid., 10.

75 See Pagliai, *Giorgio La Pira e il piano latte*, 128.

76 Piergiacomo Ferrari, *L'industria del latte in Italia* (Piacenza: Camera di commercio, industria artigianato e agricoltura di Piacenza, after 1970), 592.

12 Like Oil and Water: Food Additives and America's Food Identity Standards in the Mid-Twentieth Century

The author thanks Prof Matthew Smith, Dr Yong Chen, Dr Kavita Philip, Dr Alex Borucki and Dr Dennis Gordon for their guidance and feedback throughout the writing process, and Hugo Gordon Bettencourt for his editorial assistance.

1 Patrick Zylberman, 'Making Food Safety an Issue: Internationalized Food Politics and French Public Health from the 1870s to the Present', *Medical History* 48, no. 1 (2004), 1–28.

2 John Marchant, Bryan Reuben and Joan Alcock, *Bread: A Slice of History* (Gloustershire: The History Press, 2008), 13.

3 Ibid., 26.

4 Lorraine Swainston Goodwin, *The Pure Food, Drink, and Drug Crusaders, 1879–1914* (Jefferson: McFarland & Company, 1999); Marc T. Law, 'The Origins of State Pure Food Regulations', 1103–30, *Journal of Economic History* 63 (2003); James Harvey Young, 'The Pig That Fell into the Privy: Upton Sinclair's *The Jungle* and the Meat Inspection Amendments of 1906', *Bulletin of the History of Medicine* 59 (1985), 467–80.

5 Suzanne Junod, 'Food Standards in the United States: The Case of the Peanut Butter and Jelly Sandwich', in *Food, Science, Policy and Regulation in the Twentieth Century: International and Comparative Perspectives*, ed. David F. Smith and Jim Phillips (London: Routledge, 2000), 167–88; Richard A. Merrill and Earl M. Collier Jr., '"Like Mother Used to Make": An Analysis of FDA Food Standards of Identity', *Columbia Law Review* 74 (1974), 561–621.

6 Bee Wilson, *Swindled: The Dark History of Food Fraud, from Poisoned Candy to Counterfeit Coffee* (Princeton, NJ: Princeton University Press, 2008).

7 Matthew Smith, *An Alternative History of Hyperactivity: Food Additives and the Feingold Diet* (New Brusnwick: Rutgers University Press, 2011).

8 Deutsch, Tracey, *Building a Housewife's Paradise: Gender, Politics, and American Grocery Stores in the Twentieth Century* (Chapel Hill: University of North Carolina Press, 2010); Lizabeth Cohen, *A Consumer' Republic: The Politics of Mass Consumption in Postwar America* (New York: Vintage, 2003).

9 Aaron Bobrow-Strain, *White Bread: A Social History of the Store Bought Loaf* (Boston, MA: Beacon Press, 2012); Marchant et al., *Bread*.

10 Viggo Norn, *Emulsifiers in Food Technology* (Chichester: John Wiley and Sons, 2014), 73; Steve Ettlinger, *Ingredients: A Visual Exploration of 75 Additives and 25 Food Products* (New York: Regan Arts, 2015), 104.

11 Marchant et al., *Bread*, 174; Ettlinger, *Ingredients*, 104.

12 Norn, *Emulsifiers*, 73.

13 Marchant et al., *Bread*, 174.

14 Harvey A. Levenstein, *Revolution at the Table: The Transformation of the American Diet* (Oxford: Oxford University Press, 1988), 31–35.

15 Ibid., 37.

16 Chris Otter, 'Industrializing Diet, Industrializing Ourselves: Technology, Food and the Body since 1750', in *The Routledge History of Food*, ed. Carol Helstosky (Abingdon: Routledge, 2015), 221–22.

17 'Atlas Powder Company Records', Hagley Museum and Library, http://findingaids. hagley.org/xtf/view?docId=ead/1516.xml, accessed 4 March 2016.

18 William Bradford Williams, *History of the Manufacture of Explosives for the World War, 1917–1918* (Chicago, IL: Chicago University Press, 1920), 39.

19 Atlas Powder Company, *Better Farming with Atlas Powder* (Wilmington: Atlas Powder Company, 1919), 3.

20 Atlas Powder Company Industrial Chemicals Department, *The Nature, Suitability for and Uses in Foods and Pharmaceuticals of Sorbitol and Emulsifiers (Including Those Sold under the Trade Marks Span, Arlacel, Tween and Myrj)* (Wilmington: Atlas Chemical Company, 1949), 7.

21 Atlas Powder Company, *Food Emulsifiers* (Wilmington: Atlas Powder Company, 1948).

22 Chris Otter, 'Industrializing Diet, Industrializing Ourselves: Technology, Food and the Body since 1750', in *The Routledge History of Food*, ed. Carol Helstosky (Abingdon: Routledge, 2015), 227.

23 Bobrow-Strain, *White Bread*, 23.

24 Ibid., 32.

25 Ibid., 40.

26 Ibid., 43–44.

27 Ibid., 55.

28 Harry Snyder, *Bread: A Collection of Popular Papers on Wheat, Flour and Bread* (New York: MacMillan, 1930), 228.

29 Tracey Deutsch, *Building a Housewife's Paradise: Gender, Politics and American Grocery Stores in the Twentieth Century* (Chapel Hill: University of North Carolina Press, 2010), 9; Katherine J. Parkin, *Food Is Love* (Philadelphia: University of Pennsylvania Press, 2006), 1. Quoted text is from Parkin.

30 Bobrow-Strain, *White Bread*, 33.

31 'The Adulteration of Food', *Jeffersonian*, 19 May 1859; 'Food and It's Adulterations', *Sunbury American*, 7 July 1855; 'Adulteration of Food, Drugs', *Ottawa Free Trader*, 23 June 1855; 'Milestones in U.S. Food and Drug Law History', *US Food and Drug*

Administration, http://www.fda.gov/opacom/backgrounders/miles.html, accessed 3 March 2016; M. L. Byrn, *A Treatise on the Adulteration of Food and Drink* (Philadelphia, PA: Lippincott Grambo, 1852), 14.

32 P. H. Felker, *The Grocer's Manual* (Claremont, CA: Claremont Manufacturing Company, 1878), 1.

33 lyse D. Barkan, 'Industry Invites Regulation: The Passage of the Pure Food and Drug Act of 1906', *American Journal of Public Health* 75 (1985), 18.

34 Louise G. Baldwin and Florence Kirlin, 'Consumers Appraise the Food, Drug and Cosmetic Act', Law and Contemporary Problems 6 (1939), 146.

35 'The Federal Food Drug and Cosmetic Act', *The United States Statutes at Large*, 34 Stat. 768 (1938), http://constitution.org/uslaw/sal/052_statutes_at_large.pdf, accessed 1 March 2016.

36 Junod, 'Food Standards', 172.

37 'New Food and Drug Bill Given to House', *Los Angeles Times*, 16 April 1938; 'President Breaks Deadlock on Food and Drug Bill', *Los Angeles Times*, 12 June 1938; Merrill and Collier Jr., '"Like Mother Used to Make"', 566; Robert W. Austin, 'The Federal Food Legislation of 1938 and the Food Industry', *Law and Contemporary Problems* 6 (1939), 131.

38 'Chemicals in Food Products', House Committee to Investigate the Use of Chemicals in Food Products, HRG-1950-UCF-001, 14 September 1950.

39 Holmes Alexander, 'What Is in Some Bread? Congressmen Will Ask', *Los Angeles Times*, 27 November 1949.

40 Ibid.

41 'Utilization of Farm Crops, Fats and Oils', Subcommittee on S. Res 36; Senate Sub-Committee on Agriculture and Forestry, HRG- 1949- AFS- 0010.

42 Ibid.

43 Ibid.

44 'Senators Caution on Bread Contents', *New York Times*, 2 August 1951.

45 21 Code of Federal Regulations (CFR), Section 17 (1) (1955).

46 Bess Furman, 'New US Bread Standards Bar Chemical Softeners as Deceptive: New Standard Set for Bakers' Bread', *New York Times*, 15 May 1952.

47 The commercial name for this emulsifier was Myrj 45.

48 Harvey Levenstein, *Paradox of Plenty* (New York: Oxford University Press, 1993), 102.

49 Ibid., 110.

50 Ibid., 568.

51 Merrill and Collier Jr., '"Like Mother Used to Make"', 561.

52 21 CFR 1954 Supplement § 19.750 (7) (c).

53 21 CFR 1954 Supplement § 19.750 (a) (1).

54 21 CFR 1954 Supplement § 52.990.

55 Junod, 'Food Standards', 181.

56 Vincent A. Kleinfeld, 'The Hale Amendment- A Pyrrhic Victory', *Food Drug and Cosmetic Law Journal* 16 (1961), 155.

57 Thomas W. Christopher, 'Significant Comments', *Food, Drug, Cosmetic Law Journal* 9, no. 6 (1954), 365–68.

58 Junod, 'Food Standards', 183; Merrill and Collier Jr., '"Like Mother Used to Make"', 568.

59 John A. Osmundsen, 'Food Trade Waits Impact of U. S. Law on Additives', *New York Times*, 23 February 1959.

60   'The Delaney Clause and Other Regulatory Actions', in *Diet, Nutrition, and Cancer*, ed. Committee on Diet, Nutrition, and Cancer, National Research Council (Washington, DC: National Academies Press, 1982), https://www.ncbi.nlm.nih.gov/books/NBK216642/.

61   Osmundsen, 'Food Trade'.

62   Ibid.

63   Junod, 'Food Standards', 183; Merrill and Collier Jr., ' "Like Mother Used to Make" ', 568.

64   21 CFR § 46.1 (1962).

65   Merrill and Collier Jr., ' "Like Mother Used to Make" ', 609.

66   Frank L. Gunderson, Helen W. Gunderson and Egbert R. Ferguson, *Food Standards and Definitions in the United States: A Guidebook* (New York: Academic Press, 1963), 18.

67   Vallowe, 'Informing Consumers', 260; Austern, 'Food Standards', 447.

68   21 CFR § 37 (1964).

69   21 CFR § 31.1 (1968).

70   21 CFR § 51.1 (1962). My analysis is based on the text of the standards themselves. Further analysis of the individual hearings or framing documents is needed.

71   Elinor Lee, 'Larrick Speaks: Food Law Additions Are Urged', *Washington Post and Times Herald*, 11 April 1956; 'Scientists Agree Some Additives Are Not Safe', *Washington Post and Times Herald*, 24 August 1956.

72   Wilson, *Swindled*, 234.

73   *White House Conference on Food, Nutrition and Health: Final Report* (Washington, DC: US Government Printing Office, 1969), 103.

74   Research by scholars in the field of Critical Nutrition Studies like Charlotte Biltekoff reminds us of the subjective nature of dietary advice. While dietary advice has been shown to be deeply unstable across space and time, my analysis is meant to elucidate the persistent fear among consumers, activists and some doctors of the safety of food additives.

75   Ruth Winter, *Beware of the Food You Eat* (New York: Signet Classic, 1970), 225.

76   Richard D. Lyons, 'Do We Need All That in the Bread?', *New York Times*, 24 September 1972.

77   Peter Weaver, 'Buyer's Guide to Additives', *Washington Post*, 2 July 1972.

78   'Cancer Prevention and the Delaney Clause', Health Research Group: Public Citizen Inc., 1977, 2.

79   'Cancer Prevention and the Delaney Clause', 15.

80   Richard D. Lyons, 'Plan to Restrict Saccharin Debated', *New York Times*, 19 May 1977; Lucida Franks, 'Red Dye No. 2: The 20-Year Battle', *New York Times*, 28 February 1976. Red dye no. 2 was banned by the FDA in 1976 due to cancer concerns, but saccharine remains on the market.

81   Smith, *Hyperactivity*, 3.

82   Thomas Grubisich, 'Hyperactive Diet: A Doctor's Checklist', *Washington Post*, 17 January 1974.

83   Smith, *Hyperactivity*, 138–39.

84   Deutsch, *Building a Housewife's Paradise*, 200.

85   Helen Stone Hovey and Kay Reynolds, *The Practical Book of Food Shopping* (Philadelphia, PA: J.B. Lippincott, 1950), 261.

86   John A. Osmundsen, 'New Law Likely to Improve New Foods: Limited Use of Additives Now Totally Banned, May Aid Products', *New York Times*, 24 February 1959.

87 Deutsch, *Building a Housewife's Paradise*, 196.

88 Ettlinger, *Ingredients*, 104.

89 Will Dunham, 'Study Links Common Food Additives to Crohn's Disease', *Reuters*, 25 February 2015, http://www.reuters.com/article/us-science-emulsifiers/study-links-common-food-additives-to-crohns-disease-colitis-idUSKBN0LT26S20150225, accessed 2 September 2017.

90 Adam Drewnowski and Petra Eichelsdoerfer, 'Can Low-Income Americans Afford a Healthy Diet?', *Nutrition Today* 44, no. 6 (2010), 246–49.

91 Sonali Kohli, 'The Only Food Poor Americans Can Afford Is Making Them Unhealthy', *Atlantic*, 19 August 2014, https://www.theatlantic.com/health/archive/2014/08/the-only-food-poor-americans-can-afford-is-making-them-unhealthy/378774/.

92 David Goldman, 'Kraft Changed Its Mac & Cheese Recipe and Nobody Noticed', *CNN*, 8 March 2016, http://money.cnn.com/2016/03/08/news/companies/kraft-mac-and-cheese-recipe/index.html, accessed 2 September 2017.

93 Joanne S. Hawana, 'Food Identity Disputes Continue to Impose High-Profile Pressure on FDA', *National Law Review*, 21 August 2017, https://www.natlawreview.com/article/food-identity-disputes-continue-to-impose-high-profile-pressure-fda, accessed 1 September 2017.

94 Dan Charles, 'Americans Don't Trust Scientists' Take on Food Issues', *NPR*, 2 December 2016, http://www.npr.org/sections/thesalt/2016/12/02/504034298/americans-dont-trust-scientists-take-on-food-politicians-even-less, accessed 1 September 2017.

Bibliography

'About: *Decolonize Your Diet*'. 2018. http://decolonizeyourdiet.org/about (accessed 5 March 2018).

'Adulteration of Food, Drugs'. *Ottawa Free Trader*, 23 June 1855.

'Assistenza alimentare AAI – Programmi speciali'. *L'Alimentazione Italiana* III, no. 7 (1957).

'Atlas Powder Company Records'. Hagley Museum and Library. http://findingaids.hagley. org/xtf/view?docId=ead/1516.xml (accessed 4 March 2016).

'Breast Cancers and Other Cancers: Disease of Western Civilization?' http://thepaleodiet. com/breast-cancer-and-other-cancers-diseases-of-western-civilization/ (accessed 29 September 2017).

'Calling All Consumers'. *The Chicago Defender*, 6 May 1968.

'Cancer in Ireland: An Economical Question'. *British Medical Journal* 2 (1903): 1544.

'Cancer in the Colonies'. *British Medical Journal* 1 (1906): 812.

'Cancer Increasing at an Alarming Rate'. *Vogue* (15 April 1909): 726.

'Centrali del latte e sanità pubblica'. *Il Latte* XX, no. 8 (1946): 5–6.

'Chemicals in Food Products'. House Committee to Investigate the Use of Chemicals in Food Products. HRG-1950-UCF-001. 14 September 1950.

'Chronic Diseases Are Killing More in Poorer Countries'. https://www.nytimes. com/2014/12/04/world/asia/chronic-diseases-are-killing-more-in-poorer-countries. html?_r=0 (accessed 30 September 2017).

'Comitato Nazionale di Coordinamento Studi per il Latte e i suoi Derivati'. *Il Mondo del Latte* IV, no. 9 (1950): 485–89.

'Contro la pesca con la dinamite'. *La Vedetta d'Italia*, 2 September 1919, 6.

'Diet, Delusion and Diabetes'. 2018. https://link.springer.com/article/10.1007/s00125-008-1203-9 (accessed 3 March 2018).

'Display Ad 1 – No Title'. *New York Times*, 1915.

'Dr Loren Cordain'. http://thepaleodiet.com/dr-loren-cordain/ (accessed 29 September 2017).

'FDA Display on Food Safety Opens'. *The Chicago Defender*, 16 October 1965.

'Food and Its Adulterations'. *Sunbury American*, 7 July 1855.

'Full Text of "World's Columbian Exposition, Chicago, IL, 1893"'. 1893. https://archive. org/stream/worldscolumbian00awargoog/worldscolumbian00awargoog_djvu.txt (accessed 2 February 2018).

'Il Convegno nazionale per la valorizzazione del latte e dei suoi derivati'. *Il Latte* XXIX, no. 5 (1955): 293–302.

'Il XIV Congresso Internazionale del latte e derivati'. *Il Mondo del Latte* X, no. 9 (1956): 591–595.

'Il XIV Congresso Internazionale del latte in Italia nel 1946. Il Prof. Sabato Visco membro della FIL'. *Il Latte* XXVII, no. 8 (1953): 428.

'Insolenza dei macellai Croati'. *La Vedetta d'Italia*, 24 September 1919, 2.

'Is Race Extinction Staring Us in the Face?' *New York Times*, 15 October 1911, 11.

'La discussione e le conclusioni del convegno di Livorno'. *Il Latte* XXIX, no. 8
    (1955): 525–29.

'Lactose-Free Gains Ground Globally'. *Dairy Industries International* 77, no. 6 (2012): 8.

'Le Giornate di studio sul latte alimentare a Amalfi'. *Il Latte* XXVIII, no. 11 (1954): 637.

'Milestones in U.S. Food and Drug Law History', *Food and Drug Administration*. http://
    www.fda.gov/opacom/backgrounders/miles.html (accessed 3 March 2016).

'New Food and Drug Bill Given to House'. *Los Angeles Times*, 16 April 1938.

'Overeating and Cancer'. *British Medical Journal* 1, no. 2045 (1900): 596.

'President Breaks Deadlock on Food and Drug Bill'. *Los Angeles Times*, 12 June 1938.

'Quod superest…'. *L'Alimentazione italiana* (editorial board) II, no. 2 (1956).

'Radical New Method of Treating Diabetes: The Allen Plan, Which Upsets Old Traditions,
    Is Being Given a Thorough Test at the Rockefeller Institute – Five Salient Points of the
    System'. *New York Times*, 1916.

'Relazione del presidente sull'attività svolta dall'Associazione Italiana Lattiero-Casearia
    durante l'anno 1951'. *Il Mondo del Latte* VI, no. 6 (1952): 323–36.

'Rising Levels of Lactose Intolerance Predicted to Propel the Global Lactose Free
    Food Market Until 2020'. *Business Wire*, 4 May 2016. https://www.businesswire.
    com/news/home/20160504005106/en/Rising-Levels-Lactose-Intolerance-
    Predicted-Propel-Global.

'Senators Caution on Bread Contents'. *New York Times*, 2 August 1951.

'Sette anni di vita del Comitato Italiano del Latte nella relazione del suo illustre Presidente'.
    Il Latte XXXI, no. 8 (1957): 532–34.

'Sickly Sweetener: High Fructose Corn Syrup'. *Economist*, Saturday, 29 May 2010, issue
    8684: 69.

'Sull'eziologia della pellagra'. *Rivista Pellagrologica Italiana* 16 (1916): 17–23.

'The Adulteration of Food'. *Jeffersonian*, 19 May 1859.

'The Delaney Clause and Other Regulatory Actions'. Washington, DC: National
    Academies Press, 1982. https://www.ncbi.nlm.nih.gov/books/NBK216642/ (accessed
    15 July 2017).

'The Federal Food Drug and Cosmetic Act', *The United States Statutes at Large*, 34 Stat.
    768 (1938). http://constitution.org/uslaw/sal/052_statutes_at_large.pdf (accessed 1
    March 2016).

'Utilization of Farm Crops, Fats and Oils'. Subcommittee on S. Res 36; Senate Sub-
    committee on Agriculture and Forestry. HRG- 1949- AFS- 0010.

'XIV Congresso internazionale di latteria – Roma 24–28 settembre 1956'. *Il Mondo del
    Latte* X, no. 10 (1956): 665–74.

Abbot, Elizabeth. *Sugar: A Bittersweet History*. London: Duckworth, 2010.

Abernethy, John. *Surgical Observations on Tumours*. London: Longman, Hurst, Rees,
    Orme, and Brown, 1811.

Adams, Carol J. *The Sexual Politics of Meat (20th Anniversary Edition): A Feminist-
    Vegetarian Critical Theory*. New York: Continuum, 2010.

Affinito, Michele. *La storia della missione esplorativa dell'Unrra in Italia (1944–1945). Con,
    in appendice, il volume di Spurgeon Milton Keeny 'A mission is born. Italy July 1944-May
    1945'*. Naples: Università degli studi Suor Orsola Benincasa, 2012.

Albala, Ken. *Eating Right in the Renaissance*. Berkeley: University of California
    Press, 2002.

Albertoni, Pietro, and Pietro Tullio. *L'alimentation Maidique chez L'individu sain et chez le
    Pellagreux*. Turin: Bona, 1914.

Alexander, Holmes. 'What Is in Some Bread? Congressmen Will Ask', *Los Angeles Times*. 27 November 1949.

Allen, Frederick M. *Studies Concerning Glycosuria and Diabetes*. Cambridge: Harvard University Press, 1913. http://hdl.handle.net/2027/mdp.39015007113452.

Allen, Frederick M. *Total Dietary Regulation in the Treatment of Diabetes*. New York: Rockefeller Institute for Medical Research, 1919.

Alto Commissariato dell'Alimentazione. 'L'approvvigionamento del latte alimentare nelle singole provincie della Repubblica'. *Il Mondo del Latte* IV, no. 6 (1950): 273–80.

Alvarez, P. A., and J. I. Boyce. 'Food Production and Processing Considerations of Allergenic Food Ingredients: A Review'. *Journal of Allergy* (2012). https://www.hindawi.com/journals/ja/2012/746125/

Amministrazione per gli Aiuti Internazionali. *L'attività assistenziale dell'Amministrazione aiuti internazionali nel quadriennio 1945–48. Tavole statistiche estratte dall'Annuario Statistico Italiano 1944–48*. Rome: Istituto Poligrafico dello Stato, 1949.

Amministrazione per le Attività Assistenziali Italiane e Internazionali. *Gli alimenti e il bambino*. Brescia: La Scuola, 1961.

Amministrazione per le Attività Assistenziali Italiane e Internazionali. *Programmi di assistenza alimentare e di educazione alimentare svolti con il contributo degli Stati Uniti e la cooperazione delle Nazioni Unite. Accordi e statistiche*. Rome: Tip. F. Failli, 1961.

Andrews, Geoff. *The Slow Food Story: Politics and Pleasure*. Montreal: McGill-Queen's University Press, 2008.

Angelillo, Bruno. 'Il latte in alcuni suoi aspetti igienico-sanitari'. In *2 Convegno nazionale sul latte nel quadro alimentare dell'Italia. Milano 14 Ottobre 1968*, 41–45. Rome: FIAMCLAF, 1968.

Apple, Rima. *Mothers and Medicine: A Social History of Infant Feeding*. Madison: University of Wisconsin Press, 1987.

Apple, Rima. *Perfect Motherhood: Science and Childrearing in America*. New Brunswick, NJ: Rutgers University Press, 2006.

Apple, Rima. *Vitamania: Vitamins in American Culture*. New Brunswick, NJ: Rutgers University Press, 1996.

Armellini, Guido. *Le immagini del Fascismo nelle arti figurative*. Milan: Fabbri, 1980.

Arnaudi, Carlo. 'Aspetti del problema del latte alimentare'. *Il Latte* XXV, no. 10 (1951): 417–21.

Aronowitz, R. A. *Unnatural History: Breast Cancer and American Society*. Cambridge: Cambridge University Press, 2007.

Aronowitz, Robert A. *Making Sense of Illness: Science, Society, and Disease*. Cambridge: Cambridge University Press, 1998.

Atkins, Peter J. 'Fattening Children or Fattening Farmers? School Milk in Britain, 1921–1941'. *Economic History Review* LVIII, no. 1 (2005): 57–78.

Atkins, Peter J. 'The Milk in Schools Scheme, 1934–45: "Nationalization" and Resistance'. *History of Education* XXXIV, no. 1 (2005): 1–21.

Atlas Powder Company. *Better Farming with Atlas Powder*. Wilmington: Atlas Powder Company, 1919.

Atlas Powder Company. *Food Emulsifiers*. Wilmington: Atlas Power Company, 1948.

Atlas Powder Company Industrial Chemicals Department. *The Nature, Suitability for and Uses in Foods and Pharmaceuticals of Sorbitol and Emulsifiers (Including Those Sold under the Trade Marks Span, Arlacel, Tween and Myrj)*. Wilmington: Atlas Chemical Company, 1949.

Atwater, W. O. *The Chemical Composition of American Food Materials.*
Washington: Government Publishing Office, 1896. http://hdl.handle.net/2027/uva.
x030348906.

Atwater, Wilbur Olin. *Foods: Nutritive Value and Cost.* Washington, DC: US Dept. of
Agriculture, 1894.

Austin, Robert W. 'The Federal Food Legislation of 1938 and the Food Industry'. *Law and
Contemporary Problems* 6 (1939): 129–43.

Aziz, Imran, Federica Branchi and David Sanders. 'The Rise and Fall of Gluten!'.
Proceedings of the Nutrition Society 74 (2015): 221–26.

Babcock, J. W., and W. B. Cutting. *Pellagra.* Washington, DC: Government Printing
Office, 1911.

Babeş, Victor. *Cauzele Cancerului – Tratamentul Pelagrei [The Causes of Cancer – The
Treatment of Pellagra].* Bucharest: Institutul de Arte Grafice Carol Göbl, 1900.

Babeş, Victor. *Cercetări Nouă asupra Pelagrei [New Research on Pellagra].* Bucharest:
Librăria Socec & Comp şi C. Sfetea, 1914.

Bacchetta, Virgilio. *Alimentazione e stato di nutrizione dei bambini italiani dopo la guerra.*
Spoleto: Panetto e Petrelli, 1951.

Baima Bollone, Pier Luigi. *Cesare Lombroso ovvero il principio dell'irresponsabilità.*
Turin: Società Editrice Internazionale, 1992.

Baldwin, Louise G., and Florence Kirlin. 'Consumers Appraise the Food, Drug and
Cosmetic Act'. *Law and Contemporary Problems* 6 (1939): 144–50.

Barbaini, Luca. *Cattolicesimo, modernità, europeismo in Lodovico Montini.* Rome: Edizioni
di storia e letteratura, 2013.

Barkan, Lyse D. 'Industry Invites Regulation: The Passage of the Pure Food and Drug Act
of 1906'. *American Journal of Public Health* 75 (1985): 18–36.

Barnes Johnstone, Emm, and Joanna Baines. *The Changing Faces of Childhood
Cancer: Clinical and Cultural Visions Since 1940.* Basingstoke: Palgrave
Macmillan, 2015.

Barnett, L. Margaret. *British Food Policy during the First World War.* London: Allen and
Unwin, 1985.

Bashford, E. F., 'An Address Entitled Are the Problems of Cancer Insoluble?' *British
Medical Journal* 2 (1905): 1507–11.

Bauman, Zygmunt. *Postmodernity and Its Discontents.* Cambridge: Polity Press, 1997.

Bay, Alexander. *Beriberi in Modern Japan: The Making of a National Disease.* Rochester,
NY: University of Rochester Press, 2012.

Beil, Laura. 'Sweet Confusion: Does High Fructose Corn Syrup Deserve Such a Bad Rap?'.
Science News 183, no. 11 (2013): 22–25.

Belasco, Warren. 'Future Notes: The Meal-in-a-Pill'. *Food and Foodways* 8, no. 4
(2000): 253–71.

Belasco, Warren. *Appetite for Change: How the Counterculture Took on the Food Industry.*
Ithaca, NY: Cornell, [1989] 2007.

Beltrami, Magda, and Mara Guerra. *'Legati mani e piedi con rozze funi'. Le carte
raccontano la pellagra a Ferrara, 1859–1933.* Ferrara: Tresogni, 2015.

Bensaude-Vincent, Bernadette. *L'opinion publique et la science.* Paris: La Découverte, 2013.

Berger (abbé). *L'alimentation populaire en temps de guerre.* Enghien: Office
d'Editions, 1915.

Bernabeu-Mestre, Josep et al. 'La divulgación radiofónica de la alimentación y le higiene
infantil en la España de la Segunda Republica (1933–1935)'. *Salud Colectiva* 7, suppl. 1
(2011): 49–60.

Bernstein, Richard K. *The Diabetes Diet: Dr. Bernstein's Low-Carbohydrate Solution*, 1st edn. New York: Little, Brown, 2005.

Bernton, H. S. 'Food Allergy with Special Reference to Corn and Refined Corn Derivatives'. *Annals of Internal Medicine* 36, no. 1 (1952): 177–85.

Bevilacqua, Piero. 'Società rurale e emigrazione'. In *Storia dell'emigrazione italiana*, edited by P. Bevilacqua, A. De Clementi and E. Franzina, 1: 95–112. Rome: Donzelli, 2001.

Bigelow, George Hoyt, and Herbert Luther Lombard. *Cancer and Other Chronic Diseases in Massachusetts*. Boston, MA: Houghton Mifflin, 1933.

Biltekoff, Charlotte. 'Consumer Response: The Paradoxes of Food and Health'. *Annals of the New York Academy of Sciences* 1190, no. 1 (2010): 174–78.

Biltekoff, Charlotte. *Eating Right in America: The Cultural Politics of Food and Health*. Durham, NC: Duke University Press, 2013.

Bingham, Adrian. 'Reading Newspapers: Cultural Histories of the Popular Press in Modern Britain'. *History Compass* 10, no. 2 (2012): 140–50.

Bisaglia, Andrea. *Sulla pellagra: osservazioni*. Padua: Minerva, 1830.

Bishai, David, and Ritu Nalubola. 'The History of Food Fortification in the United States: Its Relevance for Current Fortification Efforts in Developing Countries'. *Economic Development and Cultural Change* 51, no. 1 (2002): 37–53.

Black, Maggie. *The Children and the Nations: The Story of Unicef*. New York: UNICEF, 1986.

Blair, Kirstie. '"Proved on the Pulses": Heart Disease in Victorian Culture, 1830–1860'. In *Framing and Imagining Disease in Cultural History*, edited by G. S. Rousseau, M. Gill, D. Haycock and M. Herwig, 285–302. New York: Palgrave Macmillian, 2003.

Blanc, Paul. *How Everyday Products Make People Sick: Toxins at Home and in the Workplace*. Berkeley: University of California Press, 2007.

Bliss, Michael. *Discovery of Insulin*, 25th edn. Chicago, IL: University of Chicago Press, [1982] 2013.

Blue, Rupert. 'The Problem of Pellagra in the United States'. *Transactions of the National Association for the Study of Pellagra. Second Triennial Meeting at Columbia, South Carolina, October 3 and 4, 1912*, 1–7. Columbia, SC: R. L. Bryan, 1914.

Bobrow-Strain, Aaron. *White Bread: A Social History of the Store Bought Loaf*. Boston, MA: Beacon Press, 2012.

Bock Berti, Giuseppina. 'Flippo Lussana'. *Dizionario biografico degli italiani* 66 (2006), sub voce. http://www.treccani.it/enciclopedia/filippo-lussana_(Dizionario-Biografico)/.

Bollet, Alfred Jay. 'Politics and Pellagra: The Epidemic of Pellagra in the U.S. in the Early Twentieth Century'. *Yale Journal of Biology and Medicine* 65 (1992): 211–21.

Bonadonna, Telesforo, Dino Desiderio Nai and Filippo Usuelli. 'Problemi del latte e prospettive economiche'. *Il Latte* XXIV, no. 9 (1950): 291–92.

Bonella, Anna Lia. *L'ospedale dei pazzi a Roma dai papi al '900*. Rome: Dedalo, 1994, 2 vols.

Bonfigli, Clodomiro. 'La pellagra nella provincia di Ferrara'. *Bollettino del manicomio provinciale di Ferrara* 10, no. 5 (1878): [no pagination].

Bonfigli, Clodomiro. 'Le questioni sulla pellagra … Appendice alle lettere polemiche'. *Raccoglitore Medico* series 4, 16 (1881): 3–20, 49–68, 81–95, 113–33, 177–88.

Bonfigli, Clodomiro. 'Sulla pellagra: lettere polemiche … al dott. C. Lombroso'. *Raccoglitore Medico* series 4, 11 (1879): 49–67, 105–35, 153–63, 201–23, 241–53, 305–17.

Boswel-Penc, Maia. *Tainted Milk: Breastmilk, Feminisms, and the Politics of Environmental Degradation*. New York: University of New York Press, 2006.

Braghin, Paolo. *Le diseguaglianze sociali. Analisi empirica della situazione di diseguaglianza in Italia*, vol. 1. Milan: Sapere, 1973.

Braithwaite, James. 'Excess of Salt as a Cause of Cancer'. *British Medical Journal* 2 (1902): 1376–77.

Brandt, Allan M., and Paul Rozin (eds). *Health and Morality: Interdisciplinary Perspectives*. New York: Routledge, 1997.

Brante, Thomas, and Aant Elzinga. 'Towards a Theory of Scientific Controversies'. *Social Studies* 2 (1990): 33–46.

Bravetta, Eugenio. *Vitamine e Pellagra*. Udine: Tipografia Domenico del Bianco, 1915.

Broomfield, Andrea. *Food and Cooking in Victorian England: A History*. Westport, CT: Praeger, 2007.

Brumberg, Joan J. *Fasting Girls: The History of Anorexia Nervosa*. New York: Vintage, 2000.

Bryan, Charles. *James Woods Babcock and the Red Plague of Pellagra*. Columbia: University of South Carolina Press, 2014.

Bufton, Mark W., and Virginia Berridge. 'Post-War Nutrition Science and Policy Making in Britain c. 1945–1994: The Case of Diet and Heart Disease'. In *Food, Science, Policy and Regulation in the Twentieth Century*, edited by D. F. Smith and J. Phillips, 207–21. London: Routledge, 2000.

Burg, David F. *Chicago's White City of 1893*. Lexington: University Press of Kentucky, 2015.

Burkitt, Denis. P. *Refined Carbohydrate Foods and Disease*. London: Academic Press, 1975.

Burleigh, Michael. *The Third Reich: A New History*. New York: Hill and Wang, 2000.

Buscemi, Francesco. 'Edible Lies: How Nazi Propaganda Represented Meat to Demonise the Jews'. *Media, War and Conflict* 9, no. 2 (2016): 180–97.

Buscemi, Francesco. 'From Physical Illness to Social Virtue: The Italian Way to Vegetarianism in the Newspaper *La Stampa* from 1867 to the Present'. In *Vegetarians' Dilemma: Rethinking Food Choice Throughout Time*, edited by Adam Shrintzen. Fayetteville: University of Arkansas Press (in press).

Butlin, Henry T. 'Carcinoma Is a Parasitic Disease. Being the Bradshaw Lecture Delivered before the Royal College of Surgeons of England', *British Medical Journal* 2 (1905): 1565–71.

Büttner, J. 'The Origin of Clinical Laboratories'. *European Journal of Clinical Chemistry and Clinical Biochemistry* 30 (1992): 585–93.

Byrn, M. L. *A Treatise on the Adulteration of Food and Drink*. Philadelphia, PA: Lippincott Grambo, 1852.

Bytwerk, Randall. 'The Argument for Genocide in Nazi Propaganda'. *Quarterly Journal of Speech* 91, no. 1 (2005): 37–62.

Bytwerk, Randall. *Julius Streicher: Nazi Editor of the Notorious Anti-Semitic Newspaper Der Stürmer*. Lanham, MD: Cooper Square Press/Rowman & Littlefield, 2001.

Cabanillas, B., and N. Novak. 'Effects of Daily Food Processing on Allergenicity'. *Critical Reviews in Food Science and Nutrition* 11 (2017): 1–12.

Caffaratto, Tirsi Mario. 'Lo stato della cultura e della pratica medica in Piemonte nell'ultimo periodo dell'Ottocento'. In *La scienza accademica nell'Italia post-unitaria: discipline scientifiche e ricerca universitaria*, edited by V. Ancarani, 217–55. Milan: Franco Angeli, 1989.

Callon, Michel. 'Some Elements of a Sociology of Translation: Domestication of Scallops and the Fishermen of St. Brieuc Bay'. In *The Sociological Review Monograph 32: Power Action and Belief: A New Sociology of Knowledge*, edited by John Law, 196–223. London: Routledge, 1986.

Calvi, Anna Maria. *L'alimentazione nelle collettività infantili*. Rome: F. Failli, 1966.

Calvo, Luz, and Catriona Rueda Esquibel. *Decolonize Your Diet: Plant-Based Mexican-American Recipes for Health and Healing*. Vancouver, BC: Arsenal Pulp Press, 2015.

Camurri, Vincenzo. 'L'etiologia della pellagra nel giudizio dei medici condotti in Italia'. In *Atti del quinto congresso pellagrologico italiano*, edited by G. B. Cantarutti, 220–35. Udine: Tosolini, 1912.

Cantor, David, Christian Bonah and Matthias Dörries (eds). *Meat, Medicine and Human Health in the Twentieth Century*. London: Pickering and Chatto, 2010.

Cantor, David. 'Confused Messages: Meat, Civilization and Cancer Education in the Early Twentieth Century'. In *Meat, Medicine and Human Health in the Twentieth Century*, edited by D. Cantor, C. Bonah and M. Dorries, 111–26. London: Pickering and Chatto, 2010.

Cao-Pinna, Maria. 'Le classi povere'. In *Atti della Commissione parlamentare di inchiesta sulla miseria in Italia e sui mezzi per combatterla*, edited by Camera dei Deputati, vol. 2, *Indagini tecniche. Condizioni di vita delle classi misere*, 9–111. Milan: Unione tipografica, 1953.

Cao-Pinna, Maria. 'Qualche linea di informazione sull'Accordo e di raffronto con l'Accordo Unrra'. *Assistenza d'Oggi* VI, no. 5/6 (1955): 8–19.

Capatti, Alberto. *Vegetit: le avanguardie vegetariane in Italia*. Lucca: Cinquesensi, 2016.

Carey, John. *The Intellectuals and the Masses: Pride and Prejudice among the Literary Intelligentsia, 1880–1939*. London: Faber, 1992.

Carson, R. *Silent Spring*. New York: Houghton Mifflin, 1962.

Carter, K. Codell. 'The Germ Theory, Beriberi, and the Deficiency Theory of Disease'. *Medical History* 21 (1977): 119–36.

Caso, E. K. 'Calculation of Diabetic Diets'. *Journal of the American Dietetic Association* 26 (1950): 575–83.

Cassa per Opere Straordinarie di Pubblico Interesse nell'Italia Meridionale. *Strutture e mercati dell'agricoltura meridionale*, vol. 3, edited by Carlo Aiello, *Latte e derivati. Caratteri, prospettive e fabbisogni della produzione lattiero-casearia*. Rome: Cassa per il Mezzogiorno, 1960.

Charles, Dan. 'Americans Don't Trust Scientists' Take On Food Issues', NPR, 2 December 2016. http://www.npr.org/sections/thesalt/2016/12/02/504034298/americans-dont-trust-scientists-take-on-food-politicians-even-less (accessed 1 September 2017).

Chesterton, G. K. *Irish Impressions*. London: Collins, 1919.

Christopher, Thomas W. 'Significant Comments'. *Food, Drug, Cosmetic Law Journal* 9, no. 6 (1954): 365–68.

Ciampani, Andrea. 'La costituzione dell'AAI: relazioni internazionali, ricostruzione sociale e attività assistenziali'. In *L'Amministrazione per gli Aiuti Internazionali. La ricostruzione dell'Italia tra dinamiche internazionali e attività assistenziali*, edited by Andrea Ciampani, 105–53. Milan: Franco Angeli, 2002.

Cigliana, Giorgio. 'Lodovico Montini e gli aiuti internazionali'. *Studium* 86, no. 3 (1990): 357–69.

Clarke, T. W. 'The Relation of Allergy to Character Problems in Children'. *Annals of Allergy* 8 (1950): 21–38.

Clayton, Paul, and Judith Rowbotham. 'An Unsuitable and Degraded Diet?'. *Journal of the Royal Society of Medicine* part 1, 101, no. 6 (2008): 282–89; part 2, 101, no. 7 (2008): 350–57; and part 3, 101, no. 9 (2008): 454–62.

Clementi, Antonino. *Osservazioni sugli effetti delle alimentazioni esclusive maidica e orizanica, con Speciale riguardo al problema delle vitamin*. Siena: C. Nava, 1916.

Code of Federal Regulations. Title 21. 1938–1970.

Codell Carter, K. 'Ignaz Semmelweis, Carl Mayrhofer, and the Rise of Germ Theory'. *Medical History* 29 (1985): 33–53.

Codell Carter, K. *The Rise of Causal Concepts of Disease: Case Histories.* Aldershot: Ashgate, 2003.

Cohen, Lizabeth. *A Consumer Republic: The Politics of Mass Consumption in Postwar America.* New York: Vintage, 2003

Colombelli, Carla. 'Il cibo dell'infanzia'. In *Storia d'Italia, Annali 13, L'alimentazione*, edited by A. Capatti, A. De Bernardi and A. Varni, 585–643. Turin: Einaudi, 1998.

Combs, Gerald F., Jr. *The Vitamins: Fundamental Aspects in Nutrition and Health*, 3rd edn. Amsterdam: Elsevier, 2008.

Comisso, Giovanni. *Il porto dell'amore.* Treviso: Stamperia di Antonio Vianello, 1924.

Comisso, Giovanni. *Le mie stagioni.* Treviso: Edizioni di Treviso, 1951.

Comitato Italiano Unicef (ed.). *Fondo delle nazioni unite per l'infanzia (Unicef).* Padua: Cedam, 1957.

Cone, Richard A., and Emily Martin. 'Corporeal Flows: The Immune System, Global Economies of Food, and Implications for Health'. *Ecologist* 27 (1997): 107–11.

Conford, Philip. *The Origins of the Organic Movement.* Edinburgh: Floris, 2001.

Consolato, Sandro. 'Gicomo Boni: l'archeologo vate della Terza Roma'. In *Esoterismo e Fascismo*, edited by Gianfranco De Turris, 183–96. Rome: Edizioni Mediterranee.

Coselschi, Eugenio. *La marcia di Ronchi.* Florence: Vallecchi, 1929.

Crabb, Mary Katherine. 'An Epidemic of Pride: Pellagra and the Culture of the American South'. *Anthropologica* 34 (1992): 89–103.

Cramarossa, Saladino. 'Criteri informatori della legislazione sanitaria nei paesi a più alto consumo di latte'. In *Il latte alimento per tutti nel pensiero di fisiologi, igienisti e clinici italiani*, edited by Istituto Nazionale della Nutrizione del Consiglio Nazionale delle Ricerche and Amministrazione per le Attività Assistenziali Italiane e Internazionali, 71–81. Rome: AAI, 1957.

Crofford, O. B., S. Genuth and L. Baker. 'Diabetes Control and Complications Trial (DCCT): Results of Feasibility Study'. *Diabetes Care* 10, no. 1 (1987): 1–19.

Crosby, Alfred W. *The Columbian Exchange: Biological and Cultural Consequences of 1492.* Westport, CT: Praeger, [1973] 2003.

Cullather, Nick. 'The Foreign Policy of the Calorie'. *American Historical Review* 112, no. 2 (2007): 337–64.

Curtis, L. P. *Apes and Angels: The Irishman in Victorian Caricature.* Washington, DC: Smithsonian, 1971.

Cwiertka, Katarzyna. 'Propagation of Nutritional Knowledge in Poland, 1863–1939'. In *Order and Disorder: The Health Implications of Eating and Drinking in 19th and 20th Centuries*, edited by Alexander Fenton, 96–111. East Linton: Tuckwell Press, 2000.

D'Annunzio, Gabriele. 'O Italia o morte'. *Comando di Fiume d'Italia - Bollettino Ufficiale*, 12 September 1919, year 1, n. 1.

Daston, Lorraine. 'Science Studies and the History of Science'. *Critical Inquiry* 35 (2009): 798–813.

Dawber, Thomas R. *The Framingham Heart Study.* Cambridge, MA: Harvard University Press, 1980.

Dawber, Thomas R., and William B. Kannel. 'The Framingham Study: An Epidemiological Approach to Coronary Heart Disease'. *Circulation* 34, no. 4 (1966): 553–55.

Dawber, Thomas R. et al. 'Dietary Assessment in the Epidemiologic Study of Coronary Heart Disease: The Framingham Study'. *American Journal of Clinical Nutrition* 11, no. 3 (1962): 226–34.

Dawber, Thomas R., Felix E. Moore and George V. Mann. 'Coronary Heart Disease in the Framingham Study'. *American Journal of Public Health* 47, no. 4 (1957): 4–24.

De Bernardi, Alberto. 'Pellagra, Stato e scienza medica: la curabilità impossibile'. In *Storia d'Italia. Annali 7. Malattia e medicina*, edited by Franco Della Peruta, 681–704. Turin: Einaudi, 1984.

De Bernardi, Alberto. *Il mal della rosa. Denutrizione e pellagra nelle campagne italiane fra '800 e '900*. Milan: Franco Angeli, 1984.

De Bont, Raf. '"Writing in Letters of Blood": Manners in Scientific Dispute in Nineteenth-Century Britain and the German Lands'. *History of Science* 51 (2013): 309–35.

De Felice, Renzo. *La carta del Carnaro nei testi di Alceste de Ambris e Gabriele D'Annunzio*. Bologna: il Mulino, 1973.

De Grazia, Victoria. *How Fascism Ruled Women*. Berkeley: University of California Press, 1992.

de Haan, Ido. 'Vigorous, Pure and Vulnerable: Child Health and Citizenship in the Netherlands Since the End of the Nineteenth Century'. In *Cultures of Child Health in Britain and the Netherlands in the Twentieth Century*, edited by M. Gijswijt-Hofstra and H. Marland, 31–60. Amsterdam; New York: Rodopi, 2003.

De la Pena, Carolyn. *Empty Pleasures: The Story of Artificial Sweeteners from Saccharin to Splenda*. Chapel Hill: University of North Carolina Press, 2010.

De Marzi, Guido. 'Istituito un Comitato di studio per i problemi della nutrizione'. *Assistenza d'Oggi* VI, no. 3 (1955): 60–63.

De Schaepdrijver, Sophie. 'A Civilian War Effort: The *Comité National de Secours et d'Alimentation* in Occupied Belgium, 1914–1918'. In *Remembering Herbert Hoover and the Commission for Relief in Belgium*, 24–39. Brussels: Fondation Universitaire, 2007.

Della Torre, Giovanni. *Il latte alimentare e le sue proprietà*. Milan: Hoepli, 1956.

den Hartog, Adel. 'The Role of Nutrition in Food Advertisements: The Case of the Netherlands'. In *Food Technology, Science and Marketing*, edited by Adel den Hartog, 268–80. East Linton: Tuckwell Press, 1995.

Denman, Thomas, *Observations on the Cure of Cancer, with Some Remarks upon Mr. Young's Treatment of that Disease*. London: E. Cox, 1816.

Desrosières, Alain. *The Politics of Large Numbers: A History of Statistical Reasoning*. Cambridge, MA: Harvard University Press, 1998.

Deutsch, Tracey. *Building a Housewife's Paradise: Gender, Politics and American Grocery Stores in the Twentieth Century*. Chapel Hill: University of North Carolina Press, 2010.

Dietetic and Hygienic Gazette. Gazette Publishing Company, 1896.

Diner, Hasia R. *Hungering for America: Italian, Irish and Jewish Foodways in the Age of Migration*. Cambridge, MA: Harvard University Press, 2001.

Donkin, Arthur Scott. *On the Relation between Diabetes and Food and Its Application to the Treatment of the Disease*. New York: G. P. Putnam's Sons, 1875.

'Donne, birra ed autografi'. *La Stampa*, 26 June 1931, 6.

Downham, A., and P. Collins. 'Colouring Our Foods in the Last and Next Millennium'. *International Journal of Food Science and Technology* 35, no. 1 (2000): 5–22.

Draper, H. H. 'Human Nutritional Adaptation: Biological and Cultural Aspects'. In *The Cambridge World History of Food*, edited by Kenneth F. Kiple and Kriemhild Conee Ornelas, 1466–75. Cambridge: Cambridge University Press, 2000.

Dubos, R. 'Medical Utopias'. *Daedalus* 88 (1959): 410–24.

Duden, Barbara. *The Woman beneath the Skin: A Doctor's Patients in Eighteenth-Century Germany*, trans. Thomas Dunlap. Cambridge, MA: Harvard University Press, 1991.

Dufty, William. *Sugar Blues*. New York: Warner Books, 1976.

Dunham, Will. 'Study Links Common Food Additives to Crohn's Disease'. *Reuters*, 25 February 2015. http://www.reuters.com/article/us-science-emulsifiers/study-links-common-food-additives-to-crohns-disease-colitis-idUSKBN0LT26S20150225 (accessed 2 September 2017).

Dunn, Hugh P. 'The Increase of Cancer'. *Pall Mall Gazette*, 12 May 1884.

Dupuis, Erna Melanie. *Nature's Perfect Food: How Milk Became America's Drink*. New York; London: New York University Press, 2002.

Eaton, S. Boyd, and Melvin Konner. 'Paleolithic Nutrition. A Consideration of Its Nature and Current Implications'. *New England Journal of Medicine* 312, no. 5 (1985): 283–89.

Elvehjem, Conrad A. 'Pellagra: A Deficiency Disease'. *Proceedings of the American Philosophical Society* 93 (1949): 335–39.

Emerson, Haven, and Louise D. Larimore. 'Diabetes Mellitus: A Contribution to Its Epidemiology Based Chiefly on Mortality Statistics'. *Archives of Internal Medicine* 35, no. 5 (1924): 585–630.

Engelhardt, Tristam, and Arthur Caplan (eds). *Scientific Controversies: Case Studies in the Resolution and Closure of Disputes in Science and Technology*, editors' introduction, 1–13. Cambridge: Cambridge University Press, 1987.

Epstein, J. E. 'Writing the Unspeakable: Fanny Burney's Mastectomy and the Fictive Body'. *Representations* 16, no. 1 (1986): 131–66.

Eschliman, Dwight, and Steve Ettlinger. *Ingredients: A Visual Exploration of 75 Additives & 25 Food Products*. New York: Reagan Arts, 2015.

Etheridge, Elizabeth. *The Butterfly Caste: A Social History of Pellagra in the South*. Westport, CT: Greenwood, 1972.

Eyler, John M. 'The Conceptual Origins of William Farr's Epidemiology: Numerical Methods and Social Thought in the 1830s', in *Times, Places, and Persons: Aspects of the History of Epidemiology*, ed. Abraham M. Lilienfeld (Baltimore, MD: Henry E. Sigerist Supplements to the Bulletin of the History of Medicine 4, 1980), 1–27.

Feingold, B. F. *Why Your Child Is Hyperactive*. New York: Random House, 1974.

Felice, Emanuele. 'Il settore lattiero-caseario in Italia dal dopoguerra al Duemila'. In *Una storia di qualità: Il Gruppo Granarolo fra valori etici e logiche di mercato*, edited by Giuliana Bertagnoni, 35–91. Bologna: il Mulino, 2004.

Felker, P. H. *The Grocer's Manual*. Claremont, CA: Claremont Manufacturing Company, 1878.

Fenili, Cesare. 'Filippo Lussana e la lotta alla pellagra'. In *Filippo Lussana (1820–1897): da Cenate alle neuroscienze*, edited by G. Berbenin and L. Lorusso, 97–127. Bergamo: Fondazione per la storia economica e sociale di Bergamo, 2008.

Ferrari, Massimo. 'Pellagra e pazzia nelle campagne reggiane'. *Sanità, scienza e storia* 1, no. 1 (1985): 169–212.

Ferrari, Piergiacomo. *L'industria del latte in Italia*. Piacenza: Camera di commercio, industria artigianato e agricoltura di Piacenza, after 1970.

Feudtner, Chris. 'The Want of Control: Ideas, Innovations, and Ideals in the Modern Management of Diabetes Mellitus'. *Bulletin of the History of Medicine* 69, no. 1 (1995): 66–90.

Feudtner, John Christopher. *Bittersweet: Diabetes, Insulin, and the Transformation of Illness*. Chapel Hill: University of North Carolina Press, 2013.

Fiddes, Nick. *Meat: A Natural Symbol*. London: Routledge, 1991.

Finaldi, Giuseppe. *Mussolini and Italian Fascism*. London: Routledge, 2013.

Finzi, Roberto. 'La psicosi pellagrosa in Italia fra la fine dell'800 e gli inizi del '900'. In *Follia, psichiatria e società. Istituzioni manicomiali, scienza psichiatrica e classi sociali nell'Italia moderna e contemporanea*, edited by A. De Bernardi, 284–97. Milan: Franco Angeli, 1982.

Finzi, Roberto. 'Quando e perché fu sconfitta la pellagra in Italia'. In *Salute e classi lavoratrici in Italia dall'Unità al fascismo*, edited by M. L. Betri and A. Gigli Marchetti, 391–430. Milan: Franco Angeli, 1982.

First Presbyterian Church. *The Texas Cook Book: A Thorough Treatise on the Art of Cookery*. St. Louis, MO: The Association, R. P. Studley, 1883.

Food and Drug Administration. 'Read the Label on Foods, Drugs, Devices, Cosmetics and Household Chemicals'. *US Department of Health, Education and Welfare*, FDA Publication 3 (1965): 9–13.

Forchtner, Bernhard, and Tominc, Ana. 'Kalashnikov and Cooking-Spoon: Neo-Nazism, Veganism and a Lifestyle Cooking Show on YouTube'. *Food, Culture and Society* 20, no. 3 (2017): 415–41.

Forno, Mauro. 'Scienziati e mass media: Lombroso e gli studiosi positivisti nella stampa tra Otto e Novecento'. In *Cesare Lombroso. Gli scienziati e la nuova Italia*, edited by S. Montaldo, 207–32. Bologna: il Mulino, 2010.

Foucault, Michel. 'Technologies of the self'. In *Technologies of the Self: A Seminar with Michel Foucault*, edited by Luther H. Martin, Huck Gutman and Patrick H. Hutton, 16–49. Amherst: University of Massachussets Press, 1988.

Fox, Daniel M. *Power and Illness: The Failure and Future of American Health Policy*. Berkeley: University of California Press, 1993.

Frankenfield, David. 'On Heat, Respiration, and Calorimetry'. *Nutrition* 26 (2010): 939–50.

Fraser, Henry, and A. T. Stanton. 'An Inquiry Concerning the Etiology of Beriberi'. *Lancet* 173 (1909): 451–55.

Fraser, Henry, and A. T. Stanton. 'The Etiology of Beri-beri'. *Transactions of The Royal Society of Tropical Medicine and Hygiene* 5 (1910): 257–67.

Friedman, Jeffrey M. 'A Tale of Two Hormones'. *Nature Medicine* 16, no. 10 (2010): 1100–6. https://doi.org/10.1038/nm1010-1100.

Friel, Sharon, et al., 'Shaping the Discourse: What Has the Food Industry Been Lobbying for in the Trans Pacific Partnership Trade Agreement and What Are the Implications for Dietary Health?'. *Critical Public Health* 26, no. 5 (2016): 518–29.

Frigessi, Delia. 'Cesare Lombroso tra medicina e società'. In *Cesare Lombroso cento anni dopo*, edited by S. Montalto and P. Tappero, 5–16. Turin: UTET, 2009.

Frigessi, Delia. *Cesare Lombroso*. Turin: Giulio Einaudi, 2003.

Funk, Casimir. 'On the Chemical Nature of the Substance Which Cures Polyneuritis in Birds Induced by a Diet of Polished Rice'. *Journal of Physiology* 43 (1911): 395–400.

Funk, Casimir. 'Studies on Pellagra. I. The Influence of the Milling of Maize on the Chemical Composition and the Nutritive Value of Maize-Meal'. *Journal of Physiology* 47 (1913): 389–92.

Funk, Casimir. 'The Etiology of the Deficiency Diseases. Beri-Beri, Polyneuritis in Birds, Epidemic Dropsy, Scurvy, Experimental Scurvy in Animals, Infantile Scurvy, Ship Beri-Beri, Pellagra'. *Journal of State Medicine* 20 (1912): 341–68.

Funk, Casimir. *Die Vitamine: Ihre Bedeutung für die Physiologie und Pathologie mit Besonderer Berücksichtigung der Avitaminosen: Beriberi, Skorbut, Pellagra, Rachitis*. Wiesbaden: J. F. Bergmann, 1914.

Funk, Casimir. *The Vitamines*. Baltimore, MD: Williams & Wilkins, 1922.

Galizzi, Giovanni, and Giorgio Cingolani. 'Lineamenti della produzione e del consumo di latte in Italia'. *Annali della Facoltà di Agraria* LXXVIII, no. 2 (1960): 126–59.

Garrety, Karin. 'Social Worlds, Actor-Networks and Controversy: The Case of Cholesterol, Dietary Fat and Heart Disease'. *Social Studies of Science*, 27, no. 5 (1997): 727–73.

Gatchell, Charles. '*Doctor, What Shall I Eat?*': *A Handbook of Diet in Disease, for the Profession and the People*. Milwaukee: Cramer, Aikens & Cramer, 1880. http://archive.org/details/63831160R.nlm.nih.gov.

Gazeley, Ian, and Andrew Newell. 'The First World War and Working-Class Food Consumption in Britain'. *European Review of Economic History* 17, no. 1 (2013): 72.

Gentilcore, David, and Egidio Priani. '"San Servolo Lunatic!": Segregation and Integration in the Life Cycle of Pellagra Patients at Venice's Provincial Asylums (1842–1912)'. In *Segregation and Integration in the History of the Hospital*, edited by K. Stevens Crawshaw and K. Vongsathorn. Rotterdam: Clio Medica, forthcoming.

Gentilcore, David, and Egidio Priani. *Venetian Mental Asylums Database (VMAD), 1842–1912*. UK Data Service, 2016. SN: 8058, http://doi.org/10.5255/UKDA-SN-8058-1.

Gentilcore, David. '"Italic Scurvy", "Pellarina", "Pellagra": Medical Reactions to a New Disease in Italy, 1770–1830'. In *A Medical History of Skin: Scratching the Surface*, edited by J. Reinarz and K. Siena, 57–69. London: Pickering and Chatto, 2013.

Gentilcore, David. 'Louis Sambon and the Clash of Pellagra Etiologies in Italy and the United States, 1904–15'. *Journal of the History of Medicine and Allied Sciences* 71, no. 1 (2015): 19–42.

Gentilcore, David. 'The Impact of New World Plants, 1500–1800: The Americans in Italy'. In *The New World in Early Modern Italy, 1492–1750*, edited by E. Horodowich and L. Markey, 190–205. Cambridge: Cambridge University Press, 2017.

Gentilcore, David. *Food and Health in Early Modern Europe: Diet, Medicine and Society, 1450–1800*. London: Bloomsbury, 2016.

Gentilcore, David. *Italy and the Potato: A History*. London: Continuum, 2012.

Gentilcore, David. *Pomodoro! A History of the Tomato in Italy*. New York: Columbia University Press, 2010.

Gentile, Emilio. *Le religioni della politica: tra democrazie e totalitarismi*. Bari: Laterza, 2014.

Gerra, Ferdinando. *L'impresa di Fiume*, vol. 2. Milan: Longanesi, 1974.

Giesen, Rolf. *Nazi Propaganda Films: A History and Filmography*. Jefferson, NC: McFarland, 2003.

Gifford, Kilvert. D. 'Dietary Fats, Eating Guides and Public Policy: History, Critique, and Recommendations'. *American Journal of Medicine* 113, no. 9 (2002): 80–106.

Gillespie, James A. 'International Organizations and the Problem of Child Health 1945–1960'. *Dynamis* 23 (2003): 115–42.

Gillette, Aaron. *Racial Theories in Fascist Italy*. London: Routledge, 2002.

Ginnaio, Monica. *L'impact démographique des crises sanitaires et nutritionelles des societés anciennes: le cas de la pellagre en Italie*. Villeneuve d'Ascq: Atelier national de reproduction des thèses, 2010.

Giroux, Élodie. 'The Framingham Study and the Constitution of a Restrictive Concept of Risk Factor'. *Social History of Medicine* 26, no. 1 (2013): 94–113.

Gluten-Free Products Market Size and Share, Industry Report, 2014–2025, Grandview Research, May 2017, https://www.grandviewresearch.com/industry-analysis/gluten-free-products-market.

Goldberger, Joseph, and G. A. Wheeler. 'Experimental Pellagra in the Human Subject Brought about by a Restricted Diet'. *Public Health Reports* 30 (1915): 3336–39.

Goldberger, Joseph, C. H. Waring and David G. Willets. 'The Prevention of Pellagra: A Test Diet among Institutional Inmates'. *Public Health Reports* 30 (1915): 3117–31.

Goldberger, Joseph, G. A. Wheeler and Edgar Sydenstricker. 'A Study of the Relation of Diet to Pellagra Incidence in Seven Textile-Mill Communities of South Carolina in 1916'. *Public Health Reports* 35 (1920): 648–713.

Goldberger, Joseph. 'The Treatment and Prevention of Pellagra'. *Public Health Reports* 29 (1914): 2821–25.

Goldman, David. 'Kraft Changed Its Mac & Cheese Recipe and Nobody Noticed'. *CNN*, 8 March 2016. http://money.cnn.com/2016/03/08/news/companies/kraft-mac-and-cheese-recipe/index.Html (accessed 2 September 2017).

Goodwin, Lorraine Swainston. *The Pure Food, Drink, and Drug Crusaders, 1879–1914*. Jefferson: McFarland, 1999.

Gray, Richard. *About Face: German Physiognomic Thought from Lavater to Auschwitz*. Detroit, MI: Wayne State University Press, 2004.

Gray, H., and Jean M. Stewart. 'Quantitative Diets versus Guesswork in the Treatment of Obesity and Diabetes'. *Scientific Monthly* 32, no. 1 (1931): 46–53.

Greene, Jeremy A. *Prescribing by Numbers: Drugs and the Definition of Disease*, 1st edn. Baltimore, MD: Johns Hopkins University Press, 2008.

Gregory, Adrian. *The Last Great War: British Society and the First World War*. Cambridge: Cambridge University Press, 2008.

Griffin, Roger. 'Religious Politics: A Concept Comes of Age'. *Leidschrift Historisch Tijdschrift* 26, no. 2 (2011): 7–18.

Griggs, Barbara. *The Food Factor in Disease: Why We Are What We Eat*. Harmondsworth: Penguin, 1986.

Grossman, Lev. 'Persons of the Year 2002 – TIME'. *Time*, 2002. http://content.time.com/time/specials/packages/article/0,28804,2022164_2021937_2021901,00.html (accessed 5 March 2018).

Grubisich, Thomas. 'Hyperactive Diet: A Doctor's Checklist'. *Washington Post*, 17 January 1974.

Grunert, Klaus. 'European Consumers' Acceptance of Functional Foods'. *Annals of the New York Academy of Sciences* no. 1190 (2010): 166–73.

Gunderson, Frank L., Helen W. Gunderson and Egbert R. Ferguson. *Food Standards and Definitions in the United States: A Guidebook*. New York: Academic Press, 1963.

Gwirtz, J. A., and M. N. Garcia-Casal. 'Processing Maize Flour and Corn Meal Food Products'. *Annals of the New York Academy of Sciences* 1312, no. 1 (2014): 66–75.

Hacking, Ian. *The Emergence of Probability: A Philosophical Study of the Early Ideas about Probability*. New York: Cambridge University Press, 1975.

Hacking, Ian. *The Taming of Chance*. Cambridge: Cambridge University Press, 1990.

Hardy, Anne. 'Beri-Beri, Vitamin B1 and World Food Policy, 1925–1970'. *Medical History* 39 (1995): 61–77.

Hare, F. *The Food Factor in Disease*, 2 vols. London: Longmans, Green, 1905.

Hargrove, James. 'History of the Calorie in Nutrition'. *Journal of Nutrition* 136 (2006): 2957–61.

Harris, Alexandra. *Romantic Moderns: English Writers, Artists and the Imagination from Virginia Woolf to John Piper*. London: Thames and Hudson, 2015.

Hawana, Joanne S. 'Food Identity Disputes Continue to Impose High-Profile Pressure on FDA'. *National Law Review*, 21 August 2017. https://www.natlawreview.com/article/food-identity-disputes-continue-to-impose-high-profile-pressure-fda (accessed 1 September 2017).

Haydu, Jeffrey. 'Frame Brokerage in the Pure Food Movement, 1879–1906'. *Social Movement Studies* 11 (2012): 97–112.

Helstosky, Carol. *Garlic and Oil: Politics and Food in Italy*. Oxford, NY: Berg, 2004.

Henniker, Brydges P. 'Deaths from Several Zymotic and Other Causes, and Inquest Cases, in the Divisions, Counties, and Districts of England', *Forty-Second Annual Report of the Registrar-General* (1879): 186–97.

Herasey, H. 'The Rarity of Cancer among the Aborigines of British Central Africa. Squamous Carcinoma: Acinous Carcinoma: Physiological Reasons for Immunity from Cancer of the Breast: Columnar Carcinoma'. *British Medical Journal* 2, no. 2396 (1906): 1562–63.

Herf, Jeffrey. *The Jewish Enemy: Nazi Propaganda during World War II and the Holocaust*. Harvard, MA: Harvard University Press, 2006.

Higgs, Edward. 'Registrar General's Reports for England and Wales, 1838–1858', *Online Historical Population Reports*. http://histpop.org/ (accessed 13 October 2016).

Higgs, Edward. 'The Annual Report of the Registrar-General, 1839–1920: A Textual History'. In *The Road to Medical Statistics*, edited by Eileen Magnello and Anne Hardy. Amesterdam: Brill, 2002.

Higman, Barry. W. 'The Sugar Revolution'. *Economic History Review* 3, no. 2 (2000): 213–36.

Hill-Climo, William, 'Cancer in Ireland: An Economic Question'. *The Empire Review* VI (1903): 912–34.

Hislop, P. W., and P. Clennell Fenwick. 'Cancer in New Zealand'. *British Medical Journal* 2 (1909): 1222–5.

Hoganson, Kristin L. *Consumers' Imperium: The Global Production of American Domesticity, 1865–1920*. Chapel Hill: University of North Carolina Press, 2007.

Hoobler, W. R. 'Some Early Symptoms Suggesting Protein Sensitization in Infancy'. *American Journal of Diseases of Children* 12 (1916): 129–35.

Hopkins, F. Gowland. 'Feeding Experiments Illustrating the Importance of Accessory Factors in Normal Dietaries'. *Journal of Physiology* 44 (1912): 425–60.

Hopkins, F. Gowland. *Newer Aspects of the Problem of Nutrition*. New York: Columbia University Press, 1922.

Hovey, Helen Stone, and Kay Reynolds. *The Practical Book of Food Shopping*. Philadelphia, PA: J.B. Lippincott, 1950.

Howard, John, *The Plan Adopted by the Governors of the Middlesex-Hospital for the Relief of Persons Afflicted with Cancer: With Notes and Observations*. London: H. L. Galabin, 1792.

https://www.fda.gov/Food/GuidanceRegulation/GuidanceDocumentsRegulatoryInformat ion/Allergens/ucm106187.htm (accessed 9 October 2017).

Hugo, Victor. *The Memoirs of Victor Hugo*. Project Gutenberg E-Book. http://www. gutenberg.org/files/2523/2523-h/2523-h.htm (accessed 30 September 2017).

Hunt, Karen. 'The Politics of Food and Women's Neighborhood Activism in First World War Britain'. *International Labor and Working-Class History* 77, no. 1 (2010): 8–26.

Hunter, B. T. *The Sugar Trap and How to Avoid It*. Boston, MA: Houghton Mifflin, 1982.

Hutchinson, Woods. 'The Cancer Problem: Or, Treason in the Republic of the Body'. *Contemporary Review*, July 1899.

Impiglia, Marco. 'Mussolini sportivo'. In *Sport e Fascismo*, edited by Maria Canella and Sergio Giuntini, 19–46. Milan: Franco Angeli, 2009.

Inaudi, Silvia. 'Assistenza ed educazione alimentare: l'Amministrazione per gli aiuti internazionali, 1947–1965'. *Contemporanea* XVIII, no. 3 (2015): 373–400.

Interview with Giordano Bruno Guerri. *Linea Verde*, 3 May 2015, *Rai 1* (Italian TV programme).

Jackson, M. ' "Allergy con Amore": Psychosomatic Medicine and the "Asthmogenic Home" in in the Mid-Twentieth Century'. In *Health and the Modern Home*, edited by M. Jackson, 153–74. London: Routledge, 2007.

Jackson, M. *Allergy: The History of a Modern Malady*. London: Reaktion, 2006.

Jargon, Julie. 'McDonald's to Remove High-Fructose Corn Syrup from Sandwich Buns'. *Wall Street Journal*, 2 August 2016.

John, Henry Jerry. *Diabetic Manual for Patients*. St. Louis, MO: C.V. Mosby, 1928.

Johnson, P. B. *Land Fit for Heroes: The Planning of British Reconstruction, 1916–1919*. Chicago, IL: Chicago University Press, 1968.

Johnson, R. J., L. G. Sánchez-Lozada, P. Andrews and M. A. Lanaspa . 'Perspective: A Historical and Scientific Perspective of Sugar and Its Relation with Obesity and Diabetes'. *Advances in Nutrition* 8, no. 3 (2017): 412–22.

Jones, Ashby. ' "Corn Sugar" Goes on Trial as Suit Debates High-Fructose Corn Syrup'. *Wall Street Journal*, 20 September 2011.

Jones, David S., Scott H. Podolsky and Jeremy A. Greene. 'The Burden of Disease and the Changing Task of Medicine'. *New England Journal of Medicine* 366, no. 25 (2012): 2333–38.

Jones, Thomas. *The Unbroken Front, Ministry of Food 1916–1944*. London: Everybody's Books, 1944.

Jooste, Martha E., and Andrea Overman Mackey. 'Cake Structure and Palatability as Affected by Emulsifying Agents and Temperatures'. *Journal of Food Science* 17 (1952): 185–96.

Joslin, Elliott P. 'The Treatment of Diabetes Mellitus'. *Canadian Medical Association Journal* 6, no. 8 (1916): 673–84.

Joslin, Elliott P. *A Diabetic Manual for the Mutual Use of Doctor and Patient*. Philadelphia, PA: Lea & Febiger, 1929. https://catalog.hathitrust.org/Record/001565827.

Joslin, Elliott P. *A Diabetic Manual for the Mutual Use of Doctor and Patient*. Philadelphia, PA: Lea & Febiger, 1941. https://catalog.hathitrust.org/Record/001578358.

Joslin, Elliott P. *A Diabetic Manual for the Mutual Use of Doctor and Patient*. Philadelphia, PA and New York: Lea & Febiger, 1919. https://archive.org/details/adiabeticmanual00unkngoog.

Joslin, Elliott P. *The Treatment of Diabetes Mellitus*. Philadelphia, PA: Lea & Febiger, 1946.

Junod, S. W. 'The Rise and Fall of Federal Food Standards in the United States: The Case of the Peanut and Butter Sandwich'. In *The Food and Drug Administration*, edited by M. A. Hickman, 35–48. New York: Nova, 2003.

Junod, Suzanne. 'Food Standards in the United States: The Case of the Peanut Butter and Jelly Sandwich'. In *Food, Science, Policy and Regulation in the Twentieth Century: International and Comparative Perspectives*, edited by David F. Smith and Jim Phillips. London: Routledge, 2000.

Kamminga, Harmke. ' "Axes to Grind": Popularising the Science of Vitamins, 1920s and 1930s'. In *Food, Science, Policy and Regulation in the Twentieth Century*, edited by D. F. Smith and J. Phillips, 83–100. London: Routledge, 2000.

Kamminga, Harmke. 'Nutrition for the People, or the Fate of Jacob Moleschott's Context for a Humanist Science'. In *The Science and Culture of Nutrition, 1840–1940*, edited by H. Kamminga and A. Cunningham, 15–47. Amsterdam: Rodopi, 1995.

Kannel, William B., Thomas R. Dawber, Abraham Kagan, Nicholas Revotskie and Joseph Stokes. 'Factors of Risk in the Development of Coronary Heart Disease – Six Year

Follow-Up Experience. The Framingham Study'. *Annals of Internal Medicine* 55, no. 1 (1961): 33–48.

Kaur, Navdeep, and Devinder Pal Singh. 'Deciphering the Consumer Behaviour Facets of Functional Foods: A Literature Review'. *Appetite* no. 112 (2017): 167–87.

Keller, Guido. 'Amore la nuova scuola'. *La Testa di Ferro*, 13 June 1920, 1–20.

Kellogg, John Harvey, *The New Dietetics, What to Eat and How: A Guide to Scientific Feeding in Health and Disease*. Battle Creek, MI: Modern Medicine Publishing Co., 1921.

Keys, Ancel. 'Diet and the Epidemiology of Coronary Heart Disease'. *Journal of the American Medical Association* 164, no. 17 (1957): 1912–11.

Keys, Ancel, and Margaret Keys. *Eat Well and Stay Well*. New York: Doubleday, 1959.

Kiple, K. F. 'The Question of Paleolithic Nutrition and Modern Health: From the End to the Beginning'. In *The Cambridge World History of Food*, vol. II, edited by K. F. Kiple, 1704–10. Cambridge: Cambridge University Press, 2001.

Kirwin, Gerald. 'Allied Bombing and Nazi Domestic Propaganda'. *European History Quarterly* 15, no. 3 (1985): 341–62.

Kleinfeld, Vincent A. 'The Hale Amendment: A Pyrrhic Victory'. *Food Drug and Cosmetic Law Journal* 16, no. 3 (1961): 150–63.

Krampner, J. *Creamy and Crunchy: An Informal History of Peanut Butter, the All-American Food*. New York: Columbia University Press, 2013.

Kraut, Alan. *Goldberger's War: The Life and Work of a Public Health Crusader*. New York: Hill and Wang, 2003.

Kroll-Smith, Steve, and H. Hugh Floyd. *Bodies in Protest: Environmental Illness and the Struggle over Medical Knowledge*. New York: NYU Press, 2000.

L'Amministrazione per gli aiuti internazionali. Origini, ordinamento, funzioni, attività. Rome: A.b.e.t.e., 1952.

La Banca, Domenica. *Welfare in transizione. L'esperienza dell'ONMI (1943–1950)*. Naples, Rome: Ed. Scientifiche italiane, 2013.

La Berge, Ann F. 'How the Ideology of Low Fat Conquered America'. *Journal of the History of Medicine and the Allied Sciences* 62, no. 2 (2008): 139–77.

Landau-Czajka, Anna, and A. Kreczmar. 'Diet Patterns in 19th and 20th Century School Manuals'. *Acta Poloniae Historica* 85 (2010): 265–84.

Lavinder, C. H. 'The Salient Epidemiological Features of Pellagra'. *Public Health Reports* 26 (1911): 1459–68.

Lavinder, C. H., and J. W. Babcock. *Pellagra*. Columbia, SC: State Co., 1910.

Lavinder, C. H. *Pellagra*. Washington, DC: Government Printing Office, 1908.

Law, Marc T. 'The Origins of State Pure Food Regulations'. *Journal of Economic History* 63 (2003): 458–89.

Leeden, Michael Arthur. *D'Annunzio a Fiume*. Bari: Laterza, 1975.

Leichter, Howard M. ' "Evil Habits" and "Personal Choices": Assigning Responsibility for Health in the 20th Century'. *Milbank Q.* 81, no. 4 (2003): 603–26.

Leslie, Chris. ' "Fighting an Unseen Enemy": The Infectious Paradigm in the Conquest of Pellagra'. *Journal of Medical Humanities* 23 (2002): 187–202.

Levenstein, Harvey A. *Revolution at the Table: The Transformation of the American Diet*. Oxford: Oxford University Press, 1988.

Levenstein, Harvey. *Fear of Food: A History of Why We Worry about What We Eat*. Chicago, IL: Chicago University Press, 2012.

Levenstein, Harvey. *Paradox of Plenty: A Social History of Eating in Modern America*. Berkeley: University of California Press, 2003.

Levi, Giovanni. 'L'energia disponibile'. In *Storia dell'economia italiana*, vol. 2. *L'età moderna: verso la crisi*, edited by R. Romano, 141–68. Turin: Einaudi, 1991.

Levine, Deborah. 'The Curious History of the Calorie in U.S. policy'. *American Journal of Preventive Medicine* 52, no. 1 (2017): 125–29.

Levine, Susan. *School Lunch Politics: The Surprising History of America's Favorite Welfare Program*. Princeton, NJ: Princeton University Press, 2008.

Levy, Daniel, and Susan Brink. *A Change of Heart: How the People of Framingham, Massachusetts, Helped Unravel the Mysteries of Cardiovascular Disease*. New York: Vintage, 2005.

Livarda, Alexandra, and Marijke van der Veen. 'Social Access and Dispersal of Condiments in North-West Europe from the Roman to the Medieval Period'. *Vegetation History and Archaeobotany* 17, suppl. 1 (2008): 201–9.

Lockey, S. D. 'Allergic Reactions Due to Dyes in Foods'. Speech presented to the Pennsylvania Allergy Society, 1948.

Loeb, Leo. 'The Cancer Problem'. *Interstate Medical Journal* XVII (1910): 1.

Logan, A. C., M. A. Katzman and V. Balanzá-Martínez. 'Natural Environments, Ancestral Diets, and Microbial Ecology: Is There a Modern "Paleo-Deficit Disorder"? Part I and II'. *Journal of Physiological Anthropology* 34 (2015), https://jphysiolanthropol.biomedcentral.com/articles/10.1186/s40101-015-0041-y and https://jphysiolanthropol.biomedcentral.com/articles/10.1186/s40101-014-0040-4 (accessed 20 October 2017).

Lombroso, Cesare. 'Degli ultimi studi sulla pellagra'. *Archivio di psichiatria, scienze penali e antropologia criminale* 2 (1881): 111–23.

Lombroso, Cesare. 'Sulla pellagra maniaca e sua cura'. *Giornale italiano delle malattie veneree e della pelle* 3 (1868): 31–42, 83–97, 137–54.

Lombroso, Cesare. 'Sulle cause della pellagra: lettera polemica al Prof. Lussana'. *Giornale di dermatologia* [unknown vol. number] (1872): 1–32.

Lombroso, Cesare. *La pellagra in Italia in rapporto alla pretesa insufficienza alimentare: lettera polemica … al dott. Bonfigli*. Turin: Celanza, 1880.

Lombroso, Cesare. *Studi clinici ed esperimentali sulla natura, causa e terapia della pellagra*. Bologna: Fava and Garagnani, 1869.

Lombroso, Cesare. *Trattato profilattico e clinico della pellagra*. Turin: Bocca, 1892.

Longardi, Renato. 'Una maglia di lana e una tazza di latte!'. *L'Unità*, 13 December 1951, 6.

Lorusso, Lorenzo, et al. 'Filippo Lussana (1820–1897): From Medical Practitioner to Neuroscience'. *Neurological Science* 33 (2012): 703–8.

Löwy, I., ' "Because of Their Praiseworthy Modesty, They Consult Too Late": Regimes of Hope and Cancer of the Womb, 1800–1910'. *Bulletin of the History of Medicine* 85 (2001): 356–83.

Lupton, Deborah. *Food, the Body and the Self*. London: Sage, 1996.

Lussana, Filippo, and Carlo Frua. 'Su la Pellagra'. In *Pellagra*, edited by Kenneth J. Carpenter, 13–18. Stroudsburg: Hutchinson Ross, 1981.

Lussana, Filippo, and Carlo Frua. *Su la pellagra: memoria*. Milan: Giuseppe Bernardoni, 1856.

Lussana, Filippo. 'Dottrine di G. Liebig su l'alimentazione; ed annotazioni su l'eziologia della pellagra e su la metamorfica produzione epatica dell'adipe'. *Gazzetta Medica Italiana: Lombardia* 3, no. 2 (November 1852): 406–10.

Lussana, Filippo. 'Una allucinazione del professor Lombroso'. In *Gazzetta Medica Italiana: Lombardia*. Milan: Rechiedei, 1883 [offprint].

Lussana, Filippo. *Sulle cause della pellagra*. Padua: Prosperini, 1872.

Lyons, Richard D. 'Do We Need All That in the Bread?' *New York Times*, 24 September 1972. http://search.proquest.com/docview/119569633?accountid=14509 (accessed 21 August 2017).

Macgregor, William, 'Some Problems of Tropical Medicine'. *Lancet* 156 (1900): 1055–61.

Mackarness, R. *Not All in the Mind: How Unsuspected Food Allergy Can Affect Your Body AND Your Mind*. London: Pan Books, 1976.

Mackarness, Richard. 'Stone Age Diet for Functional Disorders'. *Medical World* 91 (1959): 14–19.

Mackarness, Richard. *Eat Fat and Grow Slim*. London: Harvill Press, 1958.

Mafai, Miriam. *Pane nero*. Milan: Mondadori, 1987.

Magnello, Eileen and Anne Hardy (eds). *The Road to Medical Statistics*. Amsterdam: Brill, 2002.

Magrini, Luciano. 'India primeva e rinnovata: dove insegnano Gandhi e Tagore, e dove i missionari italiani catechizzano gli idolatri'. *La Stampa*, 23 August 1926, 3.

Mancini, Francesco. 'Il latte nella refezione scolastica'. In *Il latte alimento per tutti nel pensiero di fisiologi, igienisti e clinici italiani*, edited by Istituto Nazionale della Nutrizione del Consiglio Nazionale delle Ricerche and Amministrazione per le Attività Assistenziali Italiane e Internazionali, 97–106. Rome: AAI, 1957.

Mann, George V., Georgiana Pearson, Tavia Gordon and Thomas Dawber, 'Diet and Cardiovascular Disease in the Framingham Study I. Measurement of Dietary Intake'. *American Journal of Nutrition* 11, no. 3 (1962): 200–25.

Marchant, John, Bryan Reuben and Joan Alcock. *Bread: A Slice of History*. Gloustershire: The History Press, 2008.

Marie, Auguste. *La pellagra*. Paris: V. Giard, 1908.

Marie, Auguste. *Pellagra*, trans. C. H. Lavinder and J. W. Babcock. Columbia, SC: State Co., 1910.

Marks, Harry. 'Epidemiologists Explain Pellagra: Gender, Race, and Political Economy in the Work of Edgar Sydenstricker'. *Journal of the History of Medicine and Allied Sciences* 58 (2003): 34–55.

Marks, Harry. *The Progress of Experiment: Science and Therapeutic Reform, 1900–1990*. Cambridge: Cambridge University Press, 1997.

Marvin, Carolyn, and David W. Ingle. *Blood Sacrifice and the Nation: Totem Rituals and the American Flag*. Cambridge: Cambridge University Press, 1999.

Mattei, Rosalba, and Irene Basili. 'L'alimentazione vegetariana'. In *Manuale di nutrizione clinica*, edited by Rosalba Mattei, 543–56. Milan: Franco Angeli, 2003.

Mazur, Allan. 'Why Were "Starvation Diets" Promoted for Diabetes in the Pre-Insulin Period?' *Nutrition Journal* 10 (2011): 23. https://doi.org/10.1186/1475-2891-10-23.

McCollum, Elmer V. 'The "Vitamin" Hypothesis and the Diseases Referable to a Faulty Diet'. *Journal of the American Medical Association* 71 (1918): 937–40.

McCollum, Elmer V., and Marguerite Davis. 'The Necessity of Certain Lipins in the Diet during Growth'. *Journal of Biological Chemistry* 15 (1913): 167–75.

McCollum, Elmer V., Nina Simmonds and J. Ernestine Becker. 'Studies on Experimental Rickets. XXI. An Experimental Demonstration of the Existence of a Vitamin Which Promotes Calcium Deposition'. *Journal of Biological Chemistry* 53 (1922): 293–312.

McCollum, Elmer. *A History of Nutrition: The Sequence of Ideas in Nutrition Investigation*. Boston, MA: Houghton Mifflin, 1957.

Mediratta, S. 'Beauty and the Breast: The Poetics of Physical Absence and Narrative Presence in Frances Burney's Mastectomy Letter (1811)'. *Women: A Cultural Review* 19, no. 2 (2008): 188–207.

Mendis, Shanti. 'The Contribution of the Framingham Heart Study to the Prevention of Cardiovascular Disease: A Global Perspective'. *Progress in Cardiovascular Disease* 53, no. 1 (2010): 10–14.

Merrill Richard, A., and Earl M. Collier Jr. '"Like Mother Used to Make": An Analysis of FDA Food Standards of Identity'. *Columbia Law Review* 74 (1974): 561–621.

Messedaglia, Luigi. 'Mais e pellagra: un dramma di vita rurale'. 1927. In *La gloria del mais e altri scritti sull'alimentazione Veneta*, edited by Corrado Barberis and Ulderico Bernardi, 249–67. Castabissara: Angelo Colla, 2008.

Mexican Cookbook Collection (ed.). *El Cocinero Mexicano, ó, Coleccion de las Mejores Recetas Para Guisar Al Estilo Americano: y de las Mas Selectas Segun el Metodo de las Cocinas Española, Italiana, Francesa e Inglesa.* Mexico City: Imprenta de Galvan, 1831.

Mielke, H. W., and S. Zahran. 'The Urban Rise and Fall of Air Lead (Pb) and the Latent Surge and Retreat of Societal Violence'. *Environment International* 43 (2012): 48–55.

Mikkeli, Heikki. *Hygiene in the Early Modern Medical Tradition.* Helsinki: Academia Scientiarum Fennica, 1999.

Mikulak, Michael. *The Politics of the Pantry: Stories, Food, and Social Change.* Montreal: McGill-Queen's University Press, 2013.

Miller, Ian. *Reforming Food in Post-Famine Ireland: Medicine, Science and Improvement, 1845–1922.* Manchester: Manchester University Press, 2014.

Millward, Robert and Frances Bell. 'Economic Factors in the Decline of Mortality in Late Nineteenth Century Britain'. *European Review of Economic History* 2, no. 3 (1998): 263–88.

Mingoni, Giorgio, 'Iniziative assistenziali italiane ed internazionali'. *L'Alimentazione Italiana* II, no. 8 (1956).

Ministero di Agricoltura, Industria e Commercio. *La pellagra in Italia.* Rome: MAIC, 1880, *Annali di agricoltura*, no. 18.

Ministry of Food. *National Kitchens Handbook.* London: Stationery Office, 1917.

Mintz, Sidney W. *Sweetness and Power: The Place of Sugar in Modern History.* New York: Penguin, 1985.

Mitman, G. *Breathing Space: How Allergies Change Our Lives and Landscapes.* New Haven, CT: Yale University Press, 2007.

Montaldo, Silvano. 'Cento anni dopo: il punto della situazione'. In *Cesare Lombroso cento anni dopo*, edited by S. Montaldo and P. Tappero, ix–xvi. Turin: UTET, 2009.

Montaldo, Silvano. 'La partecipazione degli scienziati alla vita politica'. In *Cesare Lombroso. Gli scienziati e la nuova Italia*, edited by S. Montaldo, 143–73. Bologna: il Mulino, 2010.

Monti, Aldino. *I braccianti.* Bologna: il Mulino, 1998.

Montini, Lodovico. 'Introduzione'. In *Il latte alimento per tutti nel pensiero di fisiologi, igienisti e clinici italiani*, edited by Istituto Nazionale della Nutrizione del Consiglio Nazionale delle Ricerche and Amministrazione per le Attività Assistenziali Italiane e Internazionali, 5–20. Rome: AAI, 1957.

Montini, Lodovico. 'Nutrizione e assistenza in Italia'. Extract of *Quaderni della Nutrizione* XI, no. 1 (1950): 1–13.

Moore, Lauren Renée. '"But We're Not Hypochondriacs": The Changing Shape of Gluten-Free Dieting and the Contested Illness Experience'. *Social Science and Medicine* 105 (2014): 76–83.

Moore-Colyer, Richard. 'Towards "Mother Earth": Jorian Jenks, Organicism, the Right and the British Union of Fascists'. *Journal of Contemporary History* 39 (2004): 353–71.

Morgan, H. *You Can't Eat That! A Manual and Recipe Book for Those Who Suffer Either Acutely or Mildly (and Perhaps Unconsciously) from Food Allergy.* New York: Harcourt, Brace.

Mosby, Ian. ' "That Won-Ton Soup Headache": The Chinese Restaurant Syndrome, MSG and the Making of American Food, 1968–1980'. *Social History of Medicine* 22 (2009): 133–51.

Moscucci, O. 'Gender and Cancer in Britain, 1860–1910: The Emergence of Cancer as a Public Health Concern'. *American Journal of Public Health* 95, no. 8 (2005): 1312–21.

Mountin, Joseph W. 'Changing Concepts of Basic Local Public Health Services'. *American Journal of Public Health* 39, no. 11 (1949): 1417–28.

Muhammad, Elijah. *How to Eat to Live.* Chicago, IL: Muhammad Mosque of Islam no. 2, 1967.

Mukherjee, Siddhartha. *The Emperor of All Maladies: A Biography of Cancer.* New York: Scribner, 2011.

Murphy, M. *Sick Building Syndrome and the Problem of Uncertainty: Environmental Politics, Technoscience, and Women Workers.* Durham, NC: Duke University Press, 2005.

Napolitano, Valentina. *Migrant Hearts and the Atlantic Return: Transnationalism and the Roman Catholic Church.* New York, NY: Fordham University Press, 2016.

National Advisory Committee on Hyperkinesis and Food Additives. *Final Report to the Nutrition Foundation.* New York, NY: Nutrition Foundation, 1980.

Neagoe, Ioan. *Pelagra și Administrația Noastră [Pellagra and our Administration].* Bucharest: Munca, 1906.

Neagoe, Ioan. *Raportul Doctorului Ioan Neagoe asupra Misiunei Sale în Străinătate pentru a Studia Midloacele de Combatere a Pelagrei din Numitele Țeri [The Raport of Doctor Ioan Neagoe on His Mission Abroad for the Study of the Means for Combating Pellagra].* Bucharest: Statului, 1889.

Neagoe, Ioan. *Studiu asupra Pelagrei [Study on Pellagra].* Bucharest: Institutul de Arte Grafice Carol Göbl, 1900.

Nestle, Marion. *Food Politics: How the Food Industry Influences Nutrition and Health.* Berkeley and London: University of California Press, 2003.

Nguyen, Hoang. P. K., S. Lin, and P. Heidenreich. 'A Systematic Comparison of Sugar Content in Low-Fat vs Regular Versions of Food'. *Nutrition and Diabetes* 6, no. 1 (2016): 193.

Nicoud, Marilyn. *Les régimes de santé au moyen âge.* Rome: École Française de Rome, 2007.

Niles, George M. *Pellagra: An American Problem.* Philadelphia, PA: W. B. Saunders, 1912.

Nimmo, Richie. *Milk, Modernity and the Making of the Human. Purifying the Social.* Abingdon: Routledge, 2010.

Norn, Viggo. *Emulsifiers in Food Technology.* Chichester: John Wiley and Sons, 2014.

Nourrisson, Didier. 'Le lait à l'école. Pédagogie de la voie lactée'. In *À votre santé! Éducation et santé sous la IVe République,* edited by Didier Nourrisson, 85–96. Saint-Étienne: Publications de l'Université de Saint-Étienne, 2002.

Novaria, Paolo. 'Cesare Lombroso professore a Torino. Un percorso tra i documenti dell'Archivio storico dell'università'. In *Gli archivi della scienza. L'Università di Torino e altri casi italiani,* edited by S. Montaldo and P. Novaria, 40–55. Milan: Franco Angeli, 2011.

Nützenadel, Alexander. 'Dictating Food: Autarchy, Food Provision, and Consumer Politics in Fascist Italy 1922–1943'. In *Food and Conflict in Europe in the Age of the Two World*

Wars, edited by Frank Trentmann and Flemming Just, 88–108. Basingstoke: Palgrave Macmillan, 2006.

Oddy, Derek. *From Plain Fare to Fusion Food: British Diet from the 1890s to the 1990s.* Woodbridge: Boydell, 2003.

Offer, Avner. 'Body Weight and Self Control in the US and Britain since the 1950s'. *Social History of Medicine* 14, no. 1 (2001): 79–106.

Offer, Avner. *The First World War: An Agrarian Interpretation.* Oxford: Clarendon Press, 1989.

Ogilvie, H. 'Foreword' to Mackarness, R. *Eat Fat and Grow Slim.* London: Harvill Press, 1958, 1–2.

Omran, A. 'The Epidemiological Transition: A Theory of the Epidemiology of Population Change'. *Milbank Quarterly* 83, no. 4 (1971): 731–57.

Oppenheimer, Gerald M. 'Becoming the Framingham Study 1947–1950'. *American Journal of Public Health* 95, no. 4 (2005): 602–10.

Oppenheimer, Gerald M. 'Framingham Heart Study: The First 20 Years'. *Progress in Cardiovascular Disease* 53, no. 1 (2010): 55–61.

Oppenheimer, Gerald M. 'Profiling Risk: The Emergence of Coronary Heart Disease Epidemiology in the United States (1947–70)'. *International Journal of Epidemiology* 35, no. 3 (2006): 720–30.

Osborne, Thomas, and Lafayette Mendel. 'Nutritive Properties of Proteins of the Maize Kernel'. *Journal of Biological Chemistry* 18 (1914): 1–16.

Ostry, Aleck. 'The Early Development of Nutrition Policy in Canada'. In *Children's Health Issues in Historical Perspective*, edited by Cheryl Krasnick Warsh and Veronica Strong-Boag, 191–206. Waterloo: Wilfrid Laurier University Press, 2005.

Otis, Laura. 'The Metaphoric Circuit: Organic and Technological Communication in the Nineteenth Century'. *Journal of the History of Ideas* 63, no. 1 (2002): 105–28.

Otter, Chris. 'Industrializing Diet, Industrializing Ourselves: Technology, Food and the Body since 1750'. In *The Routledge History of Food*, edited by Carol Helstosky. Abingdon: Routledge, 2015.

Pagliai, Letizia. *Giorgio La Pira e il piano latte. La funzione sociale della Centrale.* Florence: Polistampa, 2010.

Paresce, Renato. 'L'arte fra gli artigli di Albione'. *La Stampa*, 9 August 1933, 3.

Park, Y., C. Sempos, C. Barton, J. Vanderveen and E. Yetley. 'Effectiveness of Food Fortification in the United States: The Case of Pellagra'. *American Journal of Public Health* 90, no. 5 (2000): 727–38.

Parkin, Katherine J. *Food Is Love.* Philadelphia: University of Pennsylvania Press, 2006.

Parr, Jessica. 'Obesity and the Emergence of Mutual Aid Groups for Weight Loss in Post-War United States'. *Social History of Medicine* 27, no. 4 (2014): 768–88.

Patel, Sejal S. 'Methods and Management: NIH Administrators, Federal Oversight, and the Framingham Heart Study'. *Bulletin of the History of Medicine* 86, no. 1 (2012): 94–121.

Peel, C. S. *Life's Enchanted Cup: An Autobiography, 1872–1933.* London: John Lane, 1933.

Pellegrini, Nicoletta, and Carlo Agostoni. 'Nutritional Aspects of Gluten-Free Products'. *Journal of the Science of Food and Agriculture* 95 (2015): 2380–85.

Perisutti, Luigi. 'La legge contro la pellagra'. In *Atti del secondo congresso pellagrologico italiano: Bologna, 26–28 Maggio 1902*, edited by Giovanni Battista Cantarutti, 303–19. Udine: Fratelli Tosolini e G. Jacob, 1902.

Perisutti, Luigi, and Giovanni Battista Cantarutti. 'Inchiesta sulla pellagra nel regno e sui provvedimenti diversi per la cura preventiva della stessa'. *Bollettino di notizie agrarie* 31 (1900): 1385–86.

Pernet, Corinne A. 'L'Unicef et la lutte contre la malnutrition en Amérique centrale dans les années 1950: entre coopération et compétition'. *Relations internationales* no. 161 (2015): 27–42.

Perroncito, Aldo. *Eziologia della Pellagra*. Florence: Societa Tipografica Fiorentina, 1913.

Petrick, G. W. 'Industrial Food'. In *The Oxford Handbook of Food History*, edited by J. M. Pilcher. Oxford: Oxford University Press, 2012.

Petty, Orlando H., and William Hoy Stoner. *Diabetes, Its Treatment by Insulin and Diet, a Handbook for the Patient*, 3rd rev. edn. Philadelphia, PA: F.A. Davis, 1926.

Philippot, Jane. 'How Healthy Are Government Dietary Guidelines? Part 1. Origin and Evolution of Dietary Guidelines'. *Nutrition Practitioner* 9, no. 1 (2009): 1–15.

Phull, Surinder. 'The Mediterranean Diet: Socio-Cultural Relevance for Contemporary Health Promotion'. *Open Public Health Journal* 8 (2015): 35–40.

Pick, Daniel. *Faces of Degeneration: A European Disorder, c. 1848–1918*. Cambridge: Cambridge University Press, 1989.

Pirquet, C. V. 'Allergie'. *Münchener Medizinische Wochenschrift* 30 (1906): 1457–58.

Plumer, B. 'A Brief History of U.S. Corn in One Chart'. *Washington Post*, 16 August 2012. https://www.washingtonpost.com/news/wonk/wp/2012/08/16/a-brief-history-of-u-s-corn-in-one-chart/?utm_term=.edbdd9da25a1 (accessed 17 October 2017).

Poen, Monte M. *Harry S. Truman versus the Medical Lobby: The Genesis of Medicare*. Columbia: University of Missouri Press, 1996.

Pollan, Michael. *In Defence of Food: The Myth of Nutrition and the Pleasures of Eating*. London: Allen Lane, 2008.

Pollan, Michael. *The Omnivore's Dilemma*. New York and Oxford: Penguin, 2006.

Pompei, Manlio. 'Una politica per il latte'. *Il Giornale d'Italia*, 30 June 1961.

Pope, Thomas. 'On Cancer'. *Association Medical Journal*, 3 (1855): 859–60.

Porisini, Giorgio. 'Agricoltura, alimentazione e condizioni sanitarie. Prime ricerche sulla pellagra in Italia dal 1880 al 1940'. *Cahiers internationaux d'histoire économique et sociale* 3 (1984): 1–50.

Porta, M. *Embedding Education into Diabetes Practice*. New York: Karger Medical and Scientific Publishers, 2005.

Porter, R. 'Civilisation and Disease: Medical Ideology in the Enlightenment'. In *Culture, Politics and Society in Britain, 1660–1800*, edited by Jeremy Black and Jeremy Gregory. Manchester: Manchester University Press, 1991.

Porter, Roy. *The Greatest Benefit to Mankind: A Medical History of Humanity from Antiquity to the Present*. London: Fontana Press, 1999.

Pozzi, Sandro. *Guido Keller: nel pensiero nelle gesta*. Milan: Mediolanum, 1933.

Priani, Egidio. ' "Shrouded in a Dark Fog": The Diagnosis of Pellagra and General Paralysis of the Insane between Italy and United Kingdom, 1840–1900'. *History of Psychiatry* 28, no. 2 (2017): 166–81.

Price John, M. et al. 'Bladder Tumours in Rats Fed Cyclohexylamine or High Doses of a Mixture of Cyclamate and Saccharin'. *Science* 167, no. 3921 (1970): 1131–32.

Raatz, Susan, LuAnn Johnson and Matthew Picklo. 'Consumption of Honey, Sucrose, and High-Fructose Corn Syrup Produces Similar Metabolic Effects in Glucose-Tolerant and Intolerant Individuals'. *Journal of Nutrition* 145, no. 10 (2015): 2265–72.

Radetsky, P. *Allergic to the Twentieth Century: The Explosion in Environmental Allergies – From Sick Buildings to Multiple Chemical Sensitivity*. Boston, MA: Little, Brown, 1997.

Ramoino, Paolo. 'Contributo allo Studio delle Alimentazioni Incomplete. Nota III. – Richerche sulle alimentazioni frugivore'. *Pathologica* 7 (April 1915): 158–61.

Randolph, T. G. 'Human Ecology and Susceptibility to the Chemical Environment'. *Annals of Allergy* 19 (1961): 518–40, 657–77, 779–99, 908–29.

Randolph, T. G., and L. B. Yeager. 'Corn Sugar as an Allergen'. *Annals of Allergy* 7 (1949): 651–61.

Randolph, T. G., and R. Moss. *Allergies: Your Hidden Enemies*. New York: Harper Collins, 1981.

Randolph, T. G. *Environmental Medicine: Beginnings and Bibliographies of Clinical Ecology*. Fort Collins, CO: Clinical Ecology, 1987.

Randolph, T. G., J. P. Rollins and C. K. Walter. 'Allergic Reactions from Ingestion or Intravenous Injection of Corn Sugar'. *Journal of Laboratory and Clinical Medicine* 24 (1949): 1741.

Randolph, T. G. 'Cornstarch as Allergen, Sources of Contact in Food Containers'. *Journal of the American Dietetic Association* 24 (1948): 841–46.

Reeves, Maud Pember. *Round about a Pound a Week*. London: Bell and Sons, 1913.

Reilly, N. R. 'The Gluten-Free Diet: Recognizing Fact, Fiction, and Fad'. *Journal of Pediatrics* 175 (2016): 206–10.

Renner, W. 'The Spread of Cancer among the Descendants of the Liberated Africans or Creoles of Sierra Leone'. *British Medical Journal* 2, no. 2075 (1910): 977–84.

Ricci, Steven. *Cinema and Fascism: Italian Film and Society, 1922–1943*. Berkeley: University of California Press, 2008.

Rinkel, H., T. G. Randolph and M. Zeller. *Food Allergy*. Springfield, IL: Charles C. Thomas, 1951.

Roberts, P. *The End of Food*. New York: Houghton Mifflin, 2008.

Roberts, Stewart R. *Pellagra: History, Distribution, Diagnosis, Prognosis, Treatment, Etiology*. St. Louis, MI: C. V. Mosby, 1913.

Roe, Daphne. 'Pellagra'. In *The Cambridge World History of Food*, edited by Kenneth F. Kiple and Kriemhild Conee Ornelas, 960–67. Cambridge: Cambridge University Press, 2000.

Roe, Daphne. *A Plague of Corn: The Social History of Pellagra*. Ithaca, NY: Cornell University Press, 1973.

Roger Williams, W. 'Cancer in Egypt and the Causation of Cancer'. *British Medical Journal* 2 (1902): 917.

Rondoni, Pietro. *Alimentazione Maidica e Vitamine (Con Dimonstrazioni)*. Florence: Fiorentona, 1915.

Rondoni, Pietro. *Ricerche sulla Alimentazione Maidica, con Speciale Riguardo alla Pellagra*. Florence: Fiorentona, 1915.

Rosenberg, Charles E. 'Banishing Risk: Continuity and Change in the Moral Management of Disease'. In *Health and Morality: Interdisciplinary Perspectives*, edited by Allan M. Brandt and Paul Rozin, 35–51. New York: Routledge, 1997.

Rosenberg, Charles. E. 'Pathologies of Progress: The Idea of Civilisation as Risk'. *Bulletin of the History of Medicine* 72, no. 4 (1998): 714–30.

Rossi, Luigi. 'L'Unrra strumento di politica estera agli albori del bipolarismo'. In *L'Amministrazione per gli Aiuti Internazionali. La ricostruzione dell'Italia tra dinamiche internazionali e attività assistenziali*, edited by Andrea Ciampani, 47–81. Milan: Franco Angeli, 2002.

Rossi, Ottorino. 'Avitaminosi e Pellagra. Dubbi e Proposte'. *Quaderni di Psichiatria* 2 (1915): 146–63.

Rothstein, William G. *Public Health and the Risk Factor: A History of an Uneven Medical Revolution*. Rochester, NY: University of Rochester Press, 2003.

Rudy, Abraham. *Practical Handbook for Diabetic Patients, with 180 International Recipes (American, Jewish, French, German, Italian, Armenian, Etc.)*. Boston, MA: M. Barrows, 1929. http://hdl.handle.net/2027/coo.31924003513623.

Ryoung Song, Mee, and Meeja Im. 'Moderating Effects of Food Type and Consumers' Attitude on the Evaluation of Food Items Labeled "Additive-free"'. *Journal of Consumer Behaviour* 17 (2018): e1–e12. https://doi.org/10.1002/cb.1671.

Salaris, Claudia. *Alla Festa della Rivoluzione: artisti e libertari con D'Annunzio a Fiume*. Bologna: il Mulino, 2002.

Salas, Ismael. 'Etiology and Prophylaxis of pellagra'. In *Pellagra*, edited by Kenneth J. Carpenter, 19–24. Stroudsburg: Hutchinson Ross, 1981.

Salvatici, Silvia. '"Not Enough Food to Feed the People". L'Unrra in Italia (1944–1945)'. *Contemporanea* XIV, no. 1 (2011): 83–100.

Sandwith, F. M. 'Can Pellagra Be a Disease Due to a Deficiency in Nutrition?' *Transactions of the National Association for the Study of Pellagra. Second Triennial Meeting at Columbia, South Carolina, October 3 and 4, 1912*. Columbia, SC: R. L. Bryan, 1914.

Sathe, S. K., and G. M. Sharma. 'Effects of Processing on Food Allergens'. *Molecular Nutrition and Food Research* 53, no. 8 (2009): 970–78.

Saunders, Eleanora B. 'The Coexistence of Pellagra and Beri-beri'. *Transactions of the National Association for the Study of Pellagra. Second Triennial Meeting at Columbia, South Carolina, October 3 and 4, 1912*. Columbia, SC: R. L. Bryan, 1914.

Sawyer, L., and E. A. M. Gale. 'Diet, Delusion and Diabetes'. *Diabetologia* 52, no. 1 (2009): 1–7. https://doi.org/10.1007/s00125-008-1203-9.

Sax, Bora. *Animals in the Third Reich: Pets, Scapegoat, and the Holocaust*. London: Continuum, 2000.

Schlenker, Ernest, and Jean Gnaedinger. 'Mono and Diglycerides in Industrial Fats'. *Journal of American Oil Chemists* 24, no. 7 (1947): 239–40.

Schneider, Herbert W. *Making the Fascist State*. New York: Oxford University Press, 1928.

Schoenberg, Bruce. 'A Program for the Conquest of Cancer: 1802'. *Journal of the History of Medicine and Allied Sciences* XXX (1975): 3–22.

Scholliers, Peter. 'Food Recommendations in Domestic Education, Belgium 1890–1940'. *Paedagogica Historica* 49, no. 5 (2013): 645–63.

Scholliers, Peter. 'Restaurants économiques à Bruxelles pendant la Grande Guerre'. In *Manger et boire entre 1914 et 1918*, edited by Caroline Poulain, 111–17. Dijon and Gand: Bibliothèque de Dijon & Editions Snoeck, 2014.

Schwartz, Richard H. *Judaism and Vegetarianism*. Herndon, VA: Lantern, 2001.

Scrinis, Gyorgy. 'On the Ideology of Nutritionism'. *Gastronomica* 8, no. 1 (2008), 39–48.

Scrinis, Gyorgy. *Nutritionism: The Science and Politics of Dietary Advice*. New York: Columbia University Press, 2013.

Scrob, Mircea. 'From Mămăligă to Bread as the "Core" Food of Romanian Villagers: A Consumer-Centered Interpretation of a Dietary Change (1900–1980)'. Budapest: Central European University, unpublished PhD dissertation.

Segers, Yves. 'Food Recommendations and Change in a Flemish Cookbook, Ons Kookboek, 1920–2000'. *Appetite* 45 (2005): 4–14.

Shapin, Steven. '"You Are What You Eat": Historical Changes in Ideas about Food and Identity'. *Historical Research* 87 (2014): 377–92.

Shortt, S. E. D. 'Physicians, Science, and Status: Issues in the Professionalization of Anglo-American Medicine in the Nineteenth Century'. *Medical History* 27 (1983): 51–68.

Shprintzen, Adam. *The Vegetarian Crusade: The Rise of an American Reform Movement, 1817–1921*. Chapel Hill: University of North Carolina Press, 2003.

Silbergeld, E. K., and A. M. Goldberg. 'Hyperactivity: A Lead-induced Behavior Disorder'. *Environmental Health Perspectives* 7 (1974): 227–32.

Skuse, Alanna. 'Wombs, Worms and Wolves: Constructing Cancer in Early Modern England'. *Social History of Medicine* 27 (2014): 632–48.

Smith, A. F. *Peanuts: The Illustrious History of the Goober Pea*. Urbana, IL: University of Illinois Press, 2002.

Smith, David (ed.). *Nutrition in Britain: Science, Scientists and Politics in the Twentieth Century*. New York: Routledge, 1996.

Smith, David F., and Jim Phillips. 'Food Policy and Regulation: A Multiplicity of Actors and Experts'. In *Food, Science, Policy and Regulation in the Twentieth Century*, edited by D. F. Smith and J. Phillips. London: Routledge, 2000.

Smith, David, and J. Philips (eds). *Food, Science, Policy and Regulation in the Twentieth Century: International and Comparative Perspectives*. Oxford: Routledge, 2000.

Smith, Matthew. *An Alternative History of Hyperactivity: Food Additives and the Feingold Diet*. New Brunswick, NJ: Rutgers University Press, 2011.

Smith, Matthew. *Another Person's Poison: A History of Food Allergy*. New York: Columbia University Press, 2015.

Smith, Matthew. *Hyperactive: The Controversial History of ADHD*. London: Reaktion, 2012.

Snijders, Aarnout J. C. *Onze voedingsmiddelen*. Zutphen: Thieme, 1889, 1896, 1911.

Snyder, Harry. *Bread: A Collection of Popular Papers on Wheat, Flour and Bread*. New York: MacMillan, 1930.

Spackman, Barbara. *Fascist Virility: Rhetoric, Ideology and Social Fantasy in Italy*. Minneapolis: University of Minnesota Press, 1996.

Spain, W. C. 'Review of *Food Allergy*'. *Quarterly Review of Biology* 28 (1953): 97–8.

Spary, Emma C. *Eating the Enlightenment: Food and the Sciences in Paris, 1670–1760*. Chicago, IL: University of Chicago Press, 2012.

Speer, F. 'Allergic Tension-Fatigue in Children'. *Annals of Allergy* 12 (1954): 168–71.

Spencer, Colin. 'The British Isles'. In *The Cambridge World History of Food*, edited by K. Kiple and K. Ornelas, 1217–26. Cambridge: Cambridge University Press, 2000.

Spencer, Colin. *The Heretic's Feast: A History of Vegetarianism*. Hanover, NH: University Press of New England, 1995.

Spiess, Maiko R. 'Doenças Cardíacas e Risco: o Framingham Heart Study'. Unpublished Doctoral Dissertation. Política Científica e Tecnológica, Universidade Estadual de Campinas, Brazil, 2014.

Steel, Frances. 'A Source of Our Wealth, Yet Adverse to Our Health? Butter and the Heart Link in New Zealand to c. 1990'. *Social History of Medicine* 18 (2005): 475–93.

Steere-Williams, Jacob. 'The Perfect Food and the Filth Disease: Milk-Borne Typhoid and Epidemiological Practice in late Victorian Britain'. *Journal of the History of Medicine and Allied Sciences* 65, no. 4 (2010): 514–45.

Stefani, Aristide. *Relazione sull'opera della Commissione pellagrologica provinciale di Padova nell'anno 1910*. Padua: Penada, 1911.

Steigmann-Gall, Richard. *The Holy Reich: Nazi Conceptions of Christianity, 1919–1945*. Cambridge: Cambridge University Press, 2003.

Stiénon, L. *Rapport sur l'alimentation*. Brussels: Hôpitaux de Bruxelles, 1902.

Strambio, Gaetano. 'Da Legnano a Mogliano Veneto: un secolo di lotta contro la pellagra'. *Memorie del Real Istituto Lombardo di Scienze e Lettere* 17 (1890): 137–551.

Susser, Mervyn. 'Epidemiology in the United States after World War II: The Evolution of Technique'. *Epidemiological Reviews* 7 (1985): 147–77.

Taccari, Egisto. 'Clodomiro Bonfigli'. *Dizionario biografico degli italiani* 12 (1971),
    sub voce. http://www.treccani.it/enciclopedia/clodomiro-bonfigli_
    (Dizionario-Biografico)/.
Taubes, Gary. *Good Calories, Bad Calories: Fats, Carbs, and the Controversial Science of
    Diet and Health*. New York: Anchor, 2008.
Taubes, Gary. 'The Soft Science of Dietary Fat'. *Science* 291, no. 5513 (2001): 2536–45.
Thorley, Virginia. 'Australian School Milk Schemes to 1974: For the Benefit of Whom?'.
    Health and History XVI, no. 2 (2014): 63–86.
Tolstoi, Edward. *The Practical Management of Diabetes*. American Lecture Series, no. 199.
    Springfield, IL: Thomas, 1953.
Trentmann, Frank, and Fleming Just (eds). *Food and Conflict in the Age of the Two World
    Wars*. London: Palgrave Macmillan, 2006.
US Department of Agriculture, *Food for Fitness – A Daily Food Guide*, leaflet
    no. 424, 1958.
U.S. Food and Drug Administration. 'Food Allergen Labeling and Consumer Protection
    Act of 2004 (FALCPA), Public Law 108–282, Title II', 2004.
Ufficio Stampa e Propaganda. 'Ai Veneti!'. *Ufficio Stampa e Propaganda del Comando città
    di Fiume, Sezione per il Veneto – Palazzo Baccich*, February 1920.
UNRRA Italian Mission, Welfare Division, Nutrition Branch. *The School Lunch Manch.*
    s.l.: s.n., 1946.
Urbeanu, Adolf. *Despre Caracteristica Alimentației Țeranului Român [On the
    Characteristics of the Romanian Peasants' Diets]*. Bucharest: Statului, 1903.
Urettini, Luigi. *Il Giovane Comisso e le sue lettere a casa (1914–1920)*. Abano
    Terme: Francisci, 1985.
Usuelli, Filippo. *Gli assillanti problemi demografici ed alimentari in Italia e nel mondo.*
    s.l.: s.n., 1953.
Van den Brandt, P. et al. 'The Contribution of Epidemiology'. *Food and Chemical
    Toxicology* 40 (2002): 387–424.
Van den Dungen, Pierre. 'Milieux de presse bruxellois pendant la Grande Guerre'. *Les
    Cahiers de la Fonderie* 32 (2005): 15–20.
Van Otterloo, Anneke. 'Dutch Food Culture and its Cookery Teachers: The Rise, Diffusion
    and Decline of a Tradition (1880–1980)'. In *The Diffusion of Food Culture in Europe
    from the Late 18th Century to the Present Day*, edited by Derek Oddy and Lydia
    Petranova, 96–106. Prague: Akademia, 2005.
Vanni, Adello, and Luigi Missiroli. 'Bonfigli contro Lombroso: della polemica sulla
    etiopatogenesi della pellagra'. *Rivista sperimentale di freniatria* 111, no. 6 (1987): 1383–
    96. http://www.rivistafreniatria.it
Vanzetto, Livio. *I ricchi e i pellagrosi: un secolo di storia dell'Istituto 'Costante Gris' di
    Mogliano Veneto*. Abano Terme: Francisci, 1992.
Vernon, James. *Hunger: A Modern History*. Cambridge, MA: Harvard University
    Press, 2007.
Vigna, Cesare. 'Sulla pellagra nella provincia di Venezia'. In *La pellagra in Italia*, 447–53.
    Rome: MAIC, 1880, *Annali di agricoltura*, no. 18.
Villani, Angela. *Dalla parte dei bambini. Italia e Unicef tra ricostruzione e sviluppo.*
    Padua: Cedam, 2016.
Visco, Sabato. 'Mezzi per favorire un maggior consumo del latte e dei derivati'. *Il Mondo
    del Latte* IX, no. 4 (1955): 224–27.
Visco, Sabato. 'Nuovi aspetti di assistenza alimentare nei programmi AAI'. *L'Alimentazione
    Italiana* II, no. 10 (1956).

Visco, Sabato. 'Problemi alimentari delle comunità'. *Assistenza d'Oggi* VI, no. 3 (1955): 16–31.

Voegelin, Eric. *Die Politische Religionen*. Vienna: Wilhelm Fink Verlag, 1996.

Voegtlin, Carl. 'Recent Work on Pellagra'. *Public Health Reports* 35 (1920): 1435–52.

Waddington, Keir, 'The Dangerous Sausage: Diet, Meat and Disease in Victorian and Edwardian Britain'. *Cultural and Social History* 8, no. 1 (2011): 51–71.

Wagner, Susan. 'FDA Warns Consumers about Pitfalls of Buying, Getting Money Worths'. *Chicago Daily Defender*, 4 October 1961.

Wagner, Susan. 'New Booklet Warns of Shopper Pitfalls'. *Washington Post*, 3 October 1961.

Waldie, Elizabeth. *Mrs Waldie's Collection of Economical Recipes Suitable for War Cookery and Notes on Meaning of Economy as Regards Food and Fuel*. Glasgow: s.n., 1917.

Walker, Charles. 'Theories and Problems of Cancer: Part III'. *Science Progress in the Twentieth Century* 7, no. 26 (1912): 223–38.

Warboys, Michael. *Spreading Germs: Disease Theories and Medical Practice in Britain, 1865–1900*. Cambridge: Cambridge University Press, 2000.

Warman, Arturo. *Corn and Capitalism: How a Botanical Bastard Grew to Global Dominance*, trans. N. Westrate. Chapel Hill: University of North Carolina Press, 2003.

Weaver, Peter. 'Buyer's Guide to Additives'. *Washington Post*, 2 July 1972.

Wedder, Edward B. 'Dietary Deficiency as the Etiological Factor in Pellagra'. *Archives of Internal Medicine* 18 (1916): 137–73.

Weinreb, Alice. *Matters of Taste: The Politics of Food and Hunger in Divided Germany 1945–1971*. PhD diss., University of Michigan, 2009.

Weinreb, Alice. *Modern Hungers: Food and Power in Twentieth-Century Germany*. New York: Oxford University Press, 2017.

Weisz, George, and Jesse Olszynko-Gryn. 'The Theory of Epidemiologic Transition: The Origins of a Citation Classic'. *Journal of the History of Medicine and Allied Sciences* 65, no. 3 (2010): 287–326.

Welch, David. 'Nazi Propaganda and the *Volksgemeinschaft*: Constructing a People's Community'. *Journal of Contemporary History* 39, no. 2 (2004): 213–38.

Welch, David. *The Third Reich: Politics and Propaganda*. Abingdon: Psychology Press, 2002.

West, C. 'Introduction of Complementary Foods to Infants'. *Annals of Nutrition and Metabolism* 70 (2017): 47–54.

Whalen, E. M., and F. J. Stare . *Panic in the Pantry*. New York: Antheum, 1975.

White House Conference on Food, Nutrition and Health: Final Report. Washington, DC: US Government Printing Office, 1969.

Willcock, Edith, and F. Gowland Hopkins. 'The Importance of Individual Amino-Acids in Metabolism. Observations on the Effect of Adding Tryptophane to a Dietary in which Zein is the sole Nitrogenous Constituent'. *Journal of Physiology* 35 (1906): 88–102.

Willet, Walter C. 'Editorial: The Dietary Pyramid: Does the Foundation Need Repair?' *American Journal of Clinical Nutrition* 68 (1998): 218–19.

Williams, William Bradford. *History of the Manufacture of Explosives for the World War, 1917–1918*. Chicago, IL: Chicago University Press, 1920.

Wilson, Bee. *Swindled: The Dark History of Food Fraud, from Poisoned Candy to Counterfeit Coffee*. Princeton, NJ: Princeton University Press, 2008.

Wilson, Robert, Jr. 'A Case of Beri-Beri Presenting an Initial Erythema Resembling Pellagra'. *Transactions of the National Association for the Study of Pellagra. Second Triennial Meeting at Columbia, South Carolina, October 3 and 4, 1912*, 321–22. Columbia, SC: R. L. Bryan, 1914.

Winter, Ruth. *Beware of the Food You Eat*. New York: Signet Classic, 1970.

Wolf, George, and Kenneth J. Carpenter. 'Early Research into the Vitamins: The Work of Wilhelm Stepp'. *Journal of Nutrition* 127 (1997): 1255–59.

Wolf, Jacqueline H. *Don't Kill Your Baby: Public Health and the Decline of Breastfeeding in the Nineteenth and Twentieth Centuries*. Columbus: Ohio State University Press, 2001.

Woloson, Wendy. *Refined Tastes: Sugar, Confectionary, and Consumers in Nineteenth Century America*. Baltimore: John Hopkins University Press, 2002.

Woods, Robert. *The Demography of Victorian England and Wales*. Cambridge: Cambridge University Press, 2000.

Wootton, David. *Bad Medicine: Doctors Doing Harm Since Hippocrates*. Oxford: Oxford University Press, 2007.

Young, James Harvey. 'The Pig That Fell into the Privy: Upton Sinclair's *The Jungle* and the Meat Inspection Amendments of 1906'. In *Bulletin of the History of Medicine* 59 (1985): 467–80.

Young, James Harvey. *Pure Food, Securing the Federal Pure Food and Drug Act of 1906*. Princeton, NJ: Princeton University Press, 1989.

Yudkin, John. *Lose Weight, Feel Great*. London: MacGibbon and Kee, 1964.

Yudkin, John. *Pure, White and Deadly*. London: Penguin, 1972.

Yudkin, John. *Pure, White and Deadly: How Sugar Is Killing Us and What We Can Do To Stop It*. London: Penguin, 1988.

Yudkin, John. *This Slimming Business*. London: MacGibbon and Kee, 1958.

Yudkin, John. 'Diet and Coronary Thrombosis: Hypothesis and Fact'. *Lancet* 270, no. 6987 (1957): 155–62.

Yudkin, John, A. M. Brown and J. C. Mackenzie . 'Knowledge of Nutrition amongst Housewives of a London Suburb'. *Nutrition* 17, no. 1 (1963): 1.

Zachman, K., and O. Østby. 'Food, Technology and Trust: An Introduction'. *History and Technology* 27, no. 1 (2011): 1–10.

Zamagni, Vera. *The Economic History of Italy, 1860–1990: Recovery after Decline*. Oxford: Clarendon Press, 1993.

Zbynek, Zeman. *Nazi Propaganda*. Oxford: Oxford University Press, 1964.

Zimmern, Helen. 'Criminal Anthropology in Italy'. *Appletons' Popular Science Monthly* 52 (April 1898): 743–60

Zingarelli, Italo. 'Dovete essere belle ma esser anche sane'. *La Stampa*, 11 October 1937, 3.

Zinman, Bernard, Jay S. Skyler, Matthew C. Riddle, and Ele Ferrannini. 'Diabetes Research and Care through the Ages'. *Diabetes Care* 40, no. 10 (2017): 1302–13. https://doi.org/10.2337/dci17-0042.

Zweiniger-Bargielowska, Ina, Rachel Duffett and Alain Drouard (eds). *Food and War in Twentieth Century Europe*. London: Routledge, 2011.

Zylberman, Patrick. 'Making Food Safety an Issue: Internationalized Food Politics and French Public Health from the 1870s to the Present'. *Medical History* 48, no. 1 (2004): 1–28.

Index